The Unofficial Guide to Surgery

Core Operations

EDITION

2

The Unofficial Guide to Surgery

Core Operations

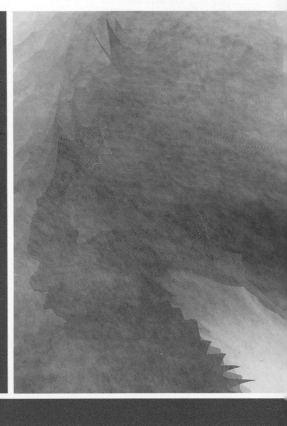

Series Editor:

Zeshan Qureshi, BM, BSc (Hons), MSc, MRCPCH, FAcadMEd, MRCPS(Glasg)

Paediatric Registrar, London Deanery, United Kingdom

Editors:

Katrina Mason, BSc, MBChB, DCH, MSc (Oxon), FRCS (ORL-HNS)

Paediatric Ear Nose & Throat Fellow, Evelina Children's Hospital, Guy's & St Thomas' NHS Foundation Trust, London, UK

Gareth Rogers, BSc (Hons), MBChB, MRCSEd

Trauma and Orthopaedics Specialist Registar, Health Education England, North West School of Surgery (East Sector), UK

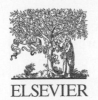

ELSEVIER

ISBN: 978-0-443-11478-6

Content Strategist: Alexandra Mortimer
Content Project Manager: Shubham Dixit
Cover Designer: Miles Hitchen
Illustrations Coordinator: Nijantha Priyadharshini
Marketing Manager: Deborah Watkins

Printed in India by Manipal Technologies Limited

Last digit is the print number: 9 8 7 6 5 4 3 2 1

Series Editor Foreword

The Unofficial Guide to Medicine is not just about helping students study; it is also about allowing those that learn to take back control of their own education. Since its inception, it has been driven by the voices of students and, through this, democratised the process of medical education, blurring the line between learners and teachers.

Medical education is an evolving process, and the latest iteration of our titles has been rewritten to bring them up to date with modern curriculums, after extensive deliberation and consultation. We have kept the series up to date, incorporating new guidelines and perspectives from a wide range of students, junior doctors and senior clinicians. There is greater consistency across the titles, more illustrations, and through these and other changes I hope the books will now be even better study aids.

These books, however, are a process of continual improvement. By reading this book, I hope that you not only get through your exams but also consider contributing to a future edition. You may be a student now, but you are also the future of medical education.

I wish you all the best with your future career and any upcoming exams.

Zeshan Qureshi
November 2022

Introduction

We are extremely proud to present the second edition of *The Unofficial Guide to Surgery*, a book designed to both inspire and support you when experiencing the operating theatre and surgical rotations. The book aims to demystify these invigorating yet intimidating environments and equip students with a comprehensive understanding of the principles of the most common operations across all surgical specialities. By fostering a foundation of knowledge that spans the entire surgical continuum, from preparation to recovery, we aim to enhance the quality of the learning experience.

For each operation, *The Unofficial Guide to Surgery* provides a concise and practical summary of the relevant indications and contraindications for surgery, detailed relevant anatomy, and a step-by-step guide on how to perform the surgery, including postoperative care, follow-up and complications. This textbook acts as an invaluable companion for students embarking on their journey into the operating theatre. Beyond the intricacies of procedures and anatomy, it equips learners with a holistic understanding of the surgical process, emphasizing not only the technical aspects but also the critical pre- and post-operative care.

Following on from the first edition, the comprehensive nature of this guide has been further amplified by ensuring each chapter is up to date with current practice and importantly included a new chapter dedicated to Oral and Maxillofacial Surgery, providing insights into a specialized field that is integral to the broader surgical landscape.

Each operation is accompanied by two high-quality images that support the understanding of the relevant clinical anatomy and the step-by-step guide on how to perform the operation. To ensure diversity in medical images, we have worked with our illustrators to represent a wide range of skin tones in our patients and surgeons.

This book reflects the collective efforts of a community dedicated to surgical education, and our partners, parents, friends, and family are integral members of this community. As we share this second edition with the world, we acknowledge and appreciate the sacrifices made by those closest to us, not only in the production of this book but also throughout the entirety of our surgical education. This is as much your achievement as it is ours, and we extend our deepest gratitude for being the silent champions behind our success.

Contributors

Ijaz Ahmad, MBBS, FRCS (Vascular Surgery), FRCS (General Surgery) — (Vascular)
Vascular Surgeon
Colchester Hospital
East Suffolk and North Essex NHS Foundation Trust
Colchester, UK

Stephen Ali, BM, MMedSc (Hons), PGCert (MedED), PGCert (Mgmt), MAcadMEd, FHEA, DMCC, MRCS (Eng) — (Anterior Resection of the Rectum, Excision of Pilonidal Sinus and Laparotomy for Necrotising Enterocolitis)
Clinical Lecturer
Institute of Life Science
Swansea University Medical School
Swansea, UK

d'Arcy Ferris Baxter, MBBS, MHLM, BInst (Development Studies) — (Obstetrics and Gynaecology)
Registrar
Obstetrics and Gynaecology
Royal North Shore Hospital
St Leonards, Australia

Alison Bradley, BSc (Hons), MBChB, MRCSEd, PGC, FRCS, PhD — (Lower Gastrointestinal)
Consultant Surgeon
University Hospital Hairmyres
Glasgow, UK

Roberta Bullingham, BMBS, BSc (Hons), BVSc, MRCS — (Useful Theatre Knowledge, Upper Gastrointestinal, Endocrine)
ST5 General Surgical Registrar
Lewisham and Greenwich Foundation Trust
London, UK

Abhishek Chitnis, MBChB, MClinEd — (Omental Patch Repair of a Perforated Duodenal Ulcer and Cholecystectomy)
Anaesthetic Registrar
Department of anaesthesia
Barts Health NHS Trust
London, UK

Luke Conway, MBChB, MRes, MRCS (Eng) — (Axillary Node Clearance, Sentinel Lymph Node Biopsy and Latissimus Dorsi Flap Reconstruction of the Breast)
Consultant Radiologist
Ipswich Hospital
Suffolk, UK

Laura Cormack, MBChB, BSc (Hons), MRCP, DTMH (Liv), FRCR — (Interventional Radiology)
Consultant Radiologist
West Suffolk Hospital
Bury Saint Edmunds, UK

Rhodri OHL Davies, MRCS, MSc, BDS, MBBS — (Orbital floor reconstruction)
StR Oral and Maxillofacial Surgery
Great Ormond Street Hospital
London, UK

Mary Patrice Eastwood, MBChB, PhD, FRCS (Paeds. Surg.) — (Paediatrics)
Paediatric Surgical Registrar
Paediatric Surgery
Royal Belfast Hospital for Sick Children
Belfast, UK

Rebecca Exley, MBChB, BDS, FRCS (OMFS), DOHNS, MFD, AKC, PGDip — (The coronal flap)
Oral and Maxillofacial Specialist Registrar – ST8
University College Hospitals London
London, UK

Angela Jane Hancock, MRCS, BDS, MBBS — (Neck dissection)
Oral and Maxillofacial Surgery Speciality Trainee
London Deanery
London, UK

Charles Jenkinson, MBBS, FRACS — (Cardiothoracics)
Department of Cardiothoracic Surgery
Sir Charles Gairdner Hospital
Perth, Australia;
The University of Western Australia
Perth, Australia

Ian Kennedy, BMSc (Hons), MBChB, MD, FRCS (Tr & Ortho) — (Lower Limb Fasciotomy)
Trauma and Orthopaedics
Queen Elizabeth University Hospital
Glasgow, UK

Mark Lawrence, MRCS, BDS, MBBS — (Le Fort 1 osteotomy and Bilateral Sagittal Split Osteotomy)
Specialty Registrar Maxillofacial Surgery
London Deanery
London, UK

**William Lo, MBBChir, FRCS (Neuro. Surg.),
    FEBNS** — (Neurosurgery)
Consultant Neurosurgeon
Birmingham Children's Hospital
Birmingham, UK

Huzaifa Malick, MbCHb, FRCOphth, PGCertMedEd —
    (Vitrectomy and Dacryocystorhinostomy)
Consultant Ophthalmologist - University Hospital of
    Leicester NHS Trust
Leicester Royal Infirmary Infirmary Square
Leicester, UK

**Katrina Mason, BSc, MBChB, DCH, MSc (Oxon),
    FRCS (ORL-HNS)** — (Surgical Positions, Ear, Nose
    and Throat, Suction Diathermy Adenoidectomy,
    Myringotomy and Tympanostomy Tube Grommet
    Insertion, Circumcision, Wedge Resection of Ingrown
    Toenail and Nail Bed Injury Repair)
Paediatric Ear, Nose & Throat Fellow
Evelina Children's Hospital
Guy's & St Thomas' NHS Foundation Trust
London, UK

Katie Nightingale, MBChB — (Breast)
General Surgery
Manchester Royal Infirmary
Manchester University Foundation Trust
Manchester, UK

Chrysavgi Oikonomou, MD, DDS, MSc —
    (Open reduction internal fixation mandible fractures
    (tooth bearing portions))
Consultant Oral and Maxillofacial Surgery
The Royal London Hospital
Barts Health NHS Trust
London, UK

Georgios Pafitanis, MD, PhD — (Plastics)
Consultant Plastic & Reconstructive Surgeon
London Reconstructive Microsurgery Unit
Department of Plastic Surgery
The Royal London Hospital
Barts Health & University College London Hospital
    NHS Trusts
London, UK

Joon Park, MBBS, MSc (Surg Sc) — (Hartmann's
    Procedure and Femoral Hernia Repair)
Principle House Officer
Gold Coast University Hospital
Gold Coast, Australia

John Pascoe, BMBS, MRCS, PgCert (ClinEd) —
    (Urology)
Specialist Registrar in Urology – South West rotation
South West Deanery, UK

Oliver Riley, MBChB, BSc Pharmacology —
    (Ophthalmology)
Ophthalmology Speciality Registrar
NHS Wales
Cardiff, UK

Gareth Rogers, BSc (Hons), MBChB, MRCSEd —
    (Orthopaedics)
Trauma and Orthopaedics Specialist Registar
Health Education England
North West School of Surgery (East Sector), UK

Farihah Tariq, BSc (Hons), MBChB, MRCGP —
    (Ophthalmology, Phacoemulsification (Cataract
    Surgery), Trabeculectomy)
NHS Scotland
Glasgow, UK

Imogen Thomson, MD — (Obstetrics and Gynaecology)
Obstetrics & Gynaecology
Royal North Shore Hospital
Sydney, Australia

**Chukwudi Uzoho, BM, BSc, BMedSci, MRCS,
    PgDip** — (Dynamic Hip Screw)
Trauma & Orthopaedic Surgery
Nottingham University Hospitals NHS Trust
Nottingham, UK

**Elizabeth Yeung, FRCS (OMFS), DOHNS, BDS, MBBS,
    BSc (Hons)** — (Maxillofacial, Bilateral Sagittal Split
    Osteotomy, The Coronal Flap, Le Fort 1 Osteotomy,
    Neck Dissection, Orbital Floor Reconstruction, Open
    Reduction and Internal Fixation of Mandibular
    Fractures (Tooth-Bearing Regions))
Consultant Oral and Maxillofacial Surgery
Northwick Park Hospital
St Mary's Hospital
London, UK

Acknowledgements

We would like to thank all of the authors, from the first and second editions, for their dedication and hard work.

CONTRIBUTORS FROM THE FIRST EDITION

Stephen Ali – Anterior Resection of the Rectum, Excision of Pilonidal Sinus, Laparotomy for Necrotising Enterocolitis

Stephanie Arrigo – Arthroscopic Rotator Cuff Tendon Repair, Intervertebral Spinal Discectomy, Total Hip Replacement (THR) Anterolateral Approach, Arthroscopic Meniscectomy

Richard D Bartlett – Carpal Tunnel Decompression Surgery

Jonathan Bialick – Scrubbing Up for Theatre

Carly Bisset – Hernia Repair, Lumbar Spinal Fusion

James Brooks – Liver Resection, Splenectomy, Burr Hole, Craniotomy, Ventriculoperitoneal (VP) Shunt Insertion

Alison Bradley – Lower Gastrointestinal

Joanna Buchan – Upper Gastrointestinal

Roberta Bullingham – Scrubbing Up for Theatre

Ivana Capin – Myringotomy and Tympanostomy Tube Grommet Insertion, Ramstedt Pyloromyotomy, Oesophageal Atresia/Tracheoesophageal Fistula Ligation with Repair

Darren KT Chan – Nephrectomy

Tyson Chan – Phacoemulsification (Cataract Surgery)

Christina Cheng – Incision and Drainage of Perianal Abscess, Thoracotomy, LADD's Procedure

Abhishek Chitnis – Omental Patch Repair of a Perforated Duodenal Ulcer, Cholecystectomy

Laura Cormack – Interventional radiology

Luke Conway – Axillary Node, Sentinel Lymph Node Biopsy, Latissimus Dorsi Flap Reconstruction of the Breast

James Cragg – Femoral Endarterectomy, Endovenous Laser Treatment for Varicose Veins (EVLT)

Alexander Dando – Lumbar Laminectomy

Kirsty Dawson – Trans-Urethral Resection of the Prostate

Ganesh Devarajan – Orthopaedics

Yasoda Dupaguntla – Left Hemicolectomy

Mary Patrice Eastwood – Paediatrics

Stephanie Eltz – Lateral Malleolus Lag Screw and Neutralisation Plate

Mathew Gallagher – Neurosurgery, Burr Hole, Craniotomy, Lumbar Laminectomy, Ventriculoperitoneal (VP) Shunt Insertion, Endoscopic Transsphenoidal Pituitary Surgery

Madelaine Gimzewska – Vascular, Carotid Endarterectomy, Open Abdominal Aortic Aneurysm Repair, Endovascular Aneurysm Repair, Radiocephalic Fistula Formation, Below Knee Amputation, Above Knee Amputation, Femoral-Popliteal Bypass Graft, Embolectomy

James Glasbey – Endocrine, Total Thyroidectomy, Parathyroidectomy, Adrenalectomy

Lisa Grundy – Gastrectomy

Louis Hainsworth – Trans-Urethral Resection of Bladder Tumour, Scrotal Exploration and Orchidopexy, Vasectomy

Nimeshi Jayakody – Endoscopic Retrograde Cholangiopancreatography, Superficial Parotidectomy

Angelina Jayakumar – Manipulation of Fractured Nasal Bones

John Kennedy – Lower Limb Fasciotomy

Maria Knöbel – Tonsillectomy

Brendan S Kelly – Interventional radiology, Angioplasty +/- Stenting, Transjugular Intrahepatic Portosystemic Shunt (TIPSS), Catheter-Directed Thrombolysis (CDT), Embolisation, Percutaneous Nephrostomy, Radiologically Inserted Gastrostomy (RIG) or Gastrojejunostomy (RIGJ)

Nicholas Leaver – Gastric Band, Thoracoscopic Pulmonary Lobectomy, Percutaneous Patent Foramen Ovale Repair

Jane Shujing Lim – Abdominoperineal Resection (APR), Mastectomy, Wide Local Excision (WLE), Hepatoportoenterostomy (Kasai Portoenterostomy), Orchidopexy

William B Lo – Neurosurgery

Nigel Tapiwa Mabvuure – Split-Thickness Skin Graft, Full-Thickness Skin Graft

Greta McLachlan – Upper Gastrointestinal

Huzaifa Malick – Vitrectomy, Dacryocystorhinostomy (DCR)

Katrina Mason – Breast, Ear nose and throat, Plastics, Endocrine, Obstetrics and gynaecology, Suction Diathermy Adenoidectomy, Myringotomy and Tympanostomy Tube Grommet Insertion, Circumcision, Nail Bed Injury Repair, Hysteroscopy, Caesarean Section, Anterior Vaginal Wall Repair, Large Loop Excision of the Transformation Zone (LLETZ), Posterior Vaginal Wall Repair, Wedge Resection of Ingrown Toenail

Andrea McCarthy – Ivor Lewis Oesophagectomy, Surgical Tracheostomy

Sameena Mohamedally – Heller Myotomy

Dariush Nikkhah – Split-Thickness Skin Graft, Full-Thickness Skin Graft

Lay Ping Ong – Cardiothoracics

Georgios Pafitanis – Deep Inferior Epigastric Perforator (DIEP) Free-Flap for Breast Reconstruction

Joon Park – Hartmann's Procedure, Femoral Hernia Repair

Esther Platt – Vascular

Conor Ramsden – Horizontal Strabismus Surgery

Paul Robinson – Dynamic Hip Screw

Jennifer Robertson – Obstetrics and gynaecology, Hysterectomy, Tension-Free Vaginal Tape (TVT), Hysteroscopy, Caesarean Section, Anterior Vaginal Wall Repair, Large Loop Excision of the Transformation Zone (LLETZ), Posterior Vaginal Wall Repair

Suhail Rokadiya – Wound Closure and Diathermy

Gareth Rogers – Orthopaedics, Cephalomedullary Femoral Nail, Cemented Hip Hemiarthroplasty, Medial Malleolus Open Reduction and Internal Fixation, Tibial Nail

Shahab Shahid – Arthroscopic ACL Reconstruction, Arthroscopic Meniscectomy

Yashashwi Sinha – Gastrectomy, Gastric Bypass, Dupuytren's Contracture Release, Total Knee Replacement (TKR)

Farihah Tariq – Ophthalmology, Phacoemulsification (Cataract Surgery), Trabeculectomy

Rebecca Telfer – Distal Radius Volar Locking Plate

Evgenia Theodorakopoulou – Urology, Nephrectomy, Local Flap Reconstruction of Soft Tissue Defects, Digital Tendon Repair

Sasha Shoba Devi Thrumurthy – Whipple's Procedure (Pancreaticoduodenectomy), Small Bowel Resection

Chukwudi Uzoho – Dynamic Hip Screw

Nicholas Wroe – Coronary Artery Bypass Grafting, Aortic Valve Repair/Replacement, Mitral Valve Repair/Replacement, Inferior Vena Cava Filter, Percutaneous Biliary Drainage

Shiying Wu – Laparoscopic Appendicectomy, Right Hemicolectomy, Haemorrhoidectomy

Alexander Yao – Ear nose and throat, Septoplasty, Functional Endoscopic Sinus Surgery (FESS)

Muhamed Zuhair – Nissen Fundoplication

Abbreviations

A&E   Accident and Emergency
AAA   abdominal aortic aneurysm
AC   alternating current
ACL   anterior cruciate ligament
ACTH   adrenocorticotrophic hormone
ADH   antidiuretic hormone
AIS   acute ischaemic stroke
AKA   above-knee amputation
ALND   axillary lymph node dissection
AMI   acute myocardial infarction
ANC   axillary node clearance
AOM   acute otitis media
AP   anterior posterior
AR   aortic regurgitation
AS   aortic stenosis
ASD   atrial septal defect
ASIS   anterior superior iliac spine
AUB   abnormal uterine bleeding
AV   arteriovenous
AVM   arteriovenous malformation
BCT   breast-conserving therapy
BKA   below-knee amputation
BMI   body mass index
BPH   benign prostatic hypertrophy
B-PT-B   bone-patellar tendon-bone
BRCA   breast cancer gene
BSS   balanced salt solution
BXO   balanitis xerotica obliterans
CABG   coronary artery bypass grafting
CBD   common bile duct
CCA   common carotid artery
CCAM   congenital cystic adenomatoid malformation
CDT   catheter-directed thrombolysis
CES   cauda equina syndrome
CFA   common femoral artery
CHA   common hepatic artery
CMLND   complete mediastinal lymph node dissection
CMV   cytomegalovirus
CNS   clinical nurse specialist
COPD   chronic obstructive pulmonary disease
CPB   cardiopulmonary bypass
CPR   cardiopulmonary resuscitation
CRPS   complex regional pain syndrome
CRS   chronic rhinosinusitis
CSF   cerebrospinal fluid
CT   computed tomography
CTP   computed tomography perfusion
CTS   carpal tunnel syndrome

CUSA   cavitron ultrasonic surgical aspirator
CXR   chest X-ray
DCIS   ductal carcinoma in situ
DCR   dacryocystorhinostomy
DHS   dynamic hip screw
DIE   deep inferior epigastric
DIEA   deep inferior epigastric artery
DIEP   deep inferior epigastric perforator
DIEV   deep inferior epigastric vein
DIPJ   distal interphalangeal joints
DJ   duodenojejunal
DPNB   dorsal penile nerve block
DVT   deep vein thrombosis
EBV   Epstein-Barr virus
ECA   external carotid artery
ECG   electrocardiogram
EDC   extensor digitorum communis
EDM   extensor digiti minimi
EEG   electroencephalogram
EI   extensor indicis
ENT   ear, nose, throat
EOM   extraocular muscles
EPB   extensor pollicis brevis
EPL   extensor pollicis longus
ERCP   endoscopic retrograde cholangiopancreatography
ET   endotracheal tube
EUS   external urethral sphincter
EVAR   endovascular aneurysm repair
EVLT   endovenous laser treatment for varicose veins
F   French [sizing]
FCR   flexor carpi radialis
FDP   flexor digitorum profundus
FDS   flexor digitorum superficialis
FESS   functional endoscopic sinus surgery
FEV_1 forced expiratory volume (first second)
FPL   flexor pollicis longus
FSH   follicle stimulating hormone
FTSG   full-thickness skin graft
GH   growth hormone
GHK   glenohumeral joint
GI   gastrointestinal
GORD   gastro-oesophageal reflux disease
GP   general practitioner
GPA   granulomatosis with polyangiitis
GSV   great saphenous vein
GT   greater trochanter
GTN   glyceryl trinitrate
H. pylori   *Helicobacter pylori*

HCC hepatocellular carcinoma
HDU high dependency unit
HIV human immunodeficiency virus
HPT hyperparathyroidism
HPV human papillomavirus
HSV herpes simplex virus
ICA internal carotid artery
IDF inferior duodenal flexure
IJV internal jugular vein
II image intensifier
IMA inferior mesenteric artery
IMV inferior mesenteric vein
INR international normalized ratio
IOP intraocular pressure
IP infundibulo-pelvic
ITU intensive treatment unit
IUD intrauterine device
IUS internal urethral sphincter
IV intravenous
IVC inferior vena cava
LAD left anterior descending
LCA left coronary artery
LCIS lobular carcinoma in situ
LD latissimus dorsi
LDA left posterior descending artery
LFT liver function test
LGA left gastric artery
LGE left gastro-epiploic
LH luteinising hormone
LLETZ large loop excision of the transformation zone
LOAF lateral lumbricals, opponens policies, abductor pollicis brevis and flexor pollicis brevis
LUTS lower urinary tract symptoms
LV left ventricular
MCL medial collateral ligament
MCP metacarpal-phalangeal
MDT multidisciplinary team
MELD model for end-stage liver disease
MEN multiple endocrine neoplasia
MI myocardial infarction
MPL medial palpebral ligament
MR mitral regurgitation
MRI magnetic resonance imaging
MRM modified radical mastectomy
MS mitral stenosis
NAVY nerve, artery, vein, Y fronts
NEC necrotising enterocolitis
NG nasogastric tube
NHS National Health Service
NICU neonatal intensive care unit
NOF neck of femur
NSS nephron sparing surgery
NSTEMI non-ST elevation myocardial infarction
NVB neurovascular bundle
OA oesophageal atresia
OME otitis media with effusion
OSA obstructive sleep apnoea
OSNA one-step nucleic amplification

PCA patient-controlled analgesia
PCI percutaneous coronary intervention
PCL posterior cruciate ligament
PDS polydioxanone
PE pulmonary embolism
PET positron emission tomography
PFA profunda femoral artery
PFO patent foramen ovale
PH potential hydrogen
PIP proximal interphalangeal
PIPJ proximal interphalangeal joints
POEM per-oral endoscopic myotomy
PR abdominoperineal resection
PTH parathyroid hormone
RBMN recurrent branch of the median nerve
RCA right coronary artery
RCC renal cell carcinoma
RGA right gastric artery
RGE right gastro-epiploic
RIG radiologically inserted gastrostomy
RIGJ radiologically inserted gastrojejunostomy
RL recurrent laryngeal nerve
RM radical mastectomy
SAM systolic anterior motion
SCM sternocleidomastoid
SDF superior duodenal flexure
SFA superior femoral artery
SFJ saphenofemoral junction
SFV superior femoral vein
SIEA superior inferior epigastric artery
SIEV superior inferior epigastric vein
SIGN Scottish Intercollegiate Guidelines Network
SIT supraspinatus, infraspinatus, and teres minor
SLNB sentinel lymph node biopsy
SM simple mastectomy
SMA superior mesenteric artery
SMV superior mesenteric vein
SPA sphenopalatine artery
SPA superior pancreaticoduodenal artery
SSV short saphenous vein
STEMI ST elevation myocardial infarction
STSG split thickness skin graft
SUI stress urinary incontinence
T3 liothyronine
TAT transanastomotic tube
TAVI transcatheter aortic valve implantation
THR total hip replacement
TKR total knee replacement
TIPSS transjugular intrahepatic portosystemic shunt
TM tympanic membrane
TME total mesorectal excision
TOE transoesophageal echocardiography
TOF tracheoesophageal fistula
tPA tissue plasminogen activator
TRAM transverse rectus abdominis muscle
TSH thyroid stimulating hormone
TUR transurethral resection
TURP transurethral resection of the prostate

TURBT transurethral resection of bladder tumour
TVT tension-free vaginal tape
TWOC trial without catheter
USP US Pharmacopoeia
VACTERL vertebral, anal atresia, cardiovascular, tracheoesophageal, renal, and limb defects
VAN vein, artery, nerve
VATS video-assisted thoracoscopic surgery
vCJD variant Creutzfeldt–Jacob disease
VP ventriculoperitoneal
VPI velopharyngeal insufficiency
VTE venous thromboembolic
WHO World Health Organisation
WLE wide local excision

Contents

Scrubbing Up for Theatre

1

Roberta Bullingham

Aim of the Surgical Scrub

A systematic washing of the hands, forearms, and nails with an antiseptic wash with the aim of:
- Removing debris and transient microorganisms.
- Reducing commensal microorganisms to a minimum.
- Inhibiting 'rebound' growth and release of bacteria under gloved hands.

  In case of puncture of the surgical glove, and the release of bacteria to the open wound, the scrub will reduce the risk of a surgical site infection (SSI) to an absolute minimum (Fig. 1.1).

CHECKLIST

- Surgical hat (often found in changing room) and hoods to cover beards.
- Mask ± eye shield (depending on the procedure).
- Sink with hand-free taps and elbow dispenser anti-septic wash.
- Hand scrubber pack (brush, sponge, and nail pick).
- Theatre gown pack.
- Sterile gloves (get to know your size—this is important for comfort and dexterity); for double gloving—your regular size for under glove and half-a-size bigger for over.
- A helpful and willing assistant

NB: for COVID-19-positive + COVID-19 pending patients: FFP3 masks + visors are required.

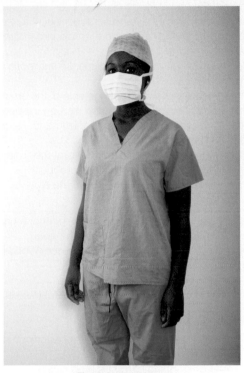

Fig. 1.1 Scrubbing.

Preparation

- Keep nails short and clean, and do not wear artificial nails or nail polish.
- Remove all jewellery or cover with plasters before entering the operating theatre.
- Wear scrubs, surgical hat, and theatre shoes to enter theatre.
- Wash hands and arms with a nonmedicated soap, and dry before entering the operating theatre.
- Tie on face mask, covering the nose and mouth (you will not be able to readjust when scrubbed).

- Open surgical gown packet, and gently tip it onto the gowning trolley so that it faces upwards.
- Open the packet by pulling the edges outwards to unfold it (maintaining sterile field of the contents).
- Open the packet containing the gloves and tip them onto the open gown packet (just to the side of the paper towels).
- Open the hand scrubber and leave it on the edge of the sink (or within easy reach).

'Scrubbing-In'

The scrub procedure should last 5 minutes (this should be timed).

PHASE 1

1. Turn on the water and regulate the flow and temperature of water (after this step, you must not touch the taps with your hands).
2. Wet hands and arms down to the elbow for a pre-scrub wash: use several drops of scrub solution, work up a heavy lather, then wash the hands and arms to the elbows (Fig. 1.2).
3. Rinse hands and arms thoroughly, allowing the water to run from the hands to the elbows.
4. Use nail pick (from the hand scrubber pack) to remove dirt from under the nails, and then discard into a sharps bin.
5. Use the elbow of one arm to dispense antiseptic wash onto the scrubber brush.
6. Lather fingertips with the sponge side of the brush; then, using the bristle side of the brush, scrub the spaces under the fingernails of the right or left hand. Repeat for the other hand (Fig. 1.3).
7. Lather fingers. Wash on all four sides of the fingers using the sponge side only. Discard the scrubber.
8. Rinse, always keeping hands above the elbows.

PHASE 2

1. Dispense antiseptic wash into the palm of one hand (using the opposite elbow to press the lever).
2. Wash hands using the six-step technique (World Health Organization (WHO) guidelines):
   a. Palm to palm
   b. Right palm over left dorsum and left palm over right dorsum
   c. Palm to palm, fingers interlaced
   d. Back of fingers to opposing palms with fingers interlocked
   e. Rotational rubbing of right thumb clasped in left palm and vice versa
   f. Rotational rubbing backwards and forwards with clasped fingers of right hand in left palm and vice versa
3. Rotationally rub the wrists, working down to the elbows with one hand and then vice versa.
4. Rinse hands and arms thoroughly from fingertip to elbow without retracing, allowing the water to drip from the elbow (Fig 1.4).

If the scrub practitioner's hands or arms accidentally touch the taps, sink, or other unsterile object during any phase of the scrub, they are considered contaminated, and the process MUST begin again.

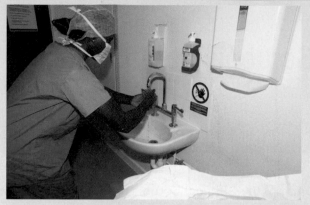

Fig. 1.2 Wetting hands.

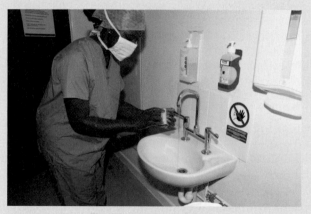

Fig. 1.3 Cleaning fingertips.

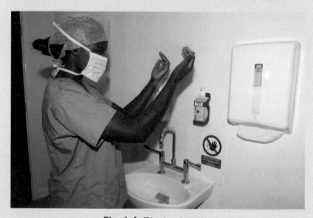

Fig. 1.4 Rinsing hands.

PHASE 3

1. Repeat phase 2 but stop halfway down the forearms.
2. Close the taps using elbows.
3. Return to the gowning trolley, pick up one hand towel from the top of the gown pack, and step back from the table. Grasp the towel and open it fully (Fig. 1.5).
4. Use an aseptic paper towel to dry using a patting motion. Start at the fingers and work down the arms; do not retrace any area. Each hand should touch only one side of the paper towel. Discard each paper towel after use (Fig. 1.6).
5. Do not retrace any areas. Discard this towel in an appropriate receptacle.
6. Repeat with the other towel from the pack for the other hand/arm.

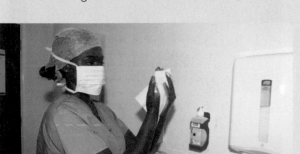

Fig. 1.5 Drying hands.

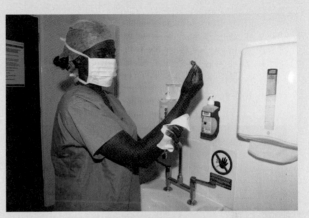

Fig. 1.6 Drying arms.

Gowning

1. Keep your hands close together with thumbs facing up and place your hands into the arms of the gown (it will be facing this way in the pack).
2. Lift it off the trolley. Taking a wide step back (making sure you have enough space that you will not touch anything by mistake), extend your elbows, moving arms apart so that the gown unfolds (Fig. 1.7).
3. Keep your hands within the sleeves (Fig. 1.8).
4. Ask an assistant to fasten the Velcro and the ties at the back.

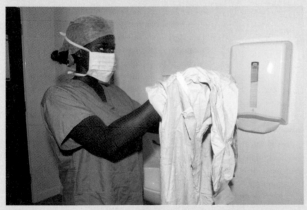

Fig. 1.7 Putting on gown.

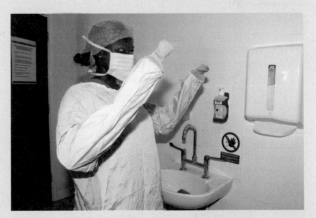

Fig. 1.8 Keeping hands within sleeves.

Donning Gloves

1. Keeping the hands tucked inside the sleeves of the gown, unfold the packet with the gloves inside.
2. Pick up one glove by the folded cuff edge with the sleeve-covered hand (opposite hand to glove labelled left or right). If you are right handed, gloving your left hand first is easiest, but either way is fine (Fig. 1.9).
3. Slip the fingers of the appropriate hand out of the sleeve of the gown into the glove (with the rest of the hand remaining covered) (Fig. 1.10).
4. Use your still-covered opposite hand to fold back the rest of the glove so that it covers the wrist.
5. Pull and adjust the sleeves of the gown so that they cover a little more than the wrists under the gloves (Fig. 1.11).
6. Follow these steps for the opposite hand.

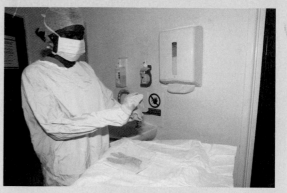

Fig. 1.10 Putting on gloves.

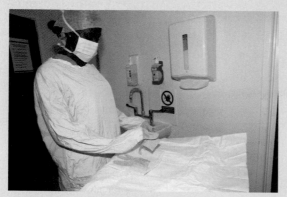

Fig. 1.9 Opening gloves.

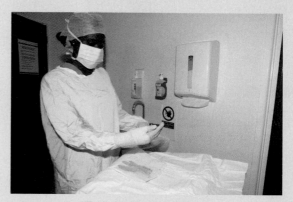

Fig. 1.11 Adjusting gloves.

Final Tie of the Gown

1. Take hold of the sterile card belt tab that secures the belt tie (Fig. 1.12).
2. Ask an assistant to take hold of the tab and walk all the way around you, ending in front of you (Fig. 1.13).
3. Then take hold of the belt tie only (being careful not to touch the tab again) and pull on the tie, leaving the assistant with only the tab in their hand (Fig. 1.14).
4. Tie the belt tie with a simple knot at the side of the gown.

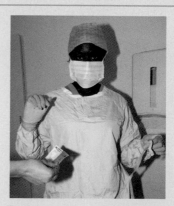

Fig. 1.13 Assistant helping with final tie.

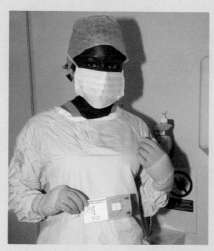

Fig. 1.12 Sterile card.

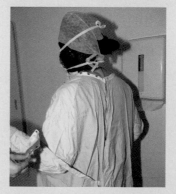

Fig. 1.14 Rotating with tie held by an assistant.

Surgeon's Top Tips

1. When waiting for the procedure to start, keep your hands raised in front of your chest to maintain your sterile field.
2. If you have any questions during the scrubbing-in procedure, ask—there are always experienced people who can help.
3. If you do accidentally make contact with an unsterile object at any time, don't be afraid to say so. The surgical team and the patient will be glad you did!
4. If you notice a scrubbed colleague breach sterility, be sure to communicate it to the team if unnoticed.

2 Wound Closure and Diathermy

Roberta Bullingham

Introduction to Sutures

- The closure of a wound with sutures is known as healing by 'primary intention' and allows for the rapid and cosmetic closure of an open wound/other tissue.
- Sutures have been around for approximately 4000 years. Linen, animal sinews, and a huge variety of other materials have been used. This chapter will help you further understand suture material types, suture examples, and their appropriate surgical uses.

Choosing the Appropriate Suture Material

- The ideal suture material should:
  - Be universally applicable
  - Be 'memory free' (i.e. limp and pliable)
  - Be inert and biocompatible
  - Have low drag when passing through tissues but good friction for knot-tying
  - Be free from stretch and not warp under tension
  - Be stable under sterilisation during manufacturing
- A suture material that is suitable for all closures does not exist. Therefore, the first question a surgeon will face when deciding on suture type is whether the suture needs to be absorbable or nonabsorbable.
- Absorbable sutures undergo natural degradation through enzymatic action followed by hydrolytic action, or through hydrolytic action alone.
- Further considerations are whether the suture material is made from natural or synthetic material. Natural suture materials such as catgut (from animal intestines—monofilament) and collagen (from bovine tendons—multifilament) were traditionally used. In the main, however, synthetic materials are now utilised.
- The choice between multifilament and monofilament sutures is based on a variety of factors:
  - Multifilament sutures run a higher potential of bacterial contamination, as bacteria can adhere more easily to the crenulations in the material. Multifilament sutures can also draw fluid into a wound increasing wound infection risk.
  - Monofilament sutures have a lower coefficient of friction, resulting in less drag than a multifilament suture. However, they are more sensitive to meticulous technique when knot-tying.
  - Thicker-grade sutures have 'suture memory', where the suture material retains the shape of its packing. Monofilament sutures often spring back to their original shape, making knot-tying more difficult.
- Recently, barbed sutures have become available in a variety of absorbable synthetic materials, with the aim of avoiding knot-tying.

Absorbable Sutures

SYNTHETIC

1. Polydioxanone or PDS:
   a. A monofilament suture hydrolysed (absorbed) in less than 1 year
   b. Has memory and is thus sometimes difficult to manipulate without practice
2. Polyglycolic acid suture (e.g. Vicryl, Polysorb, Dexon)
   a. Braided, although an ophthalmic monofilament suture is available
   b. Generally absorbed within 4 weeks
   c. Has generally good handling characteristics with little memory
3. Polyglecaprone (e.g. monocryl)
   a. Available as either a clear or a dyed (purple) monofilament suture
   b. Absorbed within 120 days. Often used in skin
   c. Has a degree of memory
4. Polyglyconate (Maxon)
   a. A long-term monofilament suture absorbed within 210 days
   b. Available as clear or green
   c. Older versions were less pliable, but the material has good knot-holding capability
5. Polyglactin 910 (Vicryl rapide)
   a. A white braided suture, absorbed fully within 6 weeks, an external component will fall off skin within 2 weeks
   b. Good handling characteristics
   c. Made from 90% polyglycolic acid combined with 10% lactic acid

NATURAL

- Despite availability and good handling characteristics, natural absorbable sutures are rarely used due to concerns regarding the possible transmission of new variant Creutzfeldt–Jakob (VCJD) causing prions in patients.

- Catgut is a monofilament, rapidly absorbed, and available either plain (fast) or chromic coated to allow faster or slower enzymatic degradation depending on the site and the patient physiology.

Nonabsorbable Sutures

SYNTHETIC

1. Nylon (e.g. Ethilon, Dafilon, Dermalon, Linex)
   a. Monofilament, good tensile strength, and minimal tissue reactivity
   b. Inexpensive and widely used
2. Polypropylene (e.g. Prolene, Surgipro)
   a. Very smooth monofilament suture but highly plastic and more difficult to tie securely than other materials
3. Polybutester (e.g. Novafil)
   a. Elastic and thus can adapt to tissue oedema
   b. Good handling and knot-tying properties
4. Polyester (e.g. Ticron, Dacron, Mersilene, Ethibond)
   a. Braided suture, very strong with good handling and low tissue reaction
5. Stainless steel
   a. Used primarily in closure of the chest following cardiothoracic surgery and in orthopaedics for cerclage and tendon repair; can also be used for abdominal wall closure
   b. High tensile strength, some elasticity, and forms a secure knot

NATURAL

1. Silk
   a. Braided treated suture
   b. Has excellent handling and knot security

Needles

DESIGN AND ANATOMY

- The needle should be made of high-quality stainless steel, be of the smallest possible cross-sectional area, and remain stable in the needle holder or hand.
- The anatomy of the needle can be separated into three parts:
  - The point
  - The body
  - The swage/eye of the needle
- Needles are available in a variety of lengths, from 75 μm to 80 mm.

POINT TYPES (FIG. 2.1)

- Cutting needles—designed to penetrate dense and thick tissues, including skin. They are triangular in cross-section and have three cutting edges, either on the inside of the curve (conventional) or the outside of the curve (reverse cutting). Reverse cutting needles have a reduced risk of cutting through tissues and are therefore used in ophthalmic and cosmetic procedures where minimal tissue trauma is vital. Spatula needles were specifically designed for ophthalmic procedures, as the needle design splits/

NEEDLE SHAPE	POINT TYPE	SYMBOL
	Taper point	
	Blunt taper point	
	Cutting edge	
	Reverse cutting edge	
	Tapercut	

Fig. 2.1 Needle types.

separates the layers of corneal tissue to create a plane through which the suture material can pass.

- Tapered point needles—useful in subcutaneous layers and abdominal viscera where tissue can be stretched and penetrated without cutting. Sharpness is dictated by the taper ratio and tip angle.
- Blunt needles—pass through friable tissue (e.g. liver and kidney) without cutting. Sometimes used to close abdominal wall to reduce risk of injury to viscera.

NEEDLE BODY TYPES (FIG. 2.2)

- Straight body—simple to use, but must be used with caution as the tissue is usually being manipulated by hand
- Curved body—can be used in tighter spaces and allow an even distribution of tension on rotation of the wrist
  - Usually represented as fractions of a circle (e.g. 3/8, 5/8)
  - Compound shape
  - J-shaped

SWAGE TYPES (THE ATTACHMENT OF THE NEEDLE TO THE SUTURE)

- Channel—These needles have a larger diameter at the swage than at the needle point (a result of crimping the needle end around the suture).
- Nonswaged—Now unlikely to be used, as they result in more tissue trauma and suture handling, these needles require passing the suture through the needle's eye (such as in tailoring).
- Drill—The end of the needle is finely removed (often with a laser) during production, allowing the swage to be a smaller diameter than the needle. This results in less tissue trauma when being pulled through.

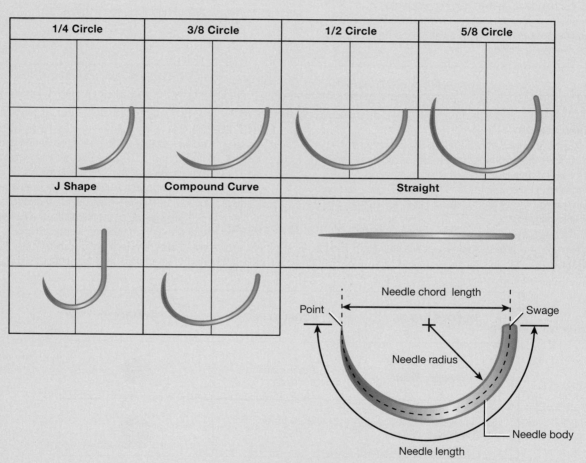

Fig. 2.2 Needle point types.

Suture Size

Sizes are listed here from smallest to largest (Fig. 2.3). Although the European units are more closely related to the actual diameter of the suture, USP (US Pharmacopoeia) units are more widely used in the UK.

USP designation	Synthetic absorbable diameter (mm)	Non-absorbable diameter (mm)	Uses
11-0		0.01	Ophthalmic surgery
10-0	0.02	0.02	Digital vessel anastomosis and nerve repair
9-0	0.03	0.03	
8-0	0.04	0.04	Vessel repair and anastomosis
7-0	0.05	0.05	Facial skin closure
6-0	0.07	0.07	Vascular grafts following endarterectomy or larger vessel repair
5-0	0.1	0.1	
4-0	0.15	0.15	Skin closure
3-0	0.2	0.2	Closure of muscle fascia/ tense skin
2-0	0.3	0.3	Bowel repair
0	0.35	0.35	Abdominal closure
1	0.4	0.4	Joint capsule repair
2	0.5	0.5	Hip and back surgery
3	0.6	0.6	Tendon repair and high-tension orthopaedic procedures
4	0.6	0.6	
5	0.7	0.7	
6		0.8	
7			

Fig. 2.3 Suture sizes.

Alternative Skin Closure

STAPLES

Staples can be applied rapidly for large scalp closures and less aesthetically demanding sites (Fig. 2.4). Used to close large abdominal wounds, e.g. laparotomy, to allow sections to be removed where there is postoperative wound collection/ infection.

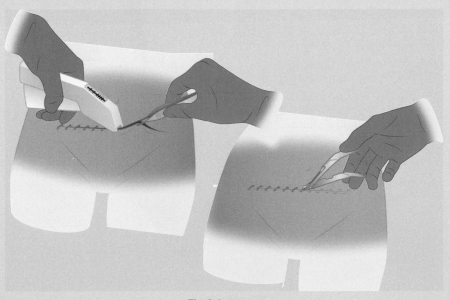

Fig. 2.4 Staples.

SKIN GLUE

Skin glue may be appropriate for small wounds with little or no wound tension or following suturing to enable a hermetic seal (Fig. 2.5).

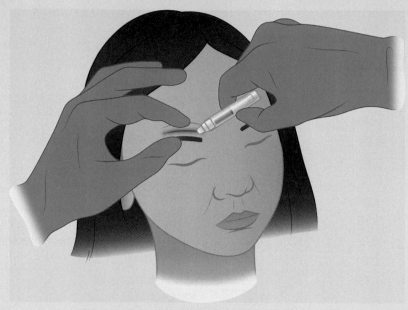

Fig. 2.5 Skin glue.

STERI-STRIPS

Wound sticky tape dressings, such as Steri-Strips, can be helpful in the apposition of skin edges following wound closure or as an adjunct to skin glue (Fig. 2.6).

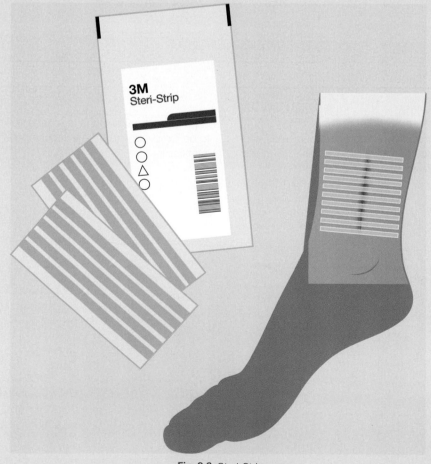

Fig. 2.6 Steri-Strips.

Diathermy

- Diathermy produces a localised heating effect through high-frequency AC electric current (400 kHz–10 MHz) by which tissue can be cut, cauterised, or destroyed.
- There are risks to the use of diathermy. To reduce these, it is important to ensure that flammable liquid (e.g. alcohol/chlorhexidine skin preparation) is allowed to dry prior to use of diathermy.
- Tissue in contact with the whole length of the metal (not just the tip) will be damaged and the thermal energy dissipates laterally, which can lead to inadvertent bystander burns.
- Electrodes should be fully in contact with the patient's skin and not overlie bony prominences.

MONOPOLAR

- From the generator, the current passes through the instrument, through the patient, and back out though a diathermy plate attached to the patient (usually the thigh) (Fig. 2.7).
- Heat is concentrated at the tip and spread over the much larger surface area of the plate (>70 cm²).
- Relatively high power and wattage are required.

BIPOLAR

- A conduction current is formed between the two limbs of the forceps so that a small amount of current passes through the tissue between the points of the forceps, locally producing heat (Fig. 2.8).
- No plate is required, and thus a smaller wattage is required.
- It is safer for patients with pacemakers for this reason.
- Employed as one of three modes—**cutting** (a constant current), **coagulation** (intermittent pulses of current), or **blend** (a combination).

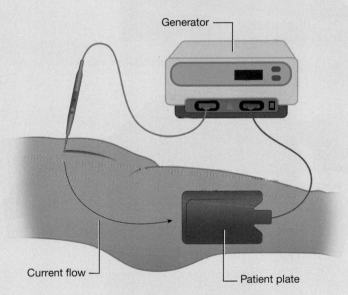

Fig. 2.7 Monopolar diathermy.

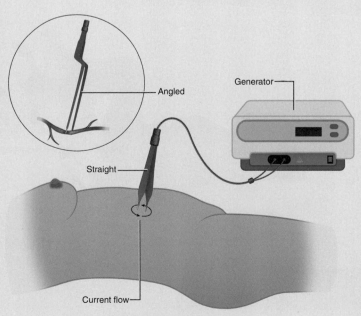

Fig. 2.8 Bipolar diathermy.

3

Surgical Positions

Katrina Mason

Figs. 3.1–3.9 demonstrate common surgical positions.

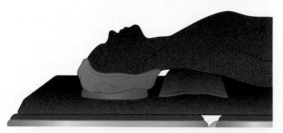

Fig. 3.1 Shoulder roll and head ring/Rose's position. Used in ENT surgery.

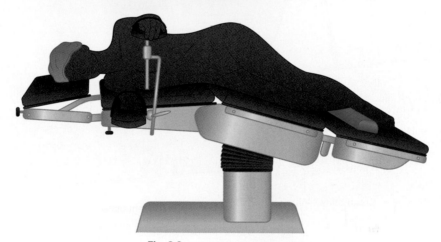

Fig. 3.2 Lateral decubitus (right).

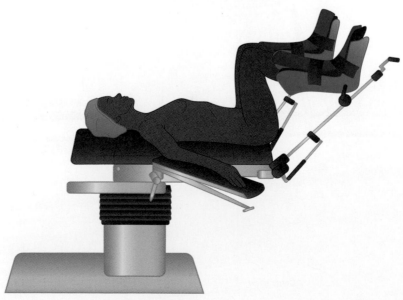

Fig. 3.3 Lithotomy.

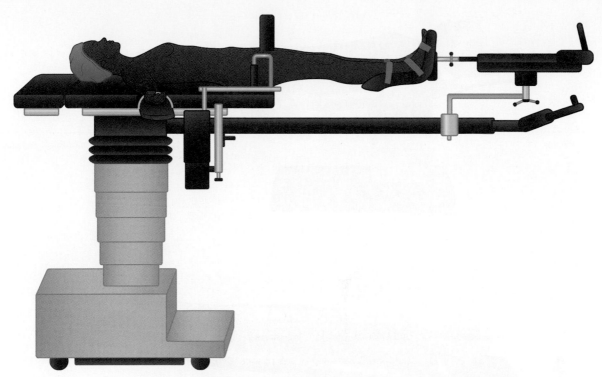

Fig. 3.4 Orthopaedic fracture table.

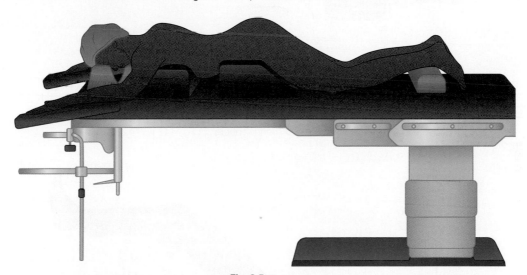

Fig. 3.5 Prone.

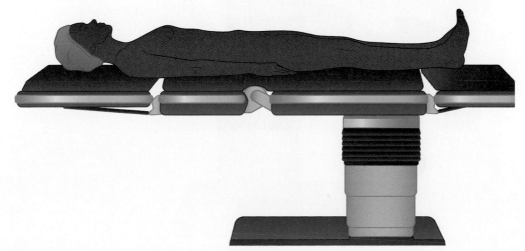

Fig. 3.6 Supine.

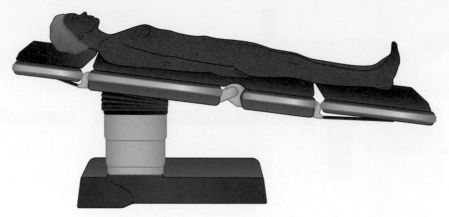

Fig. 3.7 Reverse Trendelenburg.

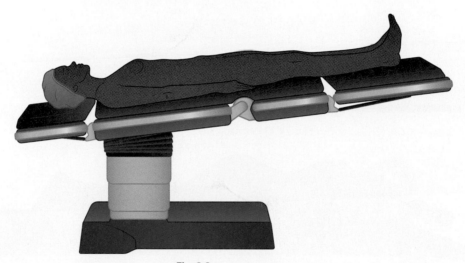

Fig. 3.8 Trendelenburg.

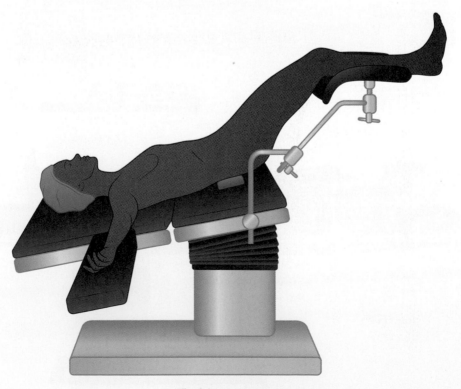

Fig. 3.9 Lloyd Davies.

Ivor Lewis Oesophagectomy

4

Roberta Bullingham

Definition

The partial removal of the oesophagus and stomach with construction of a gastric conduit through an upper midline abdominal incision and a right thoracotomy.

 ## Indications and Contraindications

INDICATIONS

- Oesophageal cancer—after multidisciplinary team (MDT) discussion and complete staging (CT of the chest, abdomen, and pelvis; staging laparoscopy; positron emission tomography (PET); endoscopic ultrasound).
- Severe strictures associated with reflux, alkali ingestion, or end-stage achalasia.
- Para-oesophageal hernia.
- Gastric cancer involving the gastro-oesophageal junction.

CONTRAINDICATIONS

- Oesophageal cancer T4b staged lesions—with invasion of the trachea, aorta, spine, or other crucial structures or with distant metastases and thus inoperable.
- Where the stomach is diseased or previously removed—other reconstructive options would need to be considered (e.g. colonic interposition).
- Those with significant comorbidities, poor performance status, or severe malnutrition.
- Poor lung function that precludes one lung ventilation.

Anatomy

GROSS ANATOMY

- The oesophagus extends from the lower border of the cricoid cartilage (C6) to the cardiac orifice of the stomach (T11).
- It is subdivided into three portions: cervical, thoracic, and abdominal.
  - The cervical portion extends from the cricopharyngeus to the suprasternal notch. Arterial supply is from the inferior thyroid artery, and venous drainage is to the inferior thyroid vein.
  - The thoracic oesophagus extends from the suprasternal notch to the diaphragm and lies in the posterior mediastinum. Arterial supply is from the bronchial and oesophageal branches of the thoracic aorta, and venous drainage is to the azygos and hemiazygos veins.
  - The abdominal portion originates at the diaphragm and runs into the cardiac portion of the stomach. Arterial supply is from the ascending branches of the left gastric artery (LGA) with contribution from the inferior phrenic artery as well, and the venous drainage is to the left gastric (coronary) vein to the portal system (site of porto-systemic anastomosis).

SURGICAL RELATIONS

- Anterior to the oesophagus; the trachea and bronchi above and the pericardium and pulmonary veins below.
- The descending aorta lies posterior to the thoracic oesophagus.
- To the right of the oesophagus, the azygos vein, formed by the union of the ascending lumbar veins and the right subcostal vein at T12, drains the posterior walls of the thorax and abdomen. The azygos vein ascends in the posterior mediastinum along the right-hand side of the thoracic vertebral column to enter the superior vena cava.
- The angle of His (the cardiac notch) is the acute angle between the cardia of the stomach and the oesophagus. It is formed by the collar sling fibres and the circular muscles surrounding the gastro-oesophageal junction. It forms a sphincter that prevents reflux.
- The thoracic duct ascends from the cisterna chyli through the oesophageal hiatus in the diaphragm between the azygos vein and the aorta.

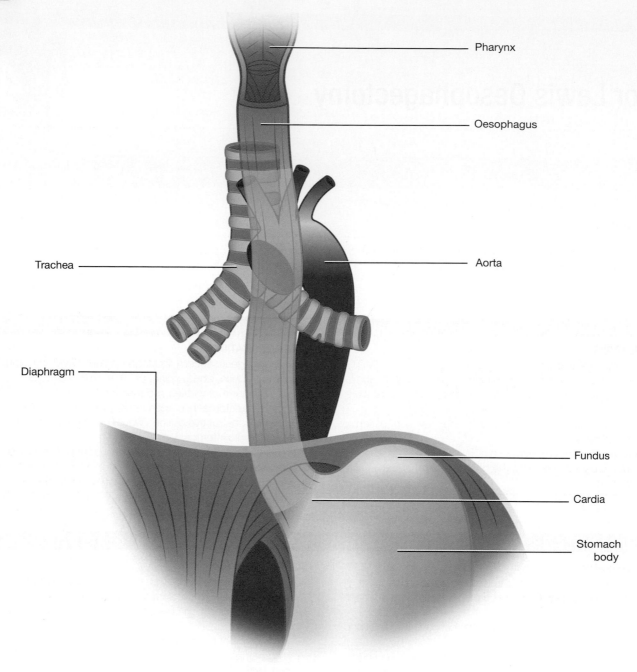

Anatomic relations of the oesophagus.

STEP-BY-STEP OPERATION

Anaesthesia: general with a double-lumen endotracheal tube to allow deflation of the right lung. An epidural is also sited and a nasogastric (NG) tube inserted.

Position: reverse Trendelenburg with the surgeon positioned between the patient's legs.

Considerations: Ivor Lewis described a two-phase oesophagectomy involving an abdominal phase (upper midline laparotomy) and a thoracic phase (right thoracotomy). This may be performed using laparoscopic and thoracoscopic approaches; many surgeons employ hybrid techniques. We describe the hybrid laparoscopic gastric and right thoracotomy below.

ABDOMINAL PHASE

1. Five ports are placed—three are placed 15 cm below the xiphisternum and the right and left midclavicular lines. One is positioned 5 cm below the costal margin, and one port for a liver retractor just below the level of the xiphisternum.
2. The stomach is mobilised along the greater curvature, taking care to preserve the gastroepiploic arcade. Omental branches and the short gastric vessels are divided with a laparoscopic energy device. The fundus is mobilised.
3. The lesser omentum is divided and the right gastric artery (RGA) divided. The left gastric artery (LGA) and vein are clipped and divided. Lymph nodes around the coeliac trunk are excised en bloc.
4. A cuff of crura is excised in continuity with the lower oesophagus and the plane developed into the mediastinum anterior to the aorta. The duodenum is mobilised as necessary to reach the diaphragm.
5. A feeding jejunostomy can be inserted at this point. Port sites are closed with absorbable sutures.

THORACIC PHASE

6. The patient is repositioned into the left lateral decubitus position. A right lateral thoracotomy is performed through the fifth intercostal space. Single-lung ventilation is used for oesophageal and mediastinal exposure.
7. The azygos vein is identified and divided; the mediastinal pleura is incised medial to the azygos vein. The thoracic duct is ligated at the level of the diaphragm. A lymphadenectomy removes the paratracheal nodes, posterior mediastinal, subcarinal, middle, and peri-oesophageal nodes en bloc with the specimen.
8. The gastro-oesophageal junction and the stomach are pulled through the oesophageal hiatus and into the chest.
9. The gastric tube is created with a linear stapler. The oesophagus is divided at least 5 cm proximal to the tumour. The specimen is removed.
10. Using a circular stapler, an anastomosis is formed between the oesophagus and the remaining stomach. The anastomosis is covered with preserved greater omentum. An NG tube is advanced into the distal stomach and two intercostal drains are placed. The ribs are approximated with non-absorbable sutures and the wound closed in layers.

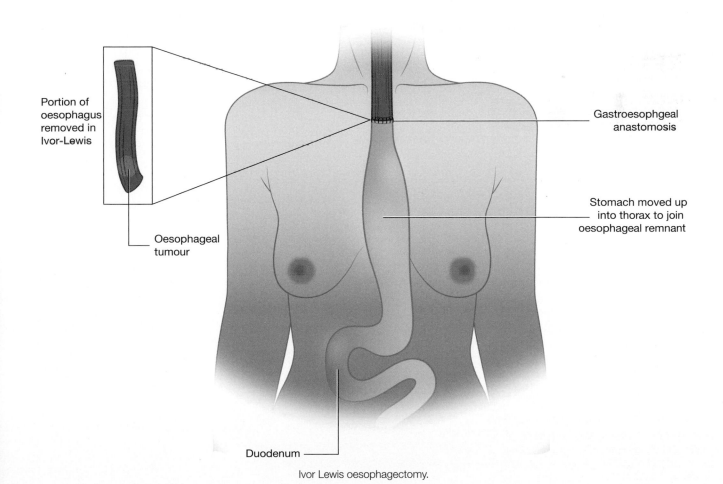

Portion of oesophagus removed in Ivor-Lewis

Oesophageal tumour

Gastroesophgeal anastomosis

Stomach moved up into thorax to join oesophageal remnant

Duodenum

Ivor Lewis oesophagectomy.

Complications

EARLY

- Haemorrhage (short gastrics, gastroepiploics, azygous vein).
- Injury to tracheobronchial tree.
- Recurrent laryngeal nerve injury—resulting in hoarseness of voice.
- Opening of the pleura during the laparoscopic phase—leading to capnothorax.
- Injury to surrounding organs—colon and splenic capsule.
- Pulmonary complications, including atelectasis, pneumonia, acute respiratory distress syndrome (ARDS).
- Thromboembolic complications.
- Cardiac complications, including arrhythmia, myocardial infarction, pericardial tamponade.
- Anastomosis leak—leading to mediastinitis or empyema.

INTERMEDIATE AND LATE

- Gastric tube necrosis.
- Chylothorax.
- Herniation of the abdominal viscera through the diaphragmatic hiatus.
- Wound dehiscence.
- Complications related to feeding jejunostomy.
- Impaired emptying of stomach.
- Anastomotic stricturing.
- Postvagotomy dumping syndrome—damage to the vagus nerve results in impaired gastric secretions and digestion. As a result, hypertonic gastric content enters the small bowel, drawing up to 25% of plasma volume into the lumen. Symptoms including bloating, nausea, diarrhoea, and dizziness.
- Reflux oesophagitis.
- Diaphragmatic hernia.
- Chronic pain in thoracotomy wound.

Postoperative Care

INPATIENT

- Nutrition via a jejunostomy tube for the first few days.
- Fluoroscopic water-soluble oral contrast swallow may be performed on day 5–7 postop to assess anastomotic integrity. Oral intake can be initiated providing there Is no anastomotic leak, commencing with liquids initially and progressing to a light diet as tolerated.
- Drains and NG tube removed when output is minimal.

OUTPATIENT

- Outpatient dietetic follow-up.
- Surgical review at 6-week and 3-month intervals for the first year.
- Multidisciplinary discussion regarding adjuvant treatment for cancer patients.

? Surgeon's Favourite Question

What provides the arterial supply to the stomach when it is relocated to the chest during an Ivor Lewis procedure?

Right gastro-epiploic artery.

Nissen Fundoplication

5

Roberta Bullingham

Definition

A procedure where the fundus of the stomach is wrapped around the gastro-oesophageal junction to strengthen the sphincter and prevent herniation of the stomach through the diaphragm. It is undertaken in conjunction with repair of the diaphragmatic crura.

Indications and Contraindications

INDICATIONS

Surgery is considered in patients with a diagnosis of gastro-oesophageal reflux disease (GORD) for whom:

- Acid suppression medication is either poorly tolerated, ineffective at controlling symptoms, or the patient not wanting to be on lifelong medication.
- The predominant symptom is volume reflux.
- Complications of GORD have developed, such as Barrett's oesophagus and peptic stricture.
- Extra-oesophageal manifestations—asthma, hoarseness, cough, chest pain, and aspiration.

CONTRAINDICATIONS

- Presence of poor gastric emptying and oesophageal hypomotility.
- Poor compliance or incomplete medical management.
- pH studies that do correlate with patient's symptom.
- Patients with excessive belching or bloating.
- Patients who qualify for bariatric surgery should be considered for this first.

Anatomy

GROSS ANATOMY

- The oesophageal hiatus is at level T10 (vena cava T8, oesophagus T10, aortic hiatus T12).
- Components of the stomach:
  - Cardia—the area of stomach adjacent to the oesophagus.
  - Fundus—the most superior aspect of the stomach.
  - Body—the main region of the stomach.
  - Pylorus—the area proximal to the duodenum.
- The lesser curvature forms the smaller concave border of the stomach and serves as the attachment of the lesser omentum.
- The lesser omentum has two separate ligaments: the gastro-hepatic ligament (connects the stomach and the liver) and the hepato-duodenal ligament (connects the first part of the duodenum and the liver and contains the hepatic artery proper, the portal vein, and the common bile duct).
- The greater curvature forms the long, convex portion of the stomach and serves as the attachment to the greater omentum, which descends anterior to the abdominal viscera and then folds back over itself to insert into the transverse colon.
- The diaphragm consists of two components: the central tendon, which fuses with the pericardium; and the peripheral muscular part that arises from the xiphisternum, the lower six costal cartilages, the vertebral column, and the arcuate ligaments.
- The crura originate from the lumbar vertebrae and arch anteriorly over the lower oesophagus with a potential space posteriorly for herniation.

- The vagus nerves lie anterior and posterior to the oesophagus as it passes through the diaphragm at T10, with branches of the left gastric vessels.
- The aorta lies posterior to the oesophagus, passing through the diaphragm with the azygos vein and the thoracic duct at T12.
- The vena cava passes through the diaphragm at T8, with the right phrenic nerve. The left phrenic nerve pierces the left dome of the diaphragm.
- These levels can be remembered using the mnemonic 'I ate ten eggs at twelve': I (IVC) ate (T8) ten (T10) eggs (oesophagus) at (aorta) twelve (T12).

NEUROVASCULATURE

- The coeliac trunk is the main blood supply to the stomach. It has three main branches: the left gastric artery, the hepatic artery proper, and the splenic artery.
- The fundus of the stomach is supplied by short gastric arteries (originating from the splenic artery).
- The pylorus of the stomach and the first part of the duodenum are supplied by the gastroduodenal artery (a branch of the hepatic artery proper).
- The lesser curvature of the stomach is supplied by the left gastric artery and the right gastric artery (a branch of the hepatic artery proper).
- The greater curvature of the stomach is supplied by an anastomosis between the right gastro-epiploic artery (a branch of the gastroduodenal artery) and the left gastro-epiploic artery (a branch of the splenic artery).

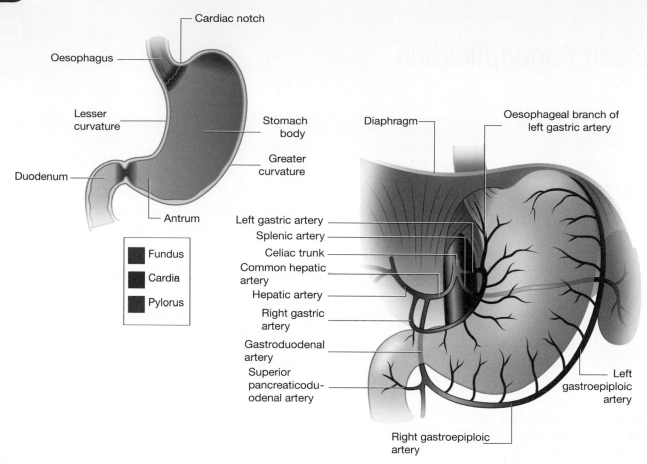

Arterial supply of the stomach.

STEP-BY-STEP OPERATION

Anaesthesia: general.

Position: reverse Trendelenburg.

Considerations: A Nissen fundoplication is a 360-degree wrap and is considered the gold standard and most widely used treatment for GORD; however, it is associated with high rates of postoperative gas bloating and dysphagia and a number of alternative 'limited' wraps between 180 and 270 degrees have been adopted.

Steps:

1. Three laparoscopic ports are required: midline camera port 15 cm below the xiphisternum and right and left upper quadrant working ports in the mid-clavicular line. A fourth port may be required below the left lateral costal margin.
2. A liver retractor is inserted through an incision below the xiphisternum to retract the left lobe of the liver.
3. The lesser omentum is incised avoiding the hepatic branch of the anterior vagus nerve, and dissection is continued towards the right crus.
4. The phreno-oesophageal ligament is divided, and the oesophagus and superior stomach are dissected to free them from surrounding structures.
5. The right and left crura of the diaphragm are defined.
6. The oesophagus is mobilised with dissection from the hiatus posteriorly to ensure that a 5 cm length is intra-abdominal (preserving all branches of the vagus nerve). Nylon tape used to retract oesophagus.
7. Non-absorbable sutures are placed to oppose the crura (closing the oesophageal hiatus).
8. Proximal short gastric vessels are identified and divided (freeing the fundus of the stomach).
9. The mobile fundus is pulled around the oesophagus at the level of the gastro-oesophageal junction to create a loose fundoplication (360 degrees) approximately 2 cm in length. Non-absorbable braided sutures through the adventitial layer are used to secure the fundoplication.
10. The 10-mm ports are closed with a figure-of-8 in the sheath. The skin of all the ports is closed with a subcuticular suture (absorbable monofilament).

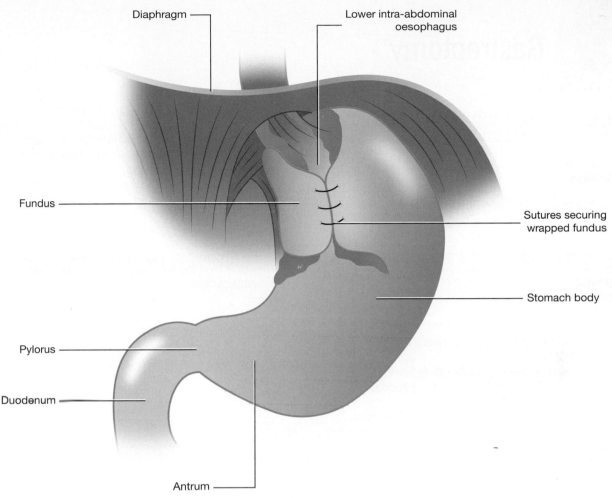

Nissen fundoplication.

Complications

EARLY
- Pneumo- or capnothorax caused by inadvertent opening of the pleura during the dissection whilst insufflating CO_2.
- Gastric or oesophageal perforation (<1%).
- Bleeding from the short gastric vessels, liver, or spleen.

INTERMEDIATE AND LATE
- Bloating—early postoperative bloating is common and occurs with 30% of patients. Long-term 'gas bloat' can occur due to difficulty belching.
- Dysphagia—caused by oedema from operative trauma, it normally resolves spontaneously over the first few weeks following surgery. Patients are advised to take a very soft diet for 3–4 weeks. A small proportion of patients have persistent dysphagia.
- Inadvertent vagal injury can cause widespread gastrointestinal dysfunction.
- Failure or recurrence of symptoms.
- 'Slipped Nissen'—the stomach can herniate upwards inside the fundoplication. This needs urgent attention, as it can lead to necrosis and perforation.

Postoperative Care

INPATIENT
- Antireflux surgery can be performed as a day-case procedure, but large hiatal hernia will require admission.
- A very soft diet is advised for 3–4 weeks.
- Avoid heavy lifting for 6 weeks.

OUTPATIENT
- Outpatient clinic follow-up 6–8 weeks postoperatively to ensure normal diet is returned and there are no postoperative complications.

Surgeon's Favourite Question

What structure is in danger during posterior repair of the crura?

The aorta.

6 Gastrectomy

Roberta Bullingham

Definition

Excision of the entire stomach (total) or a distal part of the stomach (partial or subtotal).

Indications and Contraindications

INDICATIONS
- Malignant tumours:
  - Adenocarcinoma.
  - Carcinoid (Type III).
  - Prophylactic gastrectomy in hereditary gastric cancer.
- Benign conditions:
  - Perforated or bleeding peptic ulcers, having failed conservative medical or endoscopic treatment (emergency).
  - Refractory benign ulcers that fail to heal or cause pain, anaemia, or features of gastric outlet obstruction (elective).
  - Caustic perforation.
  - Intractable reflux.

CONTRAINDICATIONS
Relative
- Malnourishment—surgery can be delayed allowing for nutritional supplementation.

Anatomy

GROSS ANATOMY
- The angle of His, also known as the cardiac notch, is the acute angle between the cardia and the oesophagus. It is formed by the collar sling fibres and the circular muscles surrounding the gastro-oesophageal junction. It contributes to the physiological prevention of reflux.
- The stomach has two curvatures (lesser and greater) and five parts (cardia, fundus, body, antrum, and pylorus).
- The stomach is attached to structures by a series of ligaments:
  - The gastrocolic ligament (part of the greater omentum)—connects the greater curvature of the stomach and the transverse colon).
  - The gastrosplenic ligament—connects the greater curvature of the stomach and the hilum of the spleen.
  - The gastrophrenic ligament—connects the fundus of the stomach to the diaphragm.
  - The hepatogastric ligament—connects the liver to the lesser curve of the stomach (forms part of the lesser omentum).
- The greater and lesser omenta are structures made of two layers of peritoneum folded on itself. The greater omentum hangs from the greater curvature of the stomach, whereas the lesser omentum attaches the stomach and duodenum to the liver.
- The omenta divide the abdominal cavity into the greater and lesser sacs, which communicate via the epiploic foramen.

NEUROVASCULATURE
- The parasympathetic nerve supply to the stomach is derived from the anterior and posterior vagus nerves.
- The sympathetic innervation is via the coeliac plexus (T6–T9).
- The blood supply is derived from the coeliac trunk, which branches from the abdominal aorta at T12.
- The left gastric artery (LGA), a direct branch of the coeliac trunk, supplies the superior lesser curvature of the stomach, whereas the right gastric artery (RGA), a branch of the common hepatic artery, supplies the inferior portion.
- The right gastro-epiploic (RGE) artery arises from the gastroduodenal artery and runs along the greater curvature from the distal aspect of the stomach.
- At the hilum of the spleen, the splenic artery divides into the short gastric arteries, which supply the fundus, and the left gastro-epiploic (LGE) artery, which supplies the proximal greater curvature.
- Gastric lymphatics run along the curvatures with the respective arteries and drain into the regional nodes.

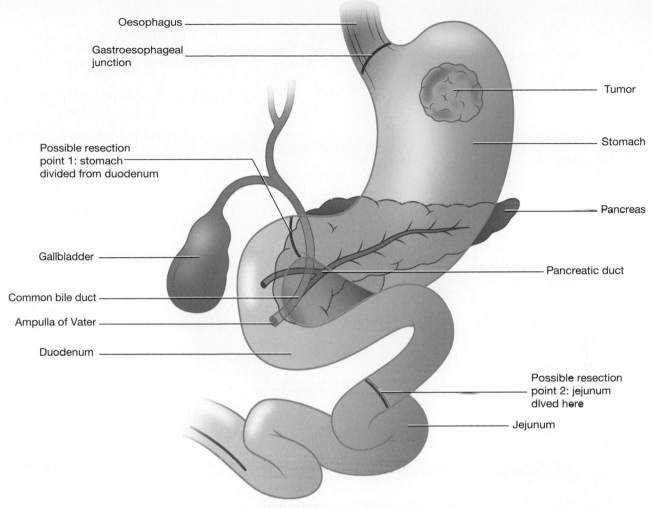

Oesophagus

Gastroesophageal junction

Possible resection point 1: stomach divided from duodenum

Gallbladder

Common bile duct

Ampulla of Vater

Duodenum

Tumor

Stomach

Pancreas

Pancreatic duct

Possible resection point 2: jejunum dived here

Jejunum

Gastrectomy points of resection.

1₂3 STEP-BY-STEP OPERATION

Anaesthesia: general.

Position: supine.

Considerations: Total gastrectomy requires Roux-en-Y reconstruction (described here); after partial gastrectomy, the proximal stomach may be anastomosed to the duodenum (Bilroth I), to a loop of jejunum (Polya), or to the Roux-en-Y (Bilroth II). Bilroth II is described here. Where appropriate, partial gastrectomy is preferred to total gastrectomy due to fewer postoperative complications and superior quality of life.

Steps:

1. Abdominal access is established (this can be either via a midline or rooftop incision, or laparoscopically).
2. Once the abdominal cavity is entered, an intraoperative assessment of resectability is performed, with the liver, the peritoneum, and the rest of the peritoneal cavity being examined for metastases.
3. The greater omentum is dissected from the transverse colon, and the lesser sac is entered.
4. The greater curvature of the stomach is mobilised up to the level of the diaphragm, and the short gastric vessels are divided.
5. The lesser omentum is divided, and the RGE artery and vein and the RGA are identified, ligated, and divided.

6. The duodenum is mobilised and divided distal to the pylorus.
7. The coeliac axis is identified by finding the plane between the superior border of the pancreas and the left gastric vessels. The left gastric (or coronary) vein and the LGA are ligated and divided. The accompanying lymph nodes are removed.
8. The dissection is continued from the ligated LGA to the oesophageal hiatus of the diaphragm. The oesophagus is mobilised and divided, and the stomach is removed. Additional resection of the lymph nodes, spleen, distal pancreas, and transverse colon is sometimes required for oncological clearance.
9. Creating a Roux-en-Y loop: The jejunum is divided approximately 20 cm distal to the duodenojejunal flexure. The distal end of the jejunum is anastomosed to the oesophagus, forming an oesophago-jejunostomy, and the proximal end of the divided jejunum is anastomosed approximately 50 cm below the oesophago-jejunostomy to the jejunum (jejunojejunostomy). The aim is to prevent bile reflux.
10. Drains around the duodenal stump and the oesophago/gastrojejunal anastomosis are left. The abdominal incision or port sites are closed.

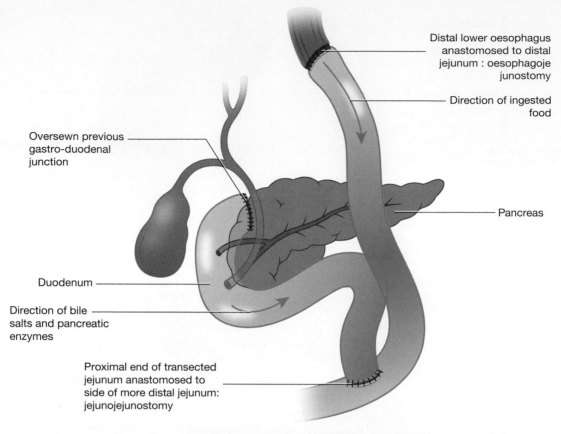

Distal lower oesophagus
anastomosed to distal
jejunum : oesophagoje
junostomy

Direction of ingested
food

Oversewn previous
gastro-duodenal
junction

Pancreas

Duodenum

Direction of bile
salts and pancreatic
enzymes

Proximal end of transected
jejunum anastomosed to
side of more distal jejunum:
jejunojejunostomy

Gastrectomy sites of anastamosis.

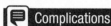 Complications

EARLY

- Bleeding from the splenic capsule—sometimes requires a splenectomy if this was not performed as part of the oncological excision.
- Anastomotic leak.
- Duodenal stump leakage.
- Pancreatitis or pancreatic fistula.
- Wound infection.
- Obstruction.

INTERMEDIATE AND LATE

- Dumping syndrome (20%), when hyperosmolar carbohydrate-rich food enters the small bowel too quickly, causing nausea, vomiting, pain, and vasomotor symptoms such as palpitation and flushing.
- Anastomotic stricture.
- Nutritional problems—anaemia (vitamin B_{12} deficiency following total gastrectomy due to removal of intrinsic factor-producing parietal cells within the stomach).
- Adhesional small bowel obstruction.
- Rapid or slow transit, causing diarrhoea or vomiting.
- Marginal ulcer.
- Internal hernia or incisional hernias.

Postoperative Care

INPATIENT

- Nutritional support through total parenteral nutrition or via a jejunostomy tube if placed.
- Drains removed when output is minimal.
- Fluoroscopic water-soluble contrast swallow study may be performed on day 5–7 postoperatively to assess for anastomotic leak. Oral intake can then be built up if intact, liquids initially, then light diet. Meals will always be smaller after total gastrectomy but should return to normal size after partial gastrectomy.
- Vitamin and mineral supplementation.

OUTPATIENT

- A dietician will be involved to help maintain nutrition.
- Follow-up depends upon the indication for surgery.

[?] Surgeon's Favourite Question

What vessel will supply the gastric remnant in a subtotal gastrectomy?

Short gastric vessels.

Omental Patch Repair of a Perforated Duodenal Ulcer

Roberta Bullingham

Definition

The repair of a perforated duodenal ulcer using a pedicle of omentum.

Indications and Contraindications

INDICATIONS
- To treat perforated peptic ulcers—prevent the leak of duodenal contents into the peritoneal cavity.
- Laparoscopic repair can be performed in haemodynamically stable patients with a history of <24 hours of acute symptoms.
- Open repair is more appropriate in patients with generalised peritonitis, those who are haemodynamically unstable, and those who have had signs of perforation for >24 hours.

CONTRAINDICATIONS
Relative
- Generalised abdominal infection.
- Duration of symptoms >24 hours.

Absolute
- Severe cardio-respiratory insufficiency.
- Haemodynamic instability.
- Major coagulopathy.

Anatomy

GROSS ANATOMY
- The duodenum is divided into four sections:
  - The first (superior part) is intraperitoneal and lies at the level of L1. It extends from the pylorus of the stomach and ends at the superior duodenal flexure (SDF). Perforated duodenal ulcers typically occur in the first part of the duodenum, on the anterior superior surface.
  - The second (descending) part is a retroperitoneal structure that runs from the SDF down to the level of L3 to end at the corner of the inferior duodenal flexure (IDF). The pancreas and common bile duct enter the second part of the duodenum through the major duodenal papilla containing the sphincter of Oddi. This point demarcates the embryological transition from foregut to midgut.
  - The third (transverse) part runs from the IDF and across the midline.
  - The fourth (ascending) part joins with the jejunum at the duodenojejunal flexure marked by the ligament of Treitz.
- The omentum:
  - The greater omentum originates from the greater curvature of the stomach and descends anterior to the abdominal viscera then folds back over itself to insert into the transverse colon.

NEUROVASCULATURE
- The duodenum:
  - Nervous supply derives from the vagus nerve and the greater and lesser splanchnic nerves.
  - The major duodenal papilla acts as a landmark between two adjacent blood supplies:
    - Proximally—the arterial supply is from the gastroduodenal artery and its branch, the superior pancreaticoduodenal artery.
    - Distally—the arterial supply is from the superior mesenteric artery and its branch, the inferior pancreaticoduodenal artery.
  - The venous drainage is into the superior pancreaticoduodenal vein (drains into the hepatic portal vein) and the inferior pancreaticoduodenal vein (drains into the superior mesenteric vein).
- The omentum:
  - The arterial supply is from the left and right gastro-epiploic arteries.
  - The venous drainage is into the left and right gastro-epiploic veins. The left gastro-epiploic vein drains into the splenic vein, whilst the right gastro-epiploic vein drains into the superior mesenteric vein.

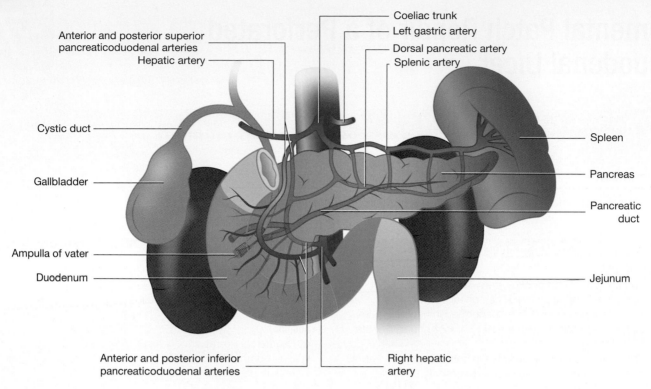

Vasculature of the duodenum and pancreas.

₁₂₃ STEP-BY-STEP OPERATION

Anaesthesia: general.

Position: supine with reverse Trendelenburg.

Considerations: This procedure can be performed via a laparotomy or laparoscopically. A nasogastric (NG) tube is required.

Steps:

1. An upper middle incision is made, which can be extended inferiorly. For the laparoscopic procedure, three or four ports are required: supraumbilical, right mid-clavicular line, left mid-clavicular line, and an epigastric port if a liver retractor is necessary.
2. The skin and fascia are dissected until the stomach and duodenum are identified.
3. Gastric contents are suctioned out of the peritoneal cavity, which is then irrigated with warm saline and the perforation is identified (most commonly located on the bulbous, first part of the duodenum).
4. If the perforation is not immediately identifiable, then the stomach and the first part of the duodenum should be mobilised to allow for full inspection.
5. Once the perforation has been identified, swabs are inserted around the perforation to prevent further leakage of gastric contents.
6. Three interrupted non-absorbable sutures are inserted across the site of the perforation.
7. A pedicle of omentum is mobilised without tension and is positioned across the perforation.
8. The previous interrupted sutures are then tied to secure the omentum in position, sealing the perforation (it is important that the sutures are strong enough to seal the perforation but not so strong that they compromise the omental blood supply).
9. The peritoneal cavity is then washed out with warm saline.
10. The skin and fascial layers are closed. A drain may be placed for 24 hours.

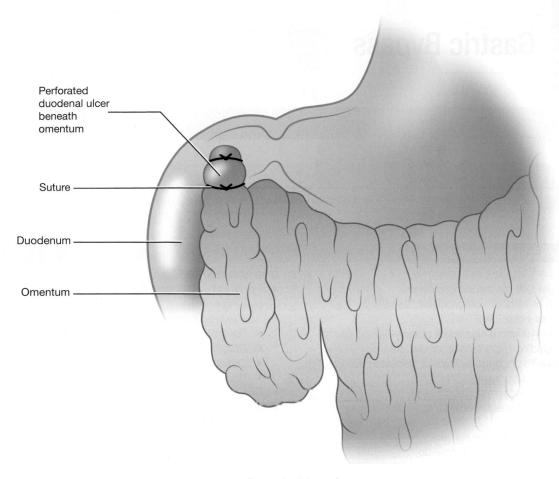

Perforated
duodenal ulcer
beneath
omentum

Suture

Duodenum

Omentum

Omental patch repair.

Complications

EARLY
- Stenosis of the duodenal lumen resulting in gastric outlet obstruction.
- Visceral injury.
- Death.

INTERMEDIATE AND LATE
- Strangulation of the omentum.
- Omental patch leak and fistula formation.
- Duodenal ulcer recurrence—in patients with no supplementary treatment (60%) and in patients with additional *Helicobacter pylori* eradication therapy (<5%).

Postoperative Care

INPATIENT
- Analgesia.
- Nil by mouth and NG tube on free drainage for 24–48 hours, after which commence oral fluids and slowly progress to a normal diet.
- Patients are commonly discharged after 5–7 days.

OUTPATIENT
- *H. pylori* eradication therapy with proton pump inhibitors and antibiotics as 90% of cases are infected with *H. pylori*.

Surgeon's Favourite Question

How do you identify the transition of the stomach to the duodenum?

Thickening of the pylorus, which underlies the pre-pyloric vein of Mayo.

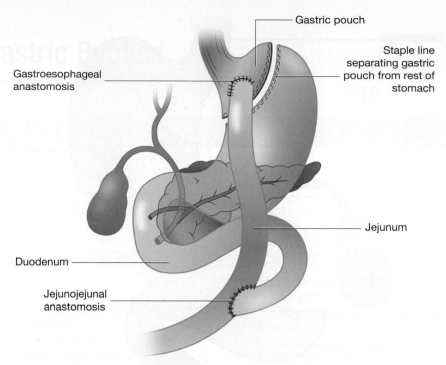

- Gastric pouch
- Staple line separating gastric pouch from rest of stomach
- Gastroesophageal anastomosis
- Jejunum
- Duodenum
- Jejunojejunal anastomosis

Gastric bypass sites of anastomosis.

Complications

EARLY

- Anastomotic leak.
- Haemorrhage.
- Iatrogenic bowel perforation.
- Wound infection.
- Internal hernia causing obstruction.
- Anastomotic leakage.

INTERMEDIATE AND LATE

- Gastric remnant distension—can be fatal if ruptures and causes peritonitis.
- Stomal stenosis—may require endoscopic balloon dilation.
- Marginal ulcers.
- Bowel obstruction due to internal herniation.
- Dumping syndrome when hyperosmolar carbohydrate-rich food enters the small bowel too quickly, causing nausea, vomiting, pain, and vasomotor symptoms such as palpitation and flushing.
- Gallstones secondary to malabsorption.
- Gastrogastric fistula.
- Incisional hernia.
- Short bowel syndrome.
- Metabolic and nutritional derangements.

Postoperative Care

INPATIENT

- If intraoperative leak test was negative, the patient can slowly build up oral intake (e.g. water, clear liquid, full liquid diet).
- IV proton pump inhibitor should be administered until oral intake is established.
- Drains, if placed, are removed when output is minimal.
- Vitamin and mineral supplementation as soon as oral intake is established (e.g. multivitamin, iron, calcium citrate).

OUTPATIENT

- Regular dietician support to ensure adequate nutrition and supplementation.
- Outpatient review at 4–6 weeks.
- Oral proton pump inhibitors for 1–3 months postoperatively.
- Depending upon weight loss, patients may develop gall-stones requiring cholecystectomy.

Surgeon's Favourite Question

What should you do if a patient with gastric bypass is admitted with abdominal pain?

After a full history and examination, the patient will most likely need an urgent CT. Due to the long biliopancreatic limb and the number of mesenteric defects, the patient can develop internal hernias and bowel obstruction. Obstruction of the biliopancreatic limb will not result in vomiting or constipation, as food does not pass down this limb.

Gastric Band

9

Roberta Bullingham

Definition

Reducing the functional size of the stomach by placement of an adjustable silicone device at the gastric cardia to aid weight loss.

Indications and Contraindications

INDICATIONS
The patient must fulfil the following criteria:
- Obesity with or without comorbidities, defined as:
  - Body mass index (BMI) ≥40.
  - BMI of 35–40 with a significant obesity-related comorbidity, including hypertension or diabetes.
  - BMI >30 with uncontrolled type 2 diabetes mellitus or metabolic syndrome.
- All nonsurgical measures unsuccessful.
- Multidisciplinary management in a specialist obesity service.
- Fit for anaesthesia and the surgery.
- Self-motivated to adhere to follow-up.
- A patient may opt for a gastric band, as it is the least invasive and is the safest weight loss procedure. As it does not reduce the actual capacity of the stomach, it still requires the patient to commit to healthy food and lifestyle choices. It requires regular adjustments, especially at the beginning, but can be removed easily if needed.

CONTRAINDICATIONS
- Inability or unwillingness to follow postoperative dietary recommendations.
- Stomach or intestinal disorders:
  - Reflux.
  - Chronic pancreatitis.
  - Oesophageal or gastric varices.
  - Portal hypertension.
- Pregnancy.
- Uncontrolled/untreated psychiatric disorder and/or suicide attempt in the last 18 months or several in the past 5 years.

Anatomy

GROSS ANATOMY
- The stomach has two curvatures (lesser and greater) and five parts (cardia, fundus, body, antrum, and pylorus).
- The acute angle between the cardia and oesophagus is known as the cardiac notch or angle of His. It is formed by collar sling fibres and the circular muscles surrounding the gastro-oesophageal junction. It forms a sphincter to prevent reflux.
- The stomach is attached to other structures by a series of ligaments:
  - Gastrocolic ligament—part of the greater omentum; connects the greater curvature of the stomach and the transverse colon.
  - Gastrosplenic ligament—connects the greater curvature of the stomach and the hilum of the spleen.
  - Gastrophrenic ligament—connects the fundus of the stomach to the diaphragm.
  - Hepatogastric ligament—connects the liver to the lesser curve of the stomach; forms part of the lesser omentum.

NEUROVASCULATURE
- The parasympathetic nerve supply to the stomach is via the vagus nerves.
- The sympathetic innervation is derived from segments T6–T9 of the spinal cord via the coeliac plexus.
- The blood supply for the stomach is derived from the coeliac trunk, which branches from the abdominal aorta (T12).
- The left gastric artery (LGA), a direct branch of the coeliac trunk, supplies the superior lesser curvature of the stomach, whereas the right gastric artery (RGA), a branch of the common hepatic artery, supplies the inferior portion of the lesser curvatures.
- The right gastro-epiploic (RGE) artery arises from the gastroduodenal artery and runs along the greater curvature from the distal aspect of the stomach.
- At the hilum of the spleen, the splenic artery divides into the short gastric arteries, which supply the fundus, and the left gastro-epiploic (LGE) artery, which supplies the proximal greater curvature of the stomach.
- Gastric lymphatics run along the curvatures with the respective arteries and drain into the regional nodes.

31

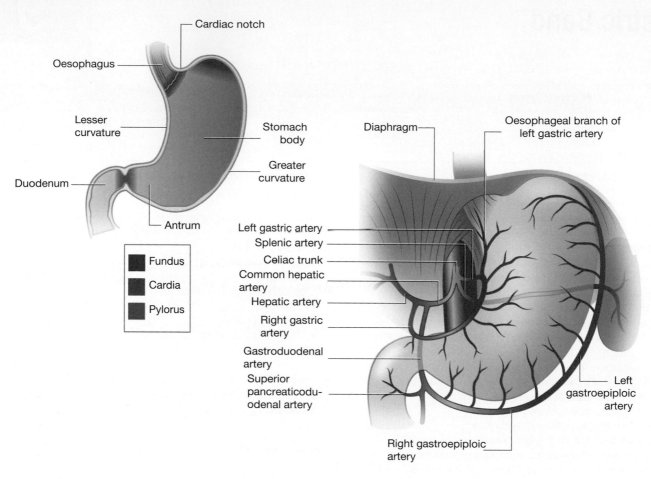

Arterial supply of the stomach.

123 STEP-BY-STEP OPERATION

Anaesthesia: general.

Position: reverse Trendelenburg.

Considerations: A low-calorie diet a week prior to surgery is advocated to reduce fat around the stomach and in the liver.

Steps:

1. One port is placed just below the left costal margin. Another is used to hold a liver retractor, and up to four more ports are placed in the epigastric, umbilical, and left hypochondriac regions.
2. A window is created in the lesser omentum, and fat is retracted to reveal the right crus of the diaphragm.
3. A window is created through the gastrophrenic ligament to reveal the stomach.
4. The band is washed in saline and tested and inserted through the largest port.
5. The band is wrapped around the fundus to create a small pouch at the top of the stomach.
6. The band may be adjusted via a port that is placed sub-cutaneously in the epigastric or left hypochondriac regions (the band can be tightened or loosened by injecting or removing saline from the bubble in the adjustment port).
7. The tubing for adjusting the band is inserted and connected to the band.
8. The adjustment port is placed under the skin by clearing a 2-cm area into which the port is inserted and sutured to the underlying muscle/fascia.
9. The system is tested and adjusted.
10. The wounds are injected with local anaesthetic and closed. Further adjustments can be made to the band at follow-up appointments.

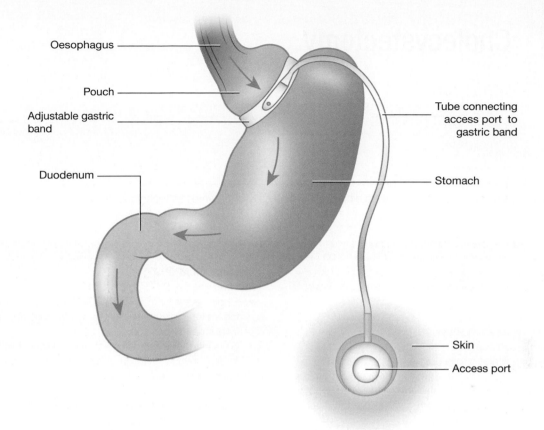

Gastric band and access port.

Complications

EARLY
- Dysphagia.
- Bleeding.
- Infection of the band or port.
- Perforation.
- Acute stomal obstruction.

INTERMEDIATE AND LATE
- Pouch or oesophageal dilation.
- Band slippage and gastric prolapse—distal stomach herniates upwards through the band; can be a surgical emergency, as it can cause gastric necrosis and leakage.
- Band failure (patient continues to eat soft foods through the band, and weight loss is negligible).
- Band erosion (band erodes into the stomach)—presents as upper abdominal pain, vomiting, and difficulty swallowing and reflux symptoms or just as increased hunger or a cessation of weight loss.
- Port tubing malfunction.
- Reflux.
- Almost 50% of patients will need surgical revision or removal of the band for the previous complications.

Postoperative Care

INPATIENT
- Most gastric bands are done as day cases, with patients being discharged once recovered from anaesthetic and eating safely.

OUTPATIENT
- A liquid diet is recommended for the first 2 weeks postoperatively, and then purees and soft solids.
- Band adjustments can be made at regular intervals (e.g., every 3 months) if required.

Surgeon's Favourite Question

What is the normal postoperative X-ray appearance of a gastric band?

The band should lie at an approximately 30- to 45-degree angle. It should not lie in the horizontal plane (indicates slippage). You should also not be able to see the open-face 'O' of the ring (indicates displacement).

10

Cholecystectomy

Roberta Bullingham

Definition

Removal of the gallbladder can be performed either laparoscopically or via an open technique.

Indications and Contraindications

INDICATIONS
- Symptomatic gallstones (cholelithiasis) with or without complications:
  - Biliary colic.
  - Acute or chronic cholecystitis.
  - Gallstone pancreatitis.
  - Choledocholithiasis (bile duct stones), which may be removed by endoscopic retrograde cholangiopancreatography (ERCP) prior to cholecystectomy or removed during the procedure via common bile duct (CBD) exploration.
  - Gallbladder polyps or porcelain gallbladder—potential for malignancy.
- Gallbladder carcinoma (may also require liver resection)—open approach favoured over laparoscopic.
- As part of a larger hepatobiliary resection (Whipple's procedure).

CONTRAINDICATIONS
Relative
- Cholecystitis of more than 48–72 hours' duration, indicating an interval cholecystectomy (typically at 6 weeks) after inflammation has subsided.
- Significant comorbidities—these patients may be suitable for less invasive alternatives such as cholecystostomy or spinal anaesthesia + laparoscopic technique.
- A laparoscopic approach may be avoided in a patient with previous abdominal surgery adhesions or where a pathology such as carcinoma is suspected.

Absolute
- Cirrhosis of the liver with portal hypertension.

Anatomy

GROSS ANATOMY
- The gallbladder is divided into the fundus, body, and neck, which follow into a narrow infundibulum and the cystic duct.
- Bile is secreted by hepatocytes and drains through the biliary tree:
  - Canniculi into intralobular ducts.
  - Intralobular ducts into collecting ducts.
  - Collecting ducts into the left and right hepatic ducts.
  - Right and left hepatic ducts unite to form the common hepatic duct.
  - The common hepatic duct is joined by the cystic duct to form the CBD.
  - The CBD is joined by the pancreatic duct to form the ampulla of Vater, which drains into the duodenum through the sphincter of Oddi.
- Calot's triangle is an anatomical space relevant for cholecystectomy. It is bordered by the cystic duct inferiorly, the lower border of the liver superiorly, and the common hepatic duct medially. The cystic artery crosses this triangle.

NEUROVASCULATURE
- Sympathetic nervous supply is via the coeliac nerve plexus (T7–T9).
- Parasympathetic nervous supply is from the right vagus nerve.
- Arterial supply is via the superficial and deep branches of the cystic artery, a branch of the right hepatic artery. Multiple cystic veins drain the neck and the cystic duct. These enter the liver directly or drain through the hepatic portal vein to the liver.
- The veins from the fundus and the body drain directly into the hepatic sinusoids.
- Lymphatic drainage is via the lymph node of Lund (also called Mascagni's lymph node) found at the neck of the gallbladder.

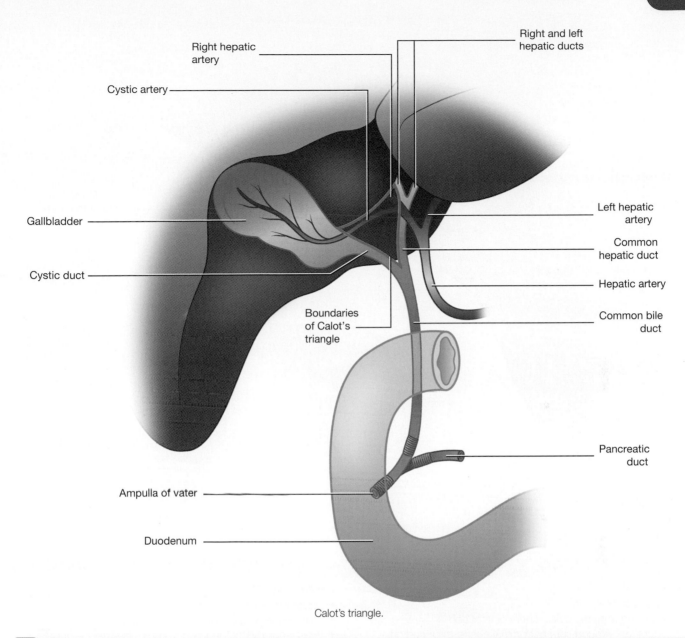

Right hepatic artery

Cystic artery

Right and left hepatic ducts

Gallbladder

Cystic duct

Boundaries of Calot's triangle

Left hepatic artery

Common hepatic duct

Hepatic artery

Common bile duct

Pancreatic duct

Ampulla of vater

Duodenum

Calot's triangle.

⅟₂₃ STEP-BY-STEP OPERATION

Anaesthesia: general.

Position: supine.

Considerations: Laparoscopic cholecystectomy (described here) is the gold-standard treatment, but open cholecystectomy may be indicated in complex pathology or suspected gallbladder cancer. Conversion to open cholecystectomy is required for significant bleeding, concern about anatomy, or injury to other structures.

Steps:

1. Three ports are placed—umbilical, right mid-clavicular line, and epigastrium—and pneumoperitoneum is established via the Hassan method. A fourth port in the right anterior axillary line is frequently added.

2. The tissue surrounding the biliary structures is dissected so that the cystic artery and cystic duct can be identified. In difficult cases, a 'fundus first' retrograde dissection approach can be used instead.

3. Prior to clipping the cystic duct and the cystic artery, a large window is created behind each of these structures. This establishes the 'critical view of safety' and minimises the risk of bile duct injury.

4. The cystic artery is clipped and divided.

5. On-table cholangiography can be performed if CBD stones are suspected (abnormal liver function tests or CBD dilatation on ultrasound scans) or to clarify the anatomy to prevent injury to the CBD. The cystic duct is clipped distally, cannulated, and injected with contrast to perform cholangiography. This displays the anatomy of the biliary ductal system, identifies ductal stones, and ensures that the contrast passes freely into the duodenum.

6. The cystic duct is then clipped and divided, ensuring that the CBD is identified to avoid injury.

7. The gallbladder is then dissected from the liver bed using diathermy.

8. Once freed, the gallbladder is removed via a retrieval bag.

9. The liver bed is observed for haemostasis and bile leakage.

10. The peritoneal cavity is deflated, the ports are removed, and port sites are closed (for larger port sites, the fascial layer is closed in addition to the skin).

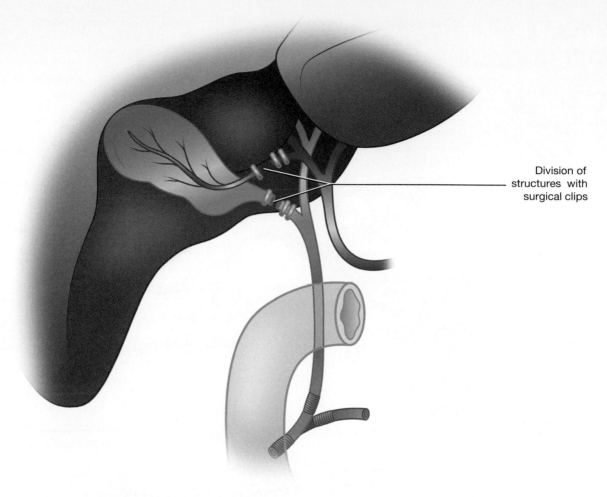

Division of
structures with
surgical clips

Division of the cystic duct and cystic artery.

Complications

EARLY
- Laparoscopic conversion to open.
- Bleeding from the cystic artery or liver bed.
- Infection—wound, intraabdominal abscess, pneumonia, and urinary tract infection.
- Bile leak resulting in biliary peritonitis, usually from the cystic duct or the duct of Luska (accessory small bile duct).
- CBD injury.
- Retained stone in the CBD.
- Damage to surrounding structures.

INTERMEDIATE AND LATE
- Incisional hernia (rare in laparoscopic surgery).
- Adhesional small bowel obstruction.
- Post-cholecystectomy syndrome—persistence of presenting symptoms postoperatively.
- Increased frequency and looser stool passage.

Postoperative Care

INPATIENT
- Eat and drink as tolerated.
- After laparoscopic cholecystectomy, patients are normally discharged the same day and normal activity is resumed within 2 weeks.
- After open cholecystectomy, patients are usually discharged after 2–4 days and normal activity is resumed within 4 weeks.

OUTPATIENT
- No routine outpatient review.

? Surgeon's Favourite Question

What is the name of the lymph node in Calot's triangle?

Lymph node of Lund.

Whipple's Procedure (Pancreaticoduodenectomy)

11

Roberta Bullingham

Definition

The removal of the following structures en bloc:
- Head of pancreas.
- Stomach antrum and pylorus.
- Duodenum.
- Proximal jejunum.
- Common bile duct (CBD).
- Gallbladder.

Indications and Contraindications

INDICATIONS
- Malignancy of the head of the pancreas, ampulla of Vater, duodenum, or distal CBD in the absence of metastasis and/or vascular involvement.
- Chronic pancreatitis causing severe pain that is refractory to medical therapy.

CONTRAINDICATIONS
- Metastatic disease.
- Nodal involvement out of the field of dissection.
- Involvement of the following structures: aorta, inferior vena cava (IVC), coeliac trunk, superior mesenteric artery (SMA), or superior mesenteric vein (SMV).

Anatomy

GROSS ANATOMY
- The pancreas is a retroperitoneal organ that lies within and is fixed to the curve of the first three parts of the duodenum.
- There are five components of the pancreas: head, uncinate process, neck, body, and tail.
- The pancreas drains via the pancreatic duct of Wirsung, which unites with the CBD to form the ampulla of Vater, which drains through the sphincter of Oddi into the second part of the duodenum.

NEUROVASCULATURE
- The pancreas is primarily supplied by the coeliac trunk and the SMA.
- The head and uncinate process are supplied by the anterior and posterior divisions of the superior pancreaticoduodenal artery (SPA), which stems from the gastroduodenal artery (a branch of the common hepatic artery (CHA)). The anterior and posterior branches of the SPA run inferiorly to anastomose with the anterior and posterior divisions of the inferior pancreaticoduodenal artery (branch of the SMA).
- The tail and body of the pancreas are supplied by the splenic artery.
- The venous drainage of the pancreas parallels the arterial supply and drains into the portal vein.
- The head of the pancreas drains into the SMV, while the body and tail of the pancreas drain into the splenic vein.
- Lymph drains via the peripancreatic and retroperitoneal nodes and into the thoracic duct, coeliac nodes, and superior mesenteric nodes.
- The pancreas is supplied by both the sympathetic system (the greater thoracic splanchnic nerves, coeliac plexus, and superior mesenteric plexus) and the parasympathetic system (the vagus nerve).

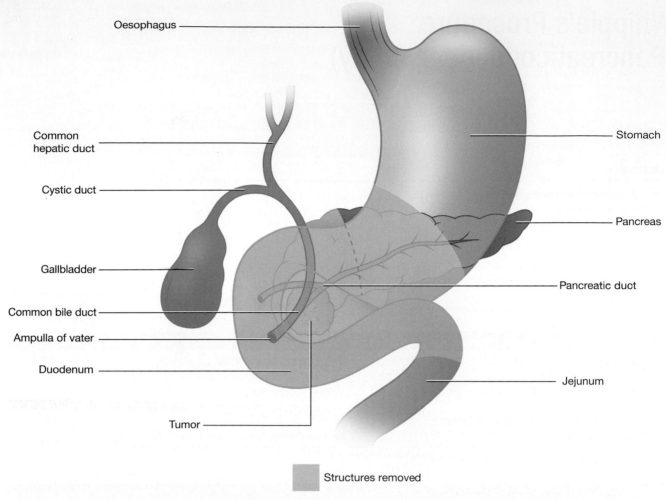

Structures removed

Structures removed en bloc in a Whipple's procedure.

123 STEP-BY-STEP OPERATION

Anaesthetic: general.
Position: supine.
Considerations: The operation can be divided into three stages: assessment of resectability, resection, and reconstruction.
Steps:
1. A vertical midline incision is made in the abdomen.
2. Assessment of resectability: the duodenum and pancreas are mobilised to ensure the absence of metastasis to either the aorta or the IVC. The SMV and neck of pancreas are inspected for the absence of tumour involvement between the two structures.
3. Resection:
   a. A cholecystectomy is performed, and the CBD is divided superior to the insertion of the cystic duct.
   b. The portal vein is dissected from its surrounding peritoneum, and the gastroduodenal artery is ligated and divided. The CHA is identified, and the surrounding lymph nodes are resected. The right gastro-epiploic vessels are then ligated and divided.
   c. The antrum and pylorus of the stomach, together with the neck of the pancreas, are subsequently excised.

d. The duodenojejunal (DJ) flexure is mobilised, and 15 cm of the jejunum that is immediately distal to the DJ flexure is excised.
   e. The uncinate process is dissected from the SMA and SMV, and all the small branches are ligated. The duodenum is then removed along with the head of the pancreas.
4. Reconstruction (consists of three main anastomosis):
   a. Pancreaticojejunostomy: the proximal part of the jejunal loop is anastomosed to the end of the pancreatic remnant.
   b. Hepaticojejunostomy: the middle of the jejunal loop is anastomosed to the end of the common hepatic duct.
   c. Gastrojejunostomy: the distal side of the jejunal loop is anastomosed to the end of the gastric remnant.
5. Drainage and closure: two percutaneous silicone drains are inserted, with one placed inferior to the left lobe of the liver and anterior to the pancreaticojejunostomy. The second drain is placed into the hepatorenal space inferior to the hepaticojejunostomy. The abdomen is irrigated with warm saline and closed in layers.

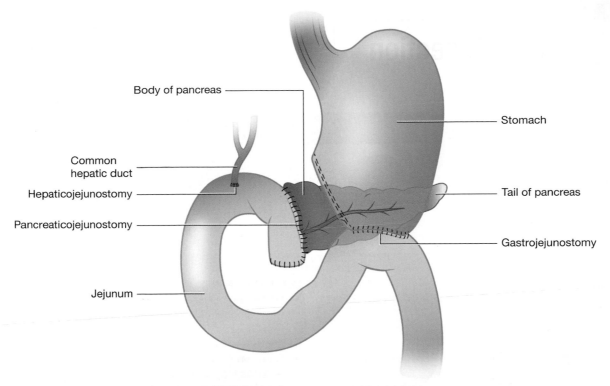

Whipple's postresection sites of anastomosis.

Complications

EARLY

- Haemorrhage.
- Delayed gastric emptying.
- Anastomotic leakage.
- Intraabdominal infection.
- Paralytic ileus.

INTERMEDIATE AND LATE

- Intraabdominal abscess—predominantly due to fistulae and/or anastomotic leaks.
- Acute pancreatitis of the remnant pancreas.
- Chyle leak.
- Pancreatic fistula.
- Dumping syndrome—loss of gastric reservoir and accelerated gastric emptying of osmotic contents; presents with diarrhoea, vomiting, and/or abdominal pain ~30 minutes after a meal.
- Pseudoaneurysm (e.g., of the gastroduodenal artery) and secondary haemorrhage (intraabdominal or gastrointestinal)—due to a ruptured pseudoaneurysm in relation to pancreatic leak, anastomotic leak, peptic ulceration, and/or sepsis.
- Pancreatic endocrine insufficiency—may cause brittle diabetes.
- Pancreatic exocrine insufficiency—may cause fat malabsorption.
- Tumour recurrence.

Postoperative Care

INPATIENT

- Average length of hospital stay: 10–14 days with the first 24–48 hours on high-dependency unit (HDU).
- IV proton pump inhibitor should be administered.
- Octreotide may be administered to reduce pancreatic secretions.
- Amylase level from abdominal drains may be checked postoperatively.

OUTPATIENT

- Patients should be reviewed regularly.
- Multidisciplinary team (MDT) involvement, including dietetic and psychosocial input, is vital.

Surgeon's Favourite Question

What structures are removed in a Whipple's operation?

- Head of pancreas.
- Stomach antrum and pylorus.
- Duodenum.
- Proximal jejunum.
- CBD.
- Gall bladder.

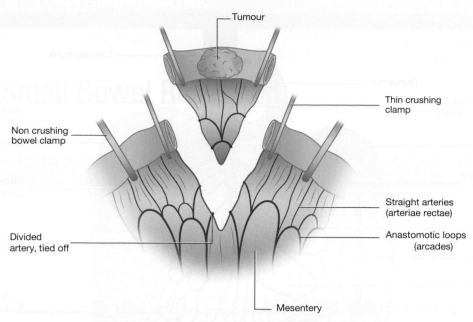

Resection of small bowel tumour.

💬 Complications

EARLY
- Bleeding.
- Paralytic ileus.

INTERMEDIATE AND LATE
- Deep vein thrombosis (DVT) and pulmonary embolism (PE).
- Infection—wound, intraabdominal abscess, pneumonia, and urinary tract infection.
- Anastomotic leak (typically 5–7 days postoperatively).
- Wound dehiscence.
- Adhesive bowel obstruction.
- Incisional hernia.
- Gallstones (after ileal resections—formation of cholesterol-rich stones is facilitated by a combination of gallbladder hypomotility and decreased bile salt concentration as a result of depletion of the body's pool of bile salts).
- Short bowel syndrome—occurs if more than 50% of small bowel is lost.

Postoperative Care

INPATIENT
- If the bowel was obstructed preoperatively, the NG tube is left on free drainage and fluids permitted. Once evidence of absorption is noted (decreased NG tube returns, and bowel activity resumes), the tube can be removed and diet introduced.
- If resection is done for a nonobstructing lesion, then normal diet can be commenced postoperation. Intravenous fluids are maintained until the patient has adequate oral intake to maintain hydration.
- If there is a prolonged period of bowel inactivity, TPN must be considered.
- Early sitting up and ambulation are encouraged with input from physiotherapy.

- Urinary catheters are removed within 48 hours of surgery to prevent infection.
- If drains are left in situ, they are removed once output is significantly reduced.

OUTPATIENT
- Patients are reviewed 2–6 weeks postoperatively with the results of pathology.
- In cases of small bowel malignancy, further treatment is decided upon by a multidisciplinary team (MDT) and depends on the results of pathology and the patient's comorbid state.

❓ Surgeon's Favourite Question

What three factors are required for an anastomosis to successfully heal?

An adequate blood supply, minimal tension, and mucosal apposition.

Laparoscopic Appendicectomy

17

Alison Bradley

Definition

A surgical procedure to resect the vermiform appendix.

Indications and Contraindications

INDICATIONS
- Acute appendicitis.
- Suspected malignancy of the appendix.

CONTRAINDICATIONS
- Contraindications to a laparoscopic procedure (laparotomy preferred):
  - Severe cardiopulmonary disease where establishing pneumoperitoneum would exert too much pressure on the cardiovascular system.
  - Extensive adhesions.
  - Patients too unstable to tolerate pneumoperitoneum.
  - Extensive contamination
- Relative
  - Pregnancy

Anatomy

GROSS ANATOMY
- The vermiform appendix is 2–20 cm long (average 9 cm), arising embryonically from the midgut.
- The three taeniae coli of the caecum converge at the caecal pole, which marks the base of the appendix.
- The position of the appendix is variable:
  - Retrocaecal: 64%
  - Pelvic: 32%
  - The remainder are paracaecal, subcaecal, preileal, postileal, or subileal.

NEUROVASCULATURE
- The appendix is supplied by the appendicular artery within the mesoappendix (a branch of the ileocolic artery, in turn a branch of the superior mesenteric artery).
- Venous drainage is via small appendicular veins leading to the posterior caecal or ileocolic vein, which drain into the superior mesenteric vein.
- Lymphatic tissue drains to ileocolic lymph nodes and then to superior mesenteric nodes.

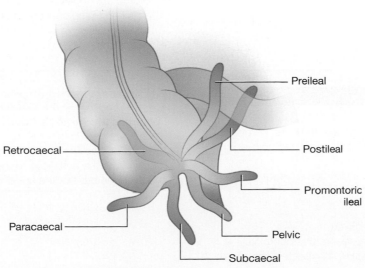

Potential anatomical locations of the appendix.

STEP-BY-STEP OPERATION

Anaesthesia: general.
Position: supine and Trendelenburg.
Considerations: A urinary catheter can be inserted, and prophylactic antibiotics are administered.
Steps:

1. Pneumoperitoneum is achieved using the Hasson technique and by inserting a port at:
   a. the umbilicus,
   b. the suprapubic region (inserted under direct vision), and
   c. the left iliac fossa (inserted under direct vision).
2. A diagnostic laparoscopy is performed (inspecting all four quadrants of the abdomen to exclude an alternative diagnosis). If purulent material is present, a sample is aspirated and sent to microbiology for culture and sensitivity.
3. The patient is placed in the Trendelenburg position with their right side tilted up to allow the small bowel to move out of the pelvis and right iliac fossa.
4. Adherent bowel loops or omentum are brushed away.
5. The appendix is grasped at its tip, and adhesions to the lateral wall are divided with diathermy, mobilising the appendix towards the appendicular base.
6. Using diathermy, a window is created in the mesoappendix (near the appendicular base).
7. The mesoappendix is dissected away from the appendix, and the appendicular artery is either clipped or cauterised and then divided.
8. The base of the appendix is secured with nooses of pre-tied sutures (two sutures are placed at the base of the appendix, and a third suture is placed slightly distally on the appendix). The appendix is then divided between the second and third sutures.
9. The appendix is removed in a specimen bag through the umbilical port.
10. The abdomen is washed out, ports are removed, and the incisions are closed.

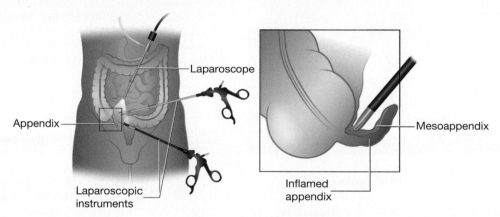

Laparoscopic appendicectomy.

Complications

EARLY
- Bleeding.
- Enteric injury.
- Paralytic ileus.

INTERMEDIATE AND LATE
- Infection—wound, intraabdominal collection, abscess, pneumonia, and urinary tract infection.
- Wound dehiscence.
- Stump appendicitis: if a long stump of the appendix is left attached to the caecum, this can be a source of ongoing appendicitis.
- Adhesions.
- Incisional hernia.

Postoperative Care

INPATIENT
- Patients are discharged within 24–48 hours—provided they are mobile and able to void urine, and pain is adequately controlled.
- In perforated appendicitis, antibiotics are continued 5 days postoperatively.

OUTPATIENT
- Routine follow-up is not required.
- Patients may be reviewed 6 weeks postoperatively with pathology results (occasionally, unexpected pathology such as carcinoid tumours are encountered).

Surgeon's Favourite Question

Where is McBurney's Point?

The point two-thirds of the way along an imaginary line drawn from the umbilicus to the anterior superior iliac spine, marking the base of the appendix.

Right Hemicolectomy

18

Alison Bradley

Definition

Removal of the terminal ileum and right colon, including the caecum, appendix, ascending colon, hepatic flexure, and a portion of the transverse colon. An extended right hemicolectomy includes removal of the transverse colon, the splenic flexure, and proximal descending colon.

Indications and Contraindications

INDICATIONS
- Tumours or inflammatory conditions of the right colon or terminal ileum, transverse colon, or splenic flexure.
- Large adenomatous polyps.
- Inflammatory bowel disease.
- Diverticular disease involving the right colon.
- Caecal volvulus.

CONTRAINDICATIONS
Contraindications to laparoscopic right hemicolectomy:
- Bowel obstruction or ileus leading to severe abdominal distension with poor operative view.
- Multiple previous abdominal surgeries.
- Dense adhesions.

Anatomy

GROSS ANATOMY
- Embryonically, the ascending colon to the proximal two-thirds of the transverse colon originates from the midgut. The distal one-third of the transverse colon to the sigmoid colon originates from the hindgut.
- The transverse colon and caecum are peritoneal structures.
- The ascending colon is retroperitoneal.

NEUROVASCULATURE
- Parasympathetic nerve supply is from the vagus nerve.
- Sympathetic nerve supply is from the thoracic splanchnic nerves via the coeliac and superior mesenteric ganglia and the superior mesenteric plexus.
- The arterial supply to the right colon comes from branches of the superior mesenteric artery (SMA):
  - Ileocolic artery—supplies the terminal ileum, appendix, and caecum.
- Right colic artery (only present in 20% of people)—supplies the ascending colon. Where absent the ascending colon is supplied by the ileocolic artery and right branch of middle colic artery.
- Middle colic artery—supplies the proximal two-thirds of the transverse colon.
- Venous drainage is from the ileocolic, right colic, and middle colic veins, which correspond to the arterial anatomical distribution and drain into the superior mesenteric vein, which converges with the splenic vein to form the hepatic portal vein posterior to the neck of the pancreas.
- The ileocolic, right colic, and middle colic lymph nodes drain into the superior mesenteric nodes, which are located at the origin of the SMA.

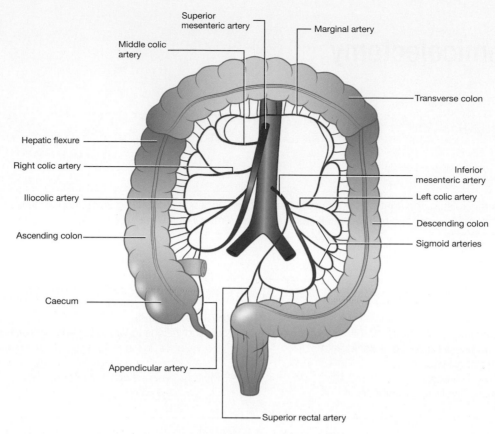

Large bowel anatomy with arterial supply.

1 2 3 STEP-BY-STEP OPERATION

Anaesthesia: general.
Position: supine.
Considerations: A urinary catheter is inserted and, in cases of obstruction, a nasogastric (NG) tube is inserted. Prophylactic antibiotics are administered.

Steps:

1. A midline laparotomy is performed and a thorough inspection of the abdominal cavity is performed. In cases of malignancy, the abdominal cavity and viscera are assessed for tumour spread.

2. Where a laparoscopic approach is being taken, port sites and patient positioning can vary. The surgeon may position themselves to the left of the patient or between the legs. The patient may also be supine or positioned with the right side elevated. A common approach to port placement is the placement of a 10–12-mm infra-umbilical port and the creation of a pneumoperitoneum. A 10–12-mm port is placed in the left lower quadrant and a 5-mm port placed in the left upper quadrant.

3. Dissection is commenced by dividing the peritoneum lateral to the right colon. The ascending colon and caecum are mobilised and retracted medially (care must be taken to identify and not injure the duodenum, right ureter, and right gonadal vessels).

4. The mesentery is palpated and inspected to identify the position of the ileocolic and the right branch of the middle colic artery, which are then ligated and divided near their origin (laparoscopically, this is achieved by applying laparoscopic clips to the vessels prior to dividing them).

5. In an extended right hemicolectomy (for tumours of the transverse colon or splenic flexure), dissection is continued to the splenic flexure or beyond as determined by the site of the lesion.

6. Dissection is continued until the bowel can be held freely, from terminal ileum to mid-transverse colon.

7. Noncrushing bowel clamps are placed on the margins of resection (5 cm resection margin of healthy bowel should be left on either side of the diseased area), one on the ileum and one one-third of the way along the transverse colon. A crushing bowel clamp is placed on the side of the bowel to be resected, and the bowel is divided at each end between the crushing and non-crushing clamps. The resected bowel is then removed and sent for histology. Alternatively, a stapling device can be used to divide the section of bowel to be removed.

8. In laparoscopic approach, a laparoscopic stapler is used and a transverse incision is made in the abdomen through which the resected bowel is removed.

9. The remaining bowel ends are inspected for viability, and an ileocolic anastomosis is fashioned (either hand sewn or with a stapling device). Alternatively, an end ileostomy may be performed.

10. The midline laparotomy is repaired, firstly, mass closure of the midline abdominal wall and then the subcutaneous tissue and skin separately. In laparoscopic approach, the transverse incision and port sites are closed.

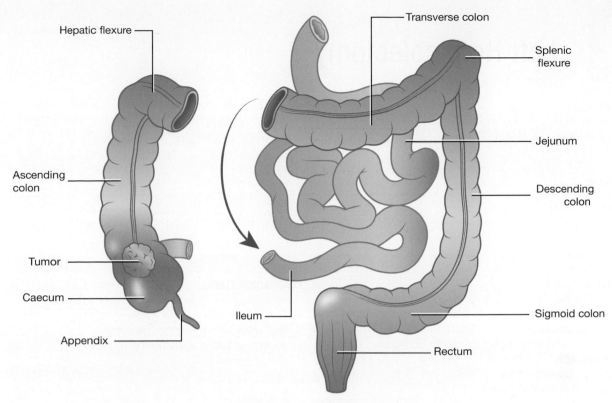

Resection of caecal tumour.

 Complications

EARLY

- Damage to surrounding structures—right ureter, gonadal vessels, duodenum.
- Paralytic ileus.
- Atelectasis.

INTERMEDIATE AND LATE

- Infection—wound, intraabdominal abscess, pneumonia, and urinary tract infection.
- Incisional hernia.
- Deep vein thrombosis (DVT) or pulmonary embolism (PE).
- Adhesive bowel obstruction.
- Anastomotic stricture.
- Change in bowel habit.
- Mortality.

Postoperative Care

INPATIENT

- If the bowel was obstructed preoperatively, the NG tube is kept in until bowel activity resumes.
- If there was evidence of perforation or sepsis, antibiotics are continued postoperatively.
- Diet is gradually built up as bowel activity resumes; in prolonged ileus, TPN must be considered.
- Early ambulation with input from physiotherapy.
- Urinary catheters are removed within 48 hours to prevent infection.
- If drains are left in situ, they are removed once output is minimal.
- DVT prophylaxis is given in-hospital and continued for 28 days for colorectal cancer patients.

OUTPATIENT

- Patients are reviewed 2–6 weeks postoperatively.
- In cases of malignancy, further treatment is decided upon by a multidisciplinary team (MDT) and depends on the results of pathology and the patient's comorbid state.

? Surgeon's Favourite Question

Describe the course of the ureter.

Ureters begin at the ureteropelvic junction (L2), posterior to the renal artery and vein, and descend anterior to the psoas as a retroperitoneal structure, coursing under the gonadal vessels at the inferior pole of the kidney. They continue medially to the sacroiliac joint. They run lateral in the pelvis, crossing anterior to the iliac vessels at the bifurcation of the common iliac artery, then medially to penetrate the base of the bladder.

19 Left Hemicolectomy

Definition

Resection of the descending left colon.

 Indications and Contraindications

INDICATIONS

- Tumours of the colon in the region supplied by the inferior mesenteric artery (IMA).
- Diverticular strictures.
- Large adenomatous polyps that cannot be resected using a colonoscope.
- Segmental Crohn's colitis.
- Trauma and ischaemic injury.

CONTRAINDICATIONS

Contraindications to laparoscopic left hemicolectomy
- Bowel obstruction or ileus leading to severe abdominal distension with poor operative view.
- Multiple previous abdominal surgeries.
- Dense adhesions.

Anatomy

GROSS ANATOMY

- The embryological hindgut develops into the distal third of the transverse colon, splenic flexure, descending and sigmoid colons, and upper rectum.
- The transverse colon and sigmoid colon are intraperitoneal and mobile on their mesenteries.
- The descending colon and upper rectum are retroperitoneal and fixed.

NEUROVASCULATURE

- Parasympathetic nerve supply comes from the pelvic splanchnic nerves (S2–4), and sympathetic from the inferior mesenteric plexus.
- The IMA branches off the descending aorta at the level of L3 and supplies the hindgut.

- Branches of the IMA:
  - Left colic artery—supplies the descending colon.
  - Sigmoid arteries (2–4)—supply the sigmoid colon.
  - Superior rectal artery—supplies the upper rectum.
- Venous drainage is from the left colic, sigmoid, and superior rectal veins, which correspond to the arterial anatomical distribution. The inferior mesenteric vein (IMV) ultimately drains into the portal venous system and terminates when it joins the splenic vein. The splenic vein joins the superior mesenteric vein to form the portal vein posterior to the neck of the pancreas.
- Lymphatic drainage of the sigmoid and the upper rectum is to the para-aortic lymph nodes.

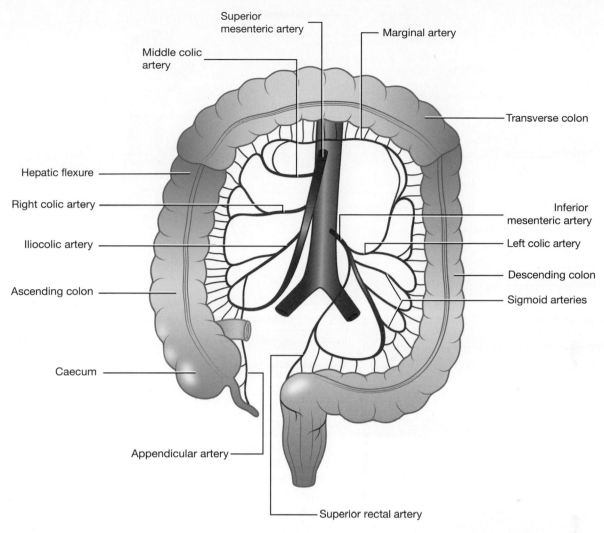

Large bowel anatomy with arterial supply.

¹²₃ STEP-BY-STEP OPERATION

Anaesthesia: general.

Position: supine or Lloyd-Davies.

Considerations: Prophylactic antibiotics are administered. An enema can be given to clear the left colon. This procedure can be performed as a laparotomy or laparoscopically.

Steps:

1. A midline laparotomy and a thorough inspection of the abdominal cavity are performed. In cases of malignancy, the abdominal cavity is assessed for tumour spread, including palpation of the liver.

2. Where a laparoscopic approach it being taken, port sites and patient positioning can vary. The surgeon may position themselves to the right of the patient or between the legs. A common approach is the placement of a 10–12-mm infraumbilical/supra umbilical port and the creation of a pneumoperitoneum, then a 10–12-mm working port in the right lower quadrant and a 5-mm right upper quadrant port.

3. Dissection is commenced by dividing the peritoneum lateral to the left colon. Care is taken to identify and preserve the left ureter and gonadal vessels.

4. The origins of the IMA and IMV are identified with palpation; they are then ligated and divided. In laparoscopic approach, these vessels are clipped.

5. Once the transverse colon, splenic flexure, and descending colon are completely mobilised, the proximal and distal points of transection are identified (5 cm resection margin of healthy bowel should be left on either side of the diseased area).

6. The bowel is divided proximally and distally, either between bowel clamps or with a linear cutting stapler, and the diseased segment is removed and sent for pathology.

7. In a laparoscopic approach, the umbilical port site incision is extended inferiorly. This allows the disease segment of the bowel to be extracted and the remaining proximal and distal bowel segments to be prepared for anastomosis.

8. The proximal and distal segments are brought together, and an end-to-end anastomosis is fashioned using staples or sutures.

9. The anastomosis is checked for any leakage before closing by submerging the anastomosis in water and inflating the colon with gas and observing for bubbles.

10. The midline laparotomy is repaired, firstly mass closure of the midline abdominal wall and then the subcutaneous tissue and skin separately.

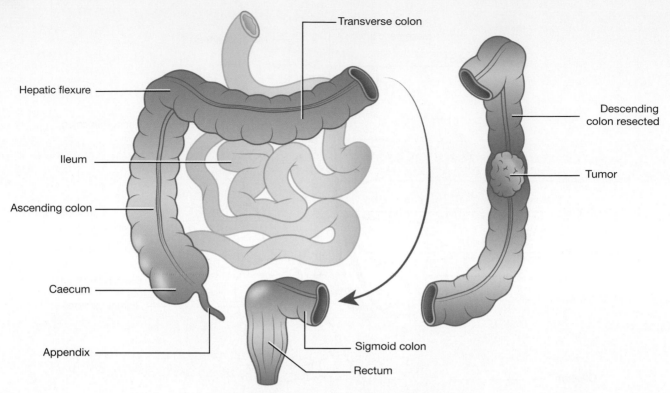

Resection of tumour of descending colon.

Complications

EARLY
- Bleeding.
- Splenic or left ureter injury.
- Ileus.

INTERMEDIATE AND LATE
- Infection—chest, urinary, and intra-abdominal collection.
- Deep vein thrombosis (DVT) or pulmonary embolism (PE).
- Anastomotic leak (typically 5–7 days postoperatively).
- Enteric fistula formation.
- Adhesive bowel obstruction.
- Incisional hernia.
- Anastomotic stricture.
- Change in bowel habit.
- Mortality.

Postoperative Care

INPATIENT
- If the bowel was obstructed preoperatively, the NG tube is kept in until bowel activity resumes.
- In cases of perforation or sepsis, antibiotics are continued postoperatively.
- Diet is gradually built up as bowel activity resumes; in prolonged ileus, TPN must be considered.
- Urinary catheters are removed within 48 hours to prevent infection.
- If drains are left in situ, they are removed once output is minimal.
- DVT prophylaxis is given in-hospital and continued for 28 days for colorectal cancer patients.

OUTPATIENT
- Patients are reviewed 2–6 weeks postoperatively.
- In cases of malignancy, further treatment is decided upon by a multidisciplinary team (MDT), and depends on the results of pathology and the patient's comorbid state.

? Surgeon's Favourite Question

What is the difference between a Hartmann's procedure and a left hemicolectomy?

In a Hartmann's procedure, an end-colostomy is fashioned, and a rectal stump is left in the pelvis; in a left hemicolectomy, a primary anastomosis is formed.

Hartmann's Procedure

Alison Bradley

Definition

An emergency procedure to remove the sigmoid colon and upper rectum, resulting in an end colostomy (colonic stoma) and an over-sewn rectal stump.

Indications and Contraindications

INDICATIONS

- Diverticular disease of the sigmoid colon with perforation, abscess, and/or peritonitis.
- Rectosigmoid cancer causing obstruction or perforation.
- Unresolved sigmoid volvulus.
- Other sigmoid pathology where a primary anastomosis would be at significant risk of breakdown:
  - Anastomotic dehiscence.
  - Ischaemia.

CONTRAINDICATIONS

- Scoring tools, such as the NELA risk calculator, can help to guide decision making by estimating 30-day mortality after emergency abdominal surgery.

Anatomy

GROSS ANATOMY

- The embryological hindgut develops into the distal third of the transverse colon, splenic flexure, descending colon, sigmoid colon, and upper rectum.
- The transverse and sigmoid colon are intraperitoneal and mobile on their mesenteries.
- The descending colon and upper rectum are retroperitoneal and fixed.

NEUROVASCULATURE

- Parasympathetic nerve supply comes from the pelvic splanchnic nerves (S2–4), and sympathetic, from the inferior mesenteric plexus.
- The inferior mesenteric artery (IMA) branches off the descending aorta at the level of L3 and supplies the hindgut.

- Branches of the IMA:
  - Left colic artery—supplies the descending colon.
  - Sigmoid arteries—supply the sigmoid colon.
  - Superior rectal artery—supplies the upper rectum.
- Venous drainage is from the left colic, sigmoid, and superior rectal veins, which correspond to the arterial anatomical distribution. The inferior mesenteric vein (IMV) ultimately drains into the portal venous system and terminates when it joins the splenic vein. The splenic vein joins the superior mesenteric vein posterior to the neck of the pancreas to form the portal vein.
- Lymphatic drainage of the sigmoid and the upper rectum is to the para-aortic lymph nodes.

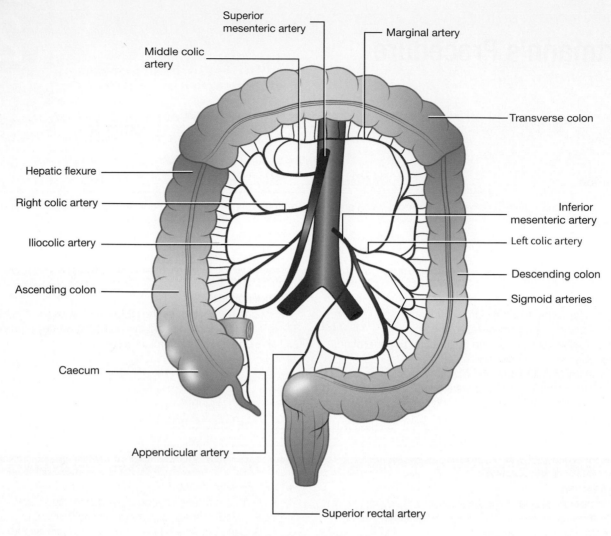

Large bowel anatomy with arterial supply.

⑫₃ STEP-BY-STEP OPERATION

Anaesthesia: general.

Position: Lloyd-Davies position.

Considerations: A urinary catheter is inserted. In cases of obstruction, a nasogastric (NG) tube is inserted, and prophylactic antibiotics are given. The stoma site is marked on the left lower quadrant.

Steps:

1. A midline laparotomy is performed.
2. The abdominal cavity is inspected, and any free fluid is sent to microbiology.
3. Dissection is commenced by dividing the peritoneum lateral to the left colon. Care is taken to identify and preserve the left ureter throughout its length.
4. The sigmoid vessels are identified within the mesentery and divided.
5. Once the sigmoid colon and descending colon are completely mobilized, the proximal and distal points of transection are identified.
6. The bowel is divided proximally and distally, either between bowel clamps or with a linear cutting stapler. Peritoneal lavage is performed using warm saline, and drains are inserted.
7. The rectal stump (either stapled or sewn over by hand) is left in situ.
8. A circular incision is made over the site of the previously marked stoma site, and the abdominal cavity is entered. The proximal colon is brought out of the abdomen and through the incision, ensuring it is not under tension.
9. The midline laparotomy is repaired, firstly mass closure of the midline abdominal wall and then the subcutaneous tissue and skin separately.
10. The protruding bowel is then fashioned into a stoma. The staple line excised and the end of colon is sutured subcuticularily to create the stoma. A stoma bag is placed over the stoma (colostomy).

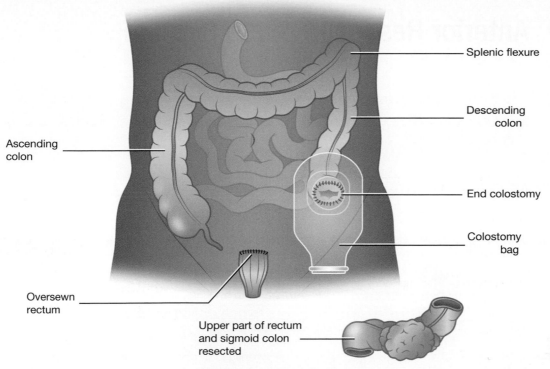

Ascending colon

Splenic flexure

Descending colon

End colostomy

Colostomy bag

Oversewn rectum

Upper part of rectum and sigmoid colon resected

Resection of tumour of sigmoid colon.

 Complications

EARLY

- Iatrogenic damage to surrounding structures—ureters and gonadal vessels.
- Paralytic ileus.
- Atelectasis.
- Stoma—retraction or ischaemia.

INTERMEDIATE AND LATE

- Infection—wound, intraabdominal abscess, pneumonia, and urinary tract infection.
- Deep vein thrombosis (DVT) or pulmonary embolism (PE).
- Incisional hernia.
- Adhesive bowel obstruction.
- Stoma—stenosis, prolapse, or para-stomal hernia.

Postoperative Care

INPATIENT

- Initial postoperative care in an intensive treatment unit (ITU)/high-dependency unit (HDU) environment.
- Antibiotics are continued for 5–7 days postoperatively.
- Full and normal diet is encouraged immediately postoperation; in prolonged ileus, parenteral nutrition must be considered.
- Urinary catheters are removed within 48 hours to prevent infection.
- If drains are left in situ, they are removed once output is minimal.
- DVT prophylaxis is given in-hospital and continued for 28 days for colorectal cancer patients.
- The patient is instructed in stoma care and must be confident with the stoma management before discharge.

OUTPATIENT

- Patients are reviewed 2–6 weeks postoperatively.
- Stoma reversal may be considered once the patient has fully recovered, usually after 6 months.
- In cases of malignancy, further treatment is decided upon by a multidisciplinary team (MDT) and depends on the results of pathology and the patient's comorbid state.

? Surgeon's Favourite Question

How do you differentiate between a colostomy and an ileostomy?

A colostomy tends to be flush with the skin, and an ileostomy is spouted. Do not simply rely on the position when attempting to differentiate between the two.

21 Anterior Resection of the Rectum

Alison Bradley

Definition

Excision of the rectum, mesorectum, and regional lymphatics via the anterior abdominal wall.

Indications and Contraindications

INDICATIONS
- Rectal cancers without invasion of the anal sphincter complex.

CONTRAINDICATIONS
Relative
- Localised, superficial, T1 rectal cancers—may be endo-scopically treated with local excision.

Absolute
- Rectal cancers very close to or involving the sphincters—managed by abdominoperineal resection.

Anatomy

GROSS ANATOMY
- The rectum arises embryologically from the hindgut.
- The upper rectum is intraperitoneal, the middle third is lined by the peritoneum anteriorly only, and the lower third, below the pelvic peritoneal reflection, is extraperitoneal.
- In males, the rectovesical pouch, base of bladder, seminal vesicles, and prostate lie anterior to the rectum, with Denonvilliers' fascia separating it from the prostate.
- In females, the posterior vaginal wall, rectovaginal sep-tum, and bladder lie anteriorly.
- For both sexes, the sacrum, coccyx, lower sacral nerves, and middle sacral artery all lie posterior to the rectum.
- The levator ani and coccygeus muscles lie lateral and inferior to the peritoneal reflection.

NEUROVASCULATURE
- Nerve supply arises from the pelvic plexus (hypogastric nerves) and splanchnic nerves (S2–S4).
- Blood supply is from the superior rectal artery (branch of the inferior mesenteric artery (IMA)), the middle rectal artery (branch of the internal iliac artery), and the inferior rectal artery (branches of the pudendal artery).
- Venous drainage is via the superior rectal vein to the infe-rior mesenteric vein (IMV), draining to the hepatic portal circulation.
- Lymphatic drainage is to the mesorectum, then the infe-rior mesenteric lymph nodes. Total mesorectal excision (TME)—removal of mesorectal fat and lymph nodes—is crucial in an oncological anterior resection.

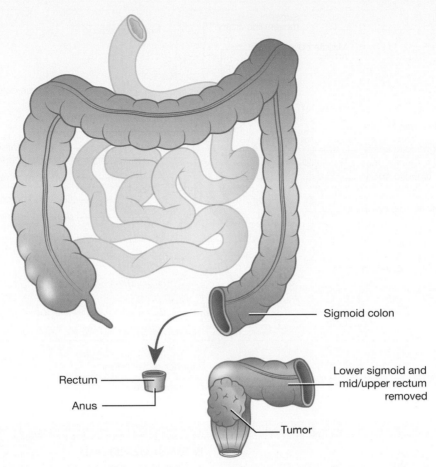

Resection of rectal tumour.

₁₂₃ STEP-BY-STEP OPERATION

Anaesthesia: general
Position: Lloyd-Davies
Considerations: A urinary catheter is inserted. Bowel preparation can be considered.
Steps:

1. A midline laparotomy is performed and the abdominal cavity is assessed for tumour spread, including palpation of the liver. This procedure can also be performed laparoscopically. Operating surgeons will have their own preferences for port placements and patient positioning.
2. Dissection is commenced by dividing the peritoneum lateral to the left colon. Care is taken to identify and preserve the left ureter throughout its length.
3. The origins of the IMA and IMV are identified with palpation. They are then ligated and divided.
4. Once the splenic flexure, descending colon, sigmoid, and rectum are completely mobilised, the proximal and distal points of transection are identified.
5. TME is then performed. Anteriorly, the dissection commences by opening the peritoneum at the rectovesical pouch in men, and between the anterior mesorectum and posterior vaginal wall in women. Dissection is then continued towards the pelvic floor, laterally and posteriorly (anterior to the coccyx).
6. After mobilisation and TME, the bowel is divided at its proximal and distal resection margins, either between bowel clamps or with a linear cutting stapler device. The specimen is excised and sent to pathology.

7. An end-to-end anastomosis is formed between the descending colon and the rectal stump, using either a circular stapling device or by hand-sewing. The anastomosis is checked for any leakage before closing. This is done by submerging the anastomosis in warmed saline and inflating the rectum with gas. There should be no leak of bubbles from the staple line.
8. A defunctioning loop ileostomy may be formed to divert faeces away from a healing anastomosis (if within 6 cm of the anal verge). A defunctioning loop ileostomy should also be considered at times if there have been technical difficulties during the construction of the anastomosis. This is placed in the right iliac fossa and can be reversed 3–6 months later.
9. To form the stoma, the loop of small bowel is delivered through the abdominal wall by excising a disc of skin. A tape or bridge is placed under the loop and the loop of bowel is opened through its anterior wall. Two lumens are therefore showing. The distal lumen is sutured to the skin. The active lumen is spouted and sutured to the skin.
10. The midline laparotomy is repaired, firstly mass closure of the midline abdominal wall and then the subcutaneous tissue and skin separately.

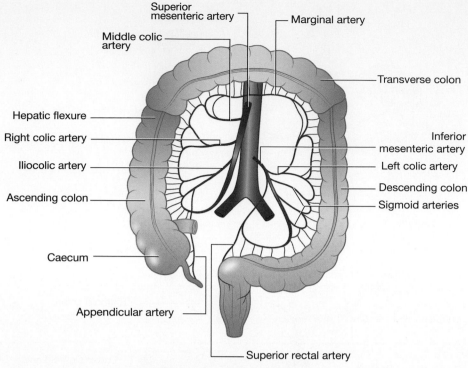

Large bowel anatomy with arterial supply.

 Complications

EARLY

- Damage to surrounding structures—the ureter and gonadal vessels.
- Paralytic ileus.
- Atelectasis.
- Stoma—retraction and ischaemia.

INTERMEDIATE AND LATE

- Infection—wound, intra-abdominal abscess, pneumonia, and urinary tract infection.
- Anastomotic leak (typically 5–7 days postoperatively).
- Anastomotic stricture.
- Bladder and sexual dysfunction.
- Deep vein thrombosis (DVT) or pulmonary embolism (PE).
- Incisional hernia.
- Adhesive bowel obstruction.
- Stoma—stenosis, prolapse, or para-stomal hernia.
- Mortality.

Postoperative Care

INPATIENT

- Diet is gradually built up as bowel activity resumes; in prolonged ileus, parenteral nutrition must be considered.
- Early ambulation with input from physiotherapy.
- Urinary catheters removed within 48 hours—attention must be paid to voiding, as bladder tone may be lost postoperatively.
- If drains are left in situ, they are removed once output is minimal.
- DVT prophylaxis is given in-hospital and continued for 28 days.
- If a loop ileostomy is formed, the patient is instructed in stoma care and must be confident with stoma management before discharge.

OUTPATIENT

- Patients are reviewed 2–6 weeks postoperatively.
- Further treatment is decided upon by a multidisciplinary team (MDT) depending on the results of pathology and the patient's comorbid state.

? **Surgeon's Favourite Question**

In what circumstances may a patient end up with an intestinal stoma after an anterior resection?

1. Anastomosis too low—they are likely to have a defunctioning loop ileostomy, which may subsequently be reversed.
2. Not technically possible—insufficient length of vascularised bowel (commonest reason), or not sensible to do so, e.g. gross examination by the naked eye shows tumour present at the resection margin or blood supply too poor, an end colostomy is performed, which would usually be permanent.
3. Anastomotic leak—the patient will likely need emergency surgery and take down of the anastomosis into an end colostomy.

Abdominoperineal Resection (APR)

Alison Bradley

Definition

Removal of the sigmoid colon, rectum, and anus with the creation of a permanent end-colostomy.

Indications and Contraindications

INDICATIONS
- Anal cancer with failed neoadjuvant therapy.
- Recurrent anal cancer.
- Low-lying rectal cancer with involvement of the anal sphincter.

CONTRAINDICATIONS
- Patients with significant morbidity may be deemed unsuitable to undergo major colorectal resection.

Anatomy

GROSS ANATOMY
- The anal canal is extraperitoneal and measures 2–4 cm.
- The anal canal is embryologically part hindgut and part proctoderm. The dentate line divides the anal canal based on this:
  - The proximal two-thirds of the anal canal lie above the dentate line. This section is hindgut in origin and is lined with columnar mucosa.
  - The distal third lies below the dentate line—this section is proctoderm in origin and is lined with squamous epithelium.

NEUROVASCULATURE
- Above the dentate line:
  - Innervated by the inferior hypogastric plexus.
  - Arterial supply is from the superior rectal artery (a branch of the inferior mesenteric artery (IMA)) and the middle rectal artery (a branch of the internal iliac artery).
  - Venous drainage is via the internal haemorrhoidal plexus to the superior rectal vein.
- Below the dentate line:
  - Innervated by the inferior rectal nerve, a branch of the pudendal nerve from the sacral plexus.
  - Arterial supply is via the inferior rectal artery from the pudendal artery.
  - Venous drainage is via the external haemorrhoidal plexus to the inferior and middle rectal veins.

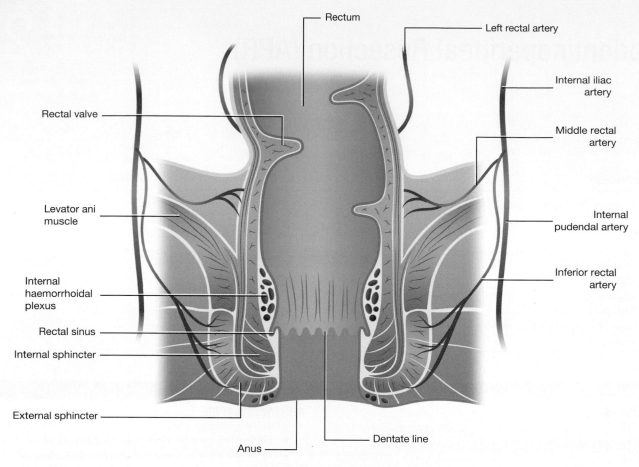

Vascular supply of the rectum.

STEP-BY-STEP OPERATION

Anaesthesia: general.

Position: supine and Lloyd-Davies.

Considerations: A urinary catheter is inserted. The abdominal and perineal components of the operation can be done concurrently if there are two surgeons.

Steps:

1. A midline laparotomy is performed. The abdominal cavity is assessed for tumour spread (including palpation of the liver). In a laparoscopic approach, the choice of port placement may vary, but as a guide, a 10-mm umbilical port is placed, followed by 5-mm right and left upper quadrant ports, a 12-mm right lower quadrant port, and a 5-mm left lower quadrant port.

2. The small bowel and sigmoid colon are retracted to the patient's right-hand side. The parietal peritoneum is dissected, starting from the junction between the sigmoid colon and the retroperitoneal descending colon. Care is taken to identify and preserve the left ureter and the left common iliac artery.

3. The IMA and vein are ligated and then the left peritoneal dissection is carried down into the total mesorectal excision plane. The peritoneum on the right is then divided and the two sides joined below the level of the bifurcation of the aorta. This allows mobilisation of the rectum and sigmoid colon.

4. The superior rectal artery is ligated. The descending colon is divided at its proximal resection margin, either between bowel clamps or with a linear cutting stapler device.

5. The proximal end of the colon is brought out through the abdominal wall and an end-colostomy is fashioned. The stoma site should ideally be marked preoperatively and a disc of skin excised in the abdominal wall through which the proximal colon is delivered. The protruding bowel is then fashioned into a stoma. The staple line is excised and the end of colon is sutured subcuticular to create the stoma. A stoma bag is placed over the stoma (colostomy).

6. Next, the perineal resection is commenced. The patient may be repositioned prone or Lloyd-Davies for this part of the procedure. An elliptical perineal incision is made from the perineal body to a point midway between the anus and coccyx.

7. The rectum is mobilised from the prostate/vagina and surrounding tissues. The inferior rectal vessels are ligated, and the rectum, sigmoid colon, and anus are removed.

8. The levator muscles are reapproximated with sutures. A mesh may be used to add extra support.

9. The perineal wound is closed in layers.

10. The midline laparotomy is repaired, firstly mass closure of the midline abdominal wall and then the subcutaneous tissue skin separately.

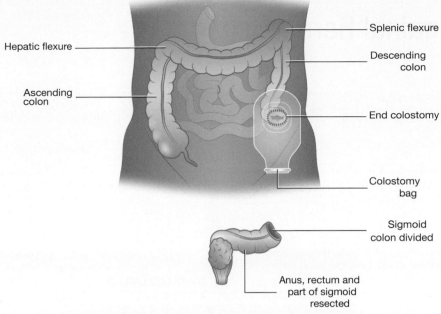

Hepatic flexure

Ascending
colon

Splenic flexure

Descending
colon

End colostomy

Colostomy
bag

Sigmoid
colon divided

Anus, rectum and
part of sigmoid
resected

Resection of rectal tumour with formation of end colostomy.

 ## Complications

EARLY
- Damage to surrounding structures—the ureters and gonadal vessels.
- Paralytic ileus.
- Atelectasis.
- Stoma problems—retraction or ischaemia.

INTERMEDIATE AND LATE
- Infection—wound, intra-abdominal abscess, pneumonia, and urinary tract infection.
- Deep vein thrombosis (DVT) or pulmonary embolism (PE).
- Wound dehiscence.
- Persistent perineal sinus (perineal wound that has not healed 6 months postoperatively).
- Bladder and sexual dysfunction.
- Incisional hernia.
- Perineal hernia.
- Adhesive bowel obstruction.
- Stoma problems—stenosis, prolapse, or para-stomal hernia.

Postoperative Care

INPATIENT
- Full and normal diet is encouraged immediately postoperation; in prolonged ileus, parenteral nutrition must be considered.
- Early ambulation with input from physiotherapy.
- Urinary catheters removed within 48 hours—attention must be paid to voiding, as bladder tone may be lost postoperatively.
- If drains are left in situ, they are removed once output is significantly reduced.
- DVT prophylaxis is given in-hospital and continued for 28 days in cases of malignancy.
- The patient is instructed in stoma care and must be confident with stoma management before discharge.

OUTPATIENT
- Patients are reviewed 2–6 weeks postoperatively.
- Further treatment is decided upon by a multidisciplinary team (MDT) and depends on the results of pathology and the patient's comorbid state.

? Surgeon's Favourite Question

When perineal defects are too large for primary repair, what are the reconstructive options available for this area?

Reconstruction can be done with either a biological mesh or a myocutaneous flap. These include a pedicled gluteus maximus, gracilis, or rectus abdominis flap.

23 Inguinal Hernia Repair

Alison Bradley

Definition

Repair of an inguinal hernia, which may be either indirect (through the deep inguinal ring) or direct (through Hesselbach's triangle)

 ## Indications and Contraindications

INDICATIONS
Elective
- Symptomatic inguinal hernia.

Emergency
- Incarcerated or strangulated hernia.

CONTRAINDICATIONS
- Pregnancy—repair should be delayed unless there are signs of an acute incarceration, strangulation, or bowel obstruction.
- Small asymptomatic hernias—can undergo watchful waiting.

Anatomy

GROSS ANATOMY
- The deep and superficial inguinal rings are the internal and external openings of the inguinal canal.
- The inguinal canal contains the ilioinguinal nerve in both sexes. In females, it contains the round ligament; in males, the spermatic cord.
- The deep ring is found deep to the midpoint of the inguinal ligament, which lies halfway between the pubic tubercle and the anterior superior iliac spine (ASIS). The superficial inguinal ring is located ~1 cm superolateral to the pubic crest.
- The borders of the inguinal canal are:
  - Anterior—aponeurosis of external and internal oblique muscles.
  - Posterior—transversalis fascia and the conjoint tendon.
  - Superior—internal oblique and transverse abdominus.
  - Inferior—inguinal and lacunar ligaments.
- Hesselbach's triangle is demarcated by:
  - Medial—rectus abdominis.
  - Lateral—inferior epigastric vessels.
  - Inferior—inguinal ligament.

PATHOLOGY
- Direct inguinal hernias arise directly through the posterior wall of the inguinal canal, medial to the inferior epigastric vessels in Hesselbach's triangle.
- Indirect inguinal hernias arise through the deep ring with the spermatic cord, lateral to the inferior epigastric vessels. Indirect hernias traverse the inguinal canal to the superficial ring and may descend into the scrotum.

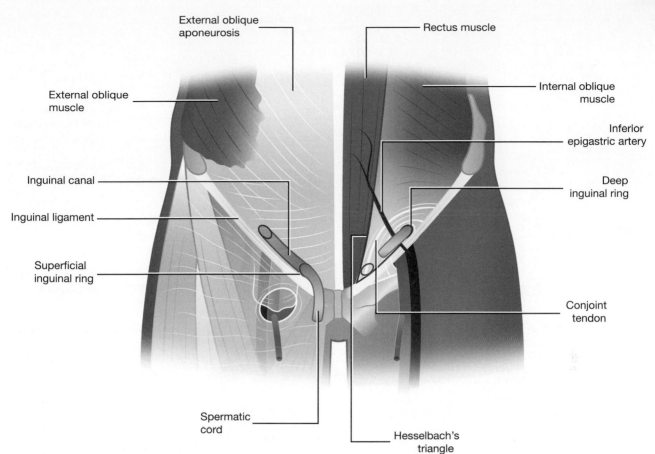

Inguinal anatomy. In a male. Note in females, the round ligament passes through the inguinal canal instead of the spermatic cord.

1 2 3 STEP-BY-STEP OPERATION

Anaesthesia: general, regional, or local.
Position: supine.
Considerations: A urinary catheter can be considered.
Steps:

1. A skin crease incision is made in the groin, running superior to, but approximately in line with, the inguinal ligament, from the pubic tubercle to the level of the deep inguinal ring.
2. Dissection is continued until the external oblique aponeurosis is visible.
3. The external oblique fibres are split as far as the superficial inguinal ring (just superior to the pubic tubercle).
4. The ilioinguinal nerve is identified and protected.
5. The contents of the inguinal canal are identified and inspected.
6. The sac is then dissected free from the cord structures, and a tape is passed around the spermatic cord (in men).

7. Sac relocation:
   a. If a direct hernia is found, the sac is pushed back into the extraperitoneal space, and non-absorbable sutures are used to plicate the posterior wall over it.
   b. If an indirect hernia is found, the sac is dissected to the deep ring and opened to determine its contents. Once emptied, it is then transfixed at its base.
8. The mesh is cut to the shape and size of the inguinal canal. The apex is sutured to the pubic tubercle with the suture being placed a short distance away from the apex, ensuring some medial overlap. A slit is made at the lateral end to create two 'tails'.
9. The inferior edge of the mesh is sutured along the inguinal ligament, and the superior edge is sutured onto the internal oblique muscle. The 'tail ends' of the mesh are sutured together around the spermatic cord lateral to the cord contents, recreating the deep inguinal ring.
10. The wound is closed in layers with absorbable sutures.

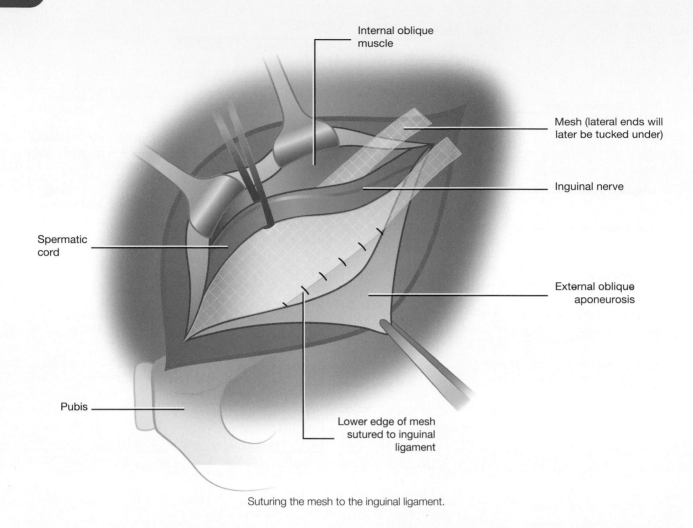

Internal oblique muscle

Mesh (lateral ends will later be tucked under)

Inguinal nerve

Spermatic cord

External oblique aponeurosis

Pubis

Lower edge of mesh sutured to inguinal ligament

Suturing the mesh to the inguinal ligament.

 Complications

EARLY
- Bleeding.
- Haematoma and seroma formation.
- Damage to vas deferens.
- Ischaemic orchitis or testicular atrophy.
- Ilioinguinal nerve damage.
- Femoral vessel damage.

INTERMEDIATE AND LATE
- Infection—wound, mesh, intra-abdominal abscess, pneumonia, and urinary tract.
- Chronic inguinal pain secondary to ilioinguinal nerve damage.
- Recurrence.
- Chronic mesh infection.

Postoperative Care

INPATIENT
- Patients can be discharged the same day, provided there were no immediate complications.

OUTPATIENT
- Avoid heavy lifting and straining for 4–6 weeks.

 Surgeon's Favourite Question

How is the difference between an indirect and direct hernia identified intraoperatively?

An indirect hernia protrudes lateral to the inferior epigastric artery; a direct hernia protrudes medial to the inferior epigastric artery.

Femoral Hernia Repair

24

Alison Bradley

Definition

Surgical closure of the femoral ring, with removal of preperitoneal fat or intestine from the femoral ring (if present).

Indications and Contraindications

INDICATIONS

Elective

- Femoral hernias are associated with a high risk of strangulation; therefore, elective repair is recommended.

Acute

- Incarcerated or strangulated hernia.

CONTRAINDICATIONS

- In patients with severe comorbidities, elective operative management may be deemed inappropriate.

Anatomy

GROSS ANATOMY

- The femoral ring forms the base of the femoral canal.
- Boundaries of the femoral canal:
  - Anterior—inguinal ligament.
  - Posterior—pectineal (Cooper's) ligament.
  - Medial—lacunar ligament.
  - Lateral—femoral vein.
- The femoral canal contains loose fatty connective tissues, lymphatic vessels, and lymph nodes (the lymph node of Cloquet).

- The relative dead space of the femoral canal allows for expansion of the femoral vein secondary to either increased lower limb venous pressure of increased intra-abdominal pressure.

PATHOLOGY

- A femoral hernia is the protrusion of pre-peritoneal fat or intestine into the femoral ring and canal.
- Femoral hernias arise inferolateral to the pubic tubercle in the anterior thigh.

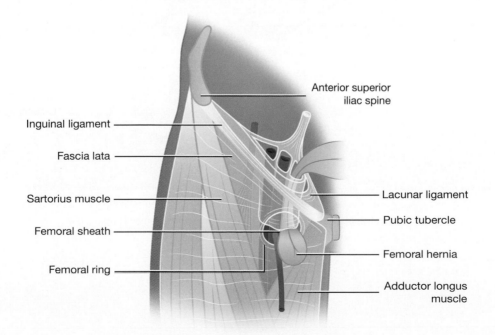

Femoral anatomy.

¹2₃ STEP-BY-STEP OPERATION

Anaesthesia: general.

Position: supine.

Considerations: A urinary catheter is inserted. Two approaches are commonly used: the low approach (elective) and the McEvedy approach (acute).

Steps:

LOW APPROACH

1. An incision is made 1 cm below and parallel to the medial inguinal ligament. The subcutaneous fat is blunt-dissected through to the level of the femoral hernia sac.
2. The hernia sac is dissected down to its neck, and the femoral and long saphenous veins are identified and preserved.
3. The sac is opened to assess contents and viability. The contents of the sac are then returned through the femoral ring to the peritoneum.

MCEVEDY APPROACH

1. An 8–10-cm incision is made over the lower abdominal wall commencing at the pubic tubercle, running obliquely and laterally.
2. The rectus sheath is opened, and the rectus muscles are retracted. The pre-peritoneal fat and areolar tissue are dissected and then peritoneum is pulled up.
3. The hernia sac is identified and dissected down to its neck and then reduced upwards through the femoral ring.
4. The sac is then opened to assess contents and their viability; any non-viable bowel should be excised.

BOTH

5. The neck of the sac is ligated as high as possible, and the femoral ring is closed with mesh sutures or interrupted non-absorbable sutures between the inguinal and pectineal ligaments.
6. The skin is closed with subcutaneous absorbable sutures.

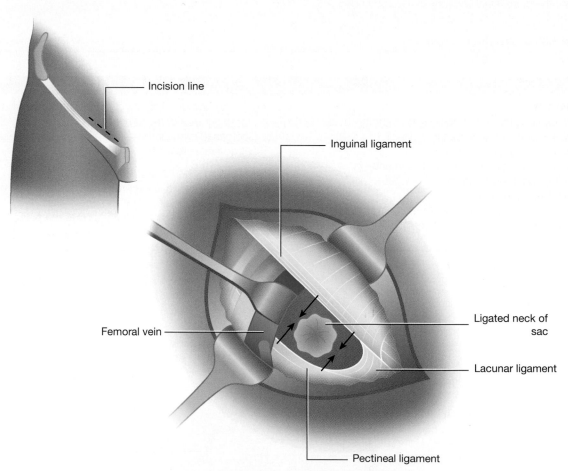

Ligation of the hernia sac and suture closure of the femoral ring.

Complications

EARLY
- Bleeding.
- Haematoma and seroma.
- Bowel injury.
- Femoral vein compression.

INTERMEDIATE AND LATE
- Infection—wound, mesh (if used), intra-abdominal abscess, pneumonia, and urinary tract infection.
- Hernia recurrence.
- Stenotic stricture of the small bowel following strangulation (stenosis of Garré).
- Persistent groin pain.

Postoperative Care

INPATIENT
- Elective patients can be discharged the same day.

OUTPATIENT
- Patients are advised to avoid heavy lifting and straining for 4–6 weeks.

 Surgeon's Favourite Question

What are the borders of the femoral ring?

Anteriorly—inguinal ligament.
Posteriorly—pectineal ligament.
Medially—lacunar ligament.
Laterally—femoral vein.

25

Haemorrhoidectomy

Alison Bradley

Definition

Surgical procedure to remove haemorrhoids (anorectal vascular cushions).

 Indications and Contraindications

INDICATIONS

External Haemorrhoids
- Symptomatic haemorrhoids refractory to conservative management.
- Large or severely symptomatic haemorrhoids.

Internal Haemorrhoids
- Prolapsed internal haemorrhoids that can be manually reduced (Grade III).
- Prolapsed and incarcerated internal haemorrhoids (Grade IV).
- Symptomatic internal haemorrhoids refractory to conservative measures.
- Combined haemorrhoids.

CONTRAINDICATIONS

Relative
- Previous operations involving the anal canal resulting in poor anal sphincter tone.
- Faecal incontinence.
- Portal hypertension with rectal varices.

Absolute
- Active disease in the anal canal or rectum, including Crohn's, colitis, and peri-anal abscess.

Anatomy

GROSS ANATOMY
- The anal canal is extraperitoneal and measures 2–4 cm.
- The anal canal is embryologically part hindgut and part proctoderm. The dentate line divides the anal canal based on this:
  - The proximal two-thirds of the anal canal lie above the dentate line. This section is hindgut in origin and is lined with columnar mucosa.
  - The distal third lies below the dentate line. This section is proctoderm in origin and is lined with squamous epithelium.

NEUROVASCULATURE
- Above the dentate line
  - Innervated by the inferior hypogastric plexus.
  - Arterial supply is from the superior rectal artery (a branch of the IMA) and the middle rectal artery (a branch of the internal iliac artery).
  - Venous drainage is via the internal haemorrhoidal plexus to the superior rectal vein.
- Below the dentate line
  - Innervated by the inferior rectal nerve, a branch of the pudendal nerve from the sacral plexus.
  - Arterial supply is via the inferior rectal arteries from the pudendal artery.
  - Venous drainage is via the external haemorrhoidal plexus to the inferior and middle rectal veins.

PATHOLOGY
- Haemorrhoids are dilated anal vascular cushions and occur due to arterial inflow from branches of the superior rectal artery in the left lateral, right anterolateral, and right posterolateral positions.
- Haemorrhoids classically arise in the 3, 7, and 11 o'clock positions in lithotomy position.
- Haemorrhoids are termed depending on whether they arise from above or below the dentate line. Haemorrhoids proximal to the dentate line are classed as internal, distal as external, and mixed if they are both proximal and distal.
- Internal haemorrhoids are classified according to the degree from which they prolapse from the anal canal:
  - Grade I—bulge into the lumen but do not prolapse below the dentate line.
  - Grade II—prolapse out of the anal canal with defecation/straining but spontaneously reduce.
  - Grade III—prolapse out of the anal canal with defecation/straining and require manual reduction.
  - Grade IV—are irreducible and therefore have the potential to strangulate.

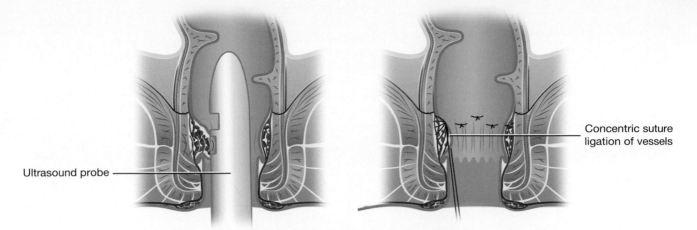

Ultrasound probe

Concentric suture ligation of vessels

Internal and external haemorrhoidal locations.

¹²₃ STEP-BY-STEP OPERATION

Anaesthesia: general.
Position: lithotomy.
Steps:

HAEMORRHOIDECTOMY

1. A digital rectal examination is performed, and an anal retractor is used to identify and examine the haemorrhoids.
2. A clip is applied to each haemorrhoid, and local anaesthetic is infiltrated into each.
3. The haemorrhoid and overlying skin are grasped and retracted. Diathermy is used to dissect the tissue off the internal anal sphincter until it remains on a pedicle.
4. The pedicle is transfixed, and the haemorrhoid is removed.
5. The skin at the anal verge can be closed or left to heal by secondary intention.

HAEMORRHOIDAL ARTERY LIGATION (HALO)

1. A probe containing bright LED lights with an integrated Doppler ultrasound is inserted into the anus. This allows direct visualisation of the mucosa of the anus and rectum by the surgeon whilst combining feedback on Doppler flow and depth perception of arteries.
2. The probe is rotated slowly until an artery is detected, and its depth assessed; safe ligation can occur on arteries up to 8 mm deep.
3. Through the window of the probe, a suture can be placed to ligate the artery; double ligation with a figure of eight knot is often used.
4. The probe is then rotated until the next artery is detected and ligated. A whole turn of the probe is made then the probe is withdrawn 1.5 cm and the process repeated. In general, five to seven arteries can be ligated but this can vary.
5. The series of suture ligations created reduce the arterial supply to the haemorrhoidal cushions which in time shrink over the next 6–8 weeks.

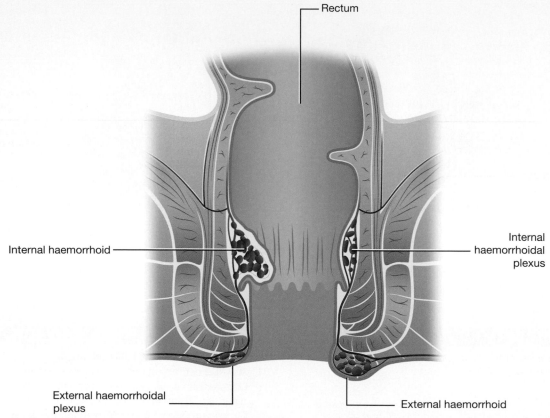

Ultrasound probe insertion and circumferential suture ligations in the HALO (haemorrhoidal artery ligation) technique.

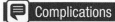 Complications

EARLY
- Pain.
- Bleeding.
- Urinary retention.

INTERMEDIATE AND LATE
- Pelvic sepsis.
- Anal canal stenosis.
- Secondary haemorrhage 10–14 days after treatment (notorious in banding).
- Faecal incontinence.
- Rectovaginal fistula (if staples are used).
- Recurrence

Postoperative Care

INPATIENT
- The patient is discharged on laxatives, analgesia, and anti-inflammatories.
- A course of oral metronidazole is prescribed postoperatively.

OUTPATIENT
- Follow-up at outpatient clinic in 4 weeks.

? Surgeon's Favourite Question

What is the grading system used for internal haemorrhoids?

Grade I—no prolapse.
Grade II—prolapse upon bearing down but reduces spontaneously.
Grade III—prolapse upon bearing down and requires reduction manually.
Grade IV—prolapsed, cannot be reduced.

Excision of Pilonidal Sinus

26

Alison Bradley

Definition

The surgical removal of a small hole or tunnel in the skin at the natal cleft.

Indications and Contraindications

INDICATIONS

- A chronic or recurrently infected pilonidal sinus.

CONTRAINDICATIONS

- Asymptomatic patients with a simple pilonidal sinus where there is a small pit or non-tender lump in the natal cleft, which may have an emergent hair—these patients do not require treatment.
- Acutely infected pilonidal sinuses—these should be drained and later return for definitive excision.

Anatomy

GROSS ANATOMY

- A pilonidal sinus is a subcutaneous sinus in the natal cleft lined by squamous epithelium and containing hair.
- The natal cleft is the groove between the buttocks extending inferiorly from the sacrum to the anus.

PATHOLOGY

- An infected sinus is usually lined with purulent material and granulation tissue.

- The sinus may be part of a deeper tract extending along the midline or to one side.
- The sinus may have one or more openings.
- Less commonly, sinuses occur in the interdigital clefts, face, and axilla.

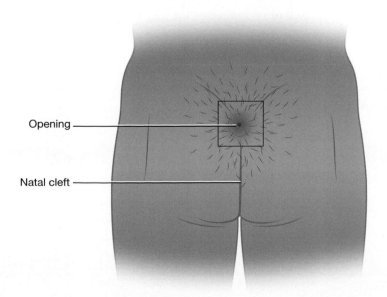

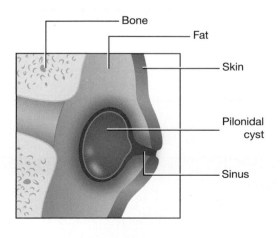

Pilonidal sinus with infected cyst.

STEP-BY-STEP OPERATION

Anaesthesia: general or local.
Position: prone with elevated hips or lateral decubitus position.
Considerations: The buttocks are taped apart to expose the sinus, and the area is shaved.
Steps:

1. The sinus is palpated, and probes are used to delineate the sinus tracts. If the sinus is difficult to palpate, methylene blue dye can be injected into the sinus tracts to delineate anatomy.
2. An elliptical incision is made around the cavity incorporating any lateral sinus tracts; an incision line lateral to the midline suture line is preferred.
3. The incision is made through the subcutaneous fat and extends down to the presacral fascia incorporating the entire sinus tract and any secondary openings.

4. The entire sinus tract with a cuff of surrounding subcutaneous fat is included in the specimen
5. The cavity is then thoroughly irrigated with normal saline and local anaesthetic can be instilled.
6. A subcutaneous fat flap is then raised by undermining the subcutaneous layer so that it is roughly 1 cm thick and 2 cm deep to allow a two-layered tension-free closure.
7. The subcutaneous layer is closed with absorbable sutures.
8. The skin is then closed with the suture line being placed laterally to the midline. A vertical mattress suture with non-absorbable sutures is preferred superiorly with absorbable sutures in the inferior natal cleft.

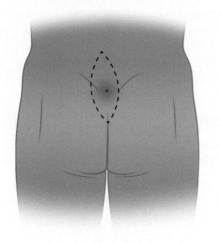
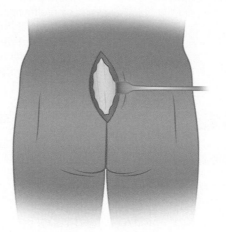
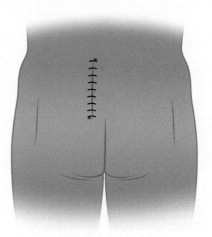
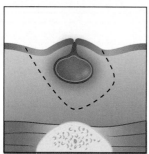
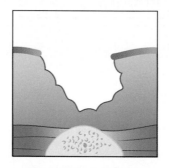
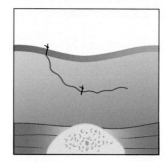

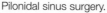
Pilonidal sinus surgery.

Complications

EARLY
- Bleeding.

INTERMEDIATE AND LATE
- Wound infection.
- Further recurrence of pilonidal sinus.
- Chronic wound and delayed wound healing.
- Scarring.
- Pain
- Paraesthesia

Postoperative Care

INPATIENT

- Patients are discharged within 24–48 hours, provided they are mobile and able to void and pain is adequately controlled.

OUTPATIENT

- If packed to heal by secondary intention, the patient is seen by the practice nurse for frequent (initially every 48 hours) dressing changes. This involves removing the ribbon gauze and repacking the cavity to allow healing by secondary intention.
- Good hygiene to keep the area clean and dry and free from any loose hairs is essential.

? Surgeon's Favourite Question

What might you expect to find lining a pilonidal sinus or cavity?

Macroscopically: hair follicles, stratified squamous epithelium with slight cornification, chronic granulation tissue, epithelial debris, and young granulation tissue.

Microscopically: lymphocytes, plasma cells, and foreign body giant cells.

27

Incision and Drainage of Perianal Abscess

Alison Bradley

Definition

The surgical washout of a localised collection of pus within the tissues situated around or near the anus.

Indications and Contraindications

INDICATIONS
- Acute perianal abscess.

CONTRAINDICATIONS
- Spontaneously ruptured perianal abscess.

Anatomy

GROSS ANATOMY
- The anal canal is extraperitoneal and measures 2–4 cm.
- The anal canal is embryologically part hindgut and part proctoderm. The dentate line divides the anal canal based on this:
  - The proximal two-thirds of the anal canal lie above the dentate line. This section is hindgut in origin and is lined with columnar mucosa.
  - The distal third lies below the dentate line. This section is proctoderm in origin and is lined with squamous epithelium.

NEUROVASCULATURE
- Above the dentate line:
  - Innervated by the inferior hypogastric plexus.
  - Arterial supply is from the superior rectal artery (a branch of the IMA) and the middle rectal artery (a branch of the internal iliac artery).
  - Venous drainage is via the internal haemorrhoidal plexus to the superior rectal vein.

- Below the dentate line:
  - Innervated by the inferior rectal nerve, a branch of the pudendal nerve from the sacral plexus.
  - Arterial supply is via the inferior rectal arteries from the pudendal artery.
  - Venous drainage is via the external haemorrhoidal plexus to the inferior and middle rectal veins.

PATHOLOGY
- Anorectal abscesses arise from infection of the anal inter-sphincteric glands.
- Anorectal abscesses are classified according to their anatomical location:
  - Perianal—around the anal orifice (60%).
  - Ischiorectal—in the ischiorectal fossa, a space between the anal canal and the levator ani muscles (30%).
  - Submucosal—deep to the anal canal mucosa (5%).
  - Pelvirectal—between the levator ani and the pelvic peritoneum (5%).

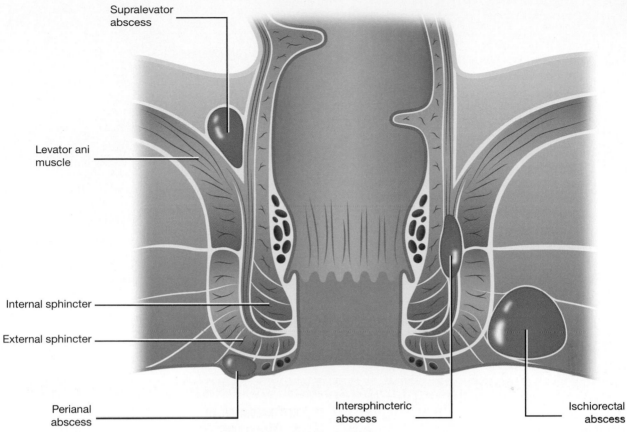

Supralevator abscess

Levator ani muscle

Internal sphincter

External sphincter

Perianal abscess

Intersphincteric abscess

Ischiorectal abscess

Perianal abscess locations.

123 STEP-BY-STEP OPERATION

Anaesthesia: general.

Position: lateral, prone, or Lloyd-Davies position.

Considerations: If there is suspicion of anal fistula, a rectal examination is performed.

Steps:

1. The abscess is palpated to delineate extension and the area of maximal fluctuance to incise.
2. An incision circumferential to the anus (not radial) is made over the abscess.
3. In large abscess, some skin may need to be de-roofed in order to prevent early closure and reformation of the abscess
4. When the abscess cavity is entered, there should be an expulsion of purulent material.
5. A swab is taken for microbiology.
6. The purulent material is expelled, and the cavity is curetted.
7. A digit is inserted and swept around the cavity to break down loculations.
8. The cavity is thoroughly irrigated with normal saline.
9. The cavity is packed with absorbent ribbon and left to heal by secondary intention.
10. A pressure dressing is applied.

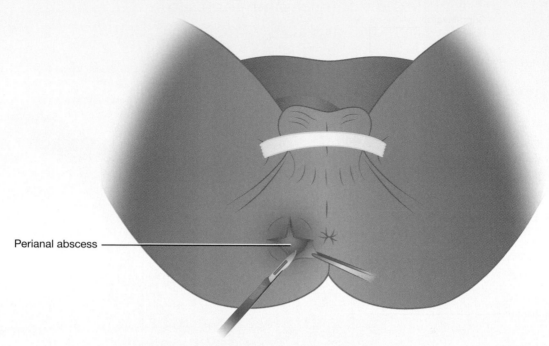

Perianal abscess

Incision of perianal abscess in the Lloyd-Davies position.

 ## Complications

EARLY
- Bleeding.

INTERMEDIATE/LATE
- Wound infection.
- Recurring abscess requiring further surgical management.
- Chronic wound and delayed wound healing.
- Scarring.

Postoperative Care

INPATIENT
- The dressing is removed after 24–48 hours.
- Patients are discharged within 24–48 hours, provided they are mobile and able to void and pain is adequately controlled.
- If there is evidence of surrounding cellulitis, antibiotics are continued for 5 days postoperatively.

OUTPATIENT
- The patient is seen by the practice nurse for frequent (initially every 48 hours) dressing changes. This involves removing the ribbon gauze and repacking the cavity to allow healing by secondary intention.
- Hygiene education—keeping the area clean, and dry.

Surgeon's Favourite Question

What is the difference between healing by primary and secondary intention?

Healing by primary intention occurs when wound edges are re-approximated and healing occurs with minimal tissue loss and scarring. Healing by secondary intention occurs when wound edges are left apart and healing occurs from the bottom of the wound upwards.

Skin-Sparing Mastectomy

28

Katie Nightingale

Definition

- Simple or total mastectomy (SM)—removal of all breast tissue and the nipple.
- Radical mastectomy (RM)—a simple mastectomy + clearance of axillary lymph nodes + removal of pectoral muscles.
- Modified radical mastectomy (MRM)—simple mastectomy + clearance of axillary lymph nodes but sparing of the pectoral muscles.
- Skin-sparing mastectomy (SSM)—removal of breast tissue and the nipple whilst preserving the skin envelope as much as possible. A new technique used for patients having mastectomy and reconstruction allowing for better cosmesis.
- Nipple-sparing mastectomy (NSM)—removal of all the breast tissue and ducts with preservation of the skin around the nipple and areola. Sometimes referred to as total skin-sparing mastectomy.

Indications and Contraindications

INDICATIONS

- Breast cancer unsuitable for breast-conserving therapy (BCT):
  - Local recurrence after previous wide local excision (WLE) and radiotherapy.
  - New primary tumour after previous BCT.
  - Multifocal disease or extensive ductal carcinoma in situ (DCIS).
  - Central tumour that involves the nipple and is not suitable for central WLE.
  - Large tumour relative to breast size.
  - Locally advanced disease with extensive skin changes.
  - Patient preference for mastectomy over BCT.
  - If BCT is inadequate and resection margins remain positive despite reexcision (generally, only one further re-excision is done).
  - Prophylactic bilateral mastectomy for women with a strong family history of breast or ovarian cancer and with high-risk gene mutations (e.g., *BRCA1* or *BRCA2* mutation).

CONTRAINDICATIONS

- Inoperable locally advanced breast cancer.
- Patient choice.

Anatomy

GROSS ANATOMY

- The breast normally extends from the second to the sixth ribs.
- The breast overlies:
  - Pectoralis major.
  - Serratus anterior.
  - External oblique.
  - The upper portion of the rectus abdominis muscle.
- Structurally, the breast parenchyma is made up of glandular tissue, arranged in lobes.
- Interspersed within the parenchyma is the fibrous stroma (Cooper's ligaments), which anchors the glandular lobes and the skin covering the breast to the pectoralis major.
- The fatty stroma makes up the rest of the breast tissue.

NEUROVASCULATURE

- The breast is innervated by the anterior and lateral cutaneous branches of the thoracic intercostal nerves (T4–T6). Sensory fibres provide innervation to the skin; autonomic fibres provide innervation to vessels and the smooth muscles of the nipple and areola.
- Arterial supply to the breast:
  - Internal mammary (thoracic) artery (60%).

- Branches of axillary artery—lateral thoracic and thoraco-acromial arteries.
  - Terminal branches of the intercostal arteries.
- The superficial veins of the breast drain into the internal thoracic vein, while the deep veins drain into the internal thoracic, intercostal, and axillary veins.
- 75% of the lymphatic drainage of the breast is into the axillary lymph nodes, with the rest to the internal mammary lymph nodes. Lymphatic vessels follow the blood supply.

PATHOLOGY
- Carcinoma in situ is a premalignant breast condition and typically found on imaging.
  - DCIS (the most common subtype) is often managed with WLE but if widespread or multifocal, a mastectomy is the treatment of choice.

- Lobular carcinoma in situ carries a higher risk of transforming into an invasive breast malignancy. If an invasive component is identified, and the individual possesses the *BRCA1/2* gene, bilateral prophylactic mastectomy is considered.
- Invasive carcinoma of the breast can be classified into invasive ductal carcinoma (80%), invasive lobular carcinoma (10%), and rarer subtypes such as medullary/colloid carcinoma.
  - Medullary carcinoma presents typically as a well-defined tumour mass often easily mistaken for a fibroadenoma.
  - Colloid carcinoma (also known as gelatinous carcinoma), like tubular carcinomas, are very rare but carry a good prognosis. They are more common in elderly/postmenopausal women.
  - Size, grade, node involvement, and receptor status influence prognosis.

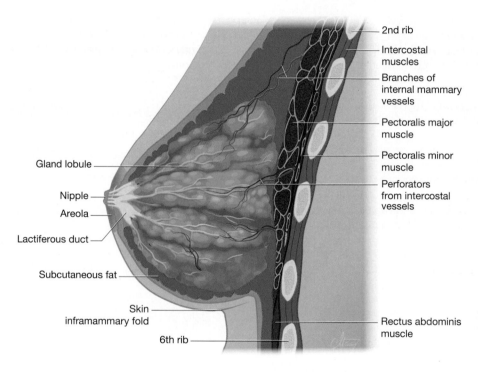

Gross anatomy of the breast.

₁₂₃ STEP-BY-STEP OPERATION

Anaesthesia: general.
Position: supine with the ipsilateral arm abducted ≤90 degrees on padded arm boards away from the breast.
Considerations: Breast reconstruction can be done at the same time as mastectomy or delayed until later. Adjuvant chemo/radiotherapy can only be started once wounds have healed. Adjuvant treatment is most effective when given within 6 weeks postoperatively, and so commonly mastectomy is performed as a first stage procedure with a delayed second stage reconstruction.
Steps:
1. An oblique or transverse elliptical incision is made (the skin ellipse should encompass both the nipple–areola complex and the skin overlying the tumour; it is important to ensure that the wound can close without tension or excess skin).

2. The incision is deepened through the subcutaneous fatty tissue, generating a skin flap 7–8 mm thick.
3. Using a combination of diathermy and blunt dissection, the skin flap is extended medially to the lateral border of the sternum, laterally to the anterior border of the latissimus dorsi muscle, superiorly to the clavicle, and inferiorly to the uppermost part of the rectus sheath.
4. The breast tissue is dissected off the pectoralis major muscle.
5. Once the dissection is complete, the breast is removed with any adherent muscle, working from the superomedial border to the inferolateral border.
6. The breast tissue sample is marked with a stitch in the axillary tail (orientation for the histopathologist).

7. Closed suction drains are inserted to prevent seroma or haematoma formation.
8. With skin-sparing mastectomy, axillary procedures are usually done through a separate counter incision.

9. The skin is closed in two layers—an absorbable dermal layer to bring the wound edges together under minimal tension and a subcuticular suture for the skin.
10. Steri-Strips can be placed over the wound and a compression dressing of gauze and tape is applied.

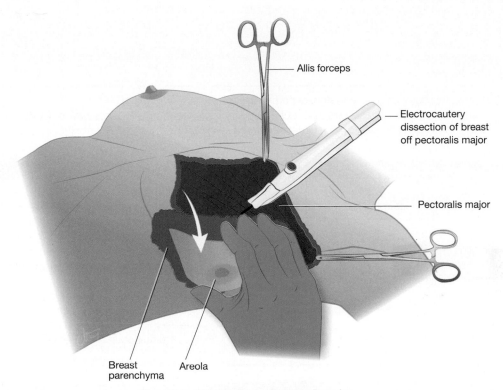

Allis forceps

Electrocautery dissection of breast off pectoralis major

Pectoralis major

Breast parenchyma

Areola

Dissection of breast tissue off pectoralis major.

Complications

EARLY
- Pneumothorax—immediate but rare
- Breast swelling
- Haematoma.
- Nerve injuries causing:
  - Postmastectomy pain syndrome (intercostobrachial nerve).
  - Phantom breast syndrome.

INTERMEDIATE AND LATE
- Infection
- Skin flap necrosis.
- Seroma—typically once drains are removed.

Postoperative Care

INPATIENT
- Patients are typically discharged the next day.

OUTPATIENT
- Breast nurse-led clinic within 1 week for wound check.
- Consultant-led clinic in 2 weeks after multidisciplinary team (MDT) review for results of histopathology and discussion of future treatment or reconstruction.
- Gentle arm and shoulder physiotherapy, starting from 1 day after the surgery, to prevent formation of significant scar tissue/fibrosis. Helps to regain the maximum range of movement and shoulder function possible.

Surgeon's Favourite Question

What is the difference between simple, radical, and modified radical mastectomy?

A radical mastectomy involves removal of the breast, axillary lymph nodes, and pectoralis muscles; modified radical is the same as radical but spares the pectoralis muscles; and simple mastectomy is removal of the breast only.

29 | Wide Local Excision (WLE)

Katie Nightingale

Definition

The removal of a breast tumour with a clear margin of normal tissue.

A margin of 5 mm is accepted in invasive disease, but a margin of at least 10 mm is necessary for DCIS when radiotherapy is not planned. Patients with a margin of <1 mm should be offered re-excision.

Indications and Contraindications

INDICATIONS

- WLE can offer a better cosmetic outcome without the need for mastectomy and reconstruction, but is only suitable in:
  - A single operable breast tumour that is small enough relative to the breast size to remove (e.g. <3 cm AND have no contraindications to further radiotherapy if required).
  - Paget's disease of the nipple (WLE of nipple–areolar complex).
  - Multifocal disease restricted to a single breast quadrant.

CONTRAINDICATIONS

- Mastectomy ± reconstruction is preferred over WLE in the following situations:
  - Multifocal breast cancer with two or more primary tumours in separate breast quadrants.
  - Diffuse malignant calcifications shown on breast mammogram.
  - If radiotherapy after WLE is contraindicated (e.g. in the first two trimesters of pregnancy, or connective tissue disease).
  - Positive resection margins after multiple re-excisions.

Anatomy

GROSS ANATOMY

- The breast normally extends from the second to the sixth ribs.
- The breast overlies:
  - Pectoralis major.
  - Serratus anterior.
  - External oblique.
  - The upper portion of the rectus abdominis muscle.
- Structurally, the breast parenchyma is made up of glandular tissue, arranged in lobes.
- Interspersed within the parenchyma is the fibrous stroma (Cooper's ligaments), which anchors the glandular lobes and the skin covering the breast to the pectoralis major.
- The fatty stroma makes up the rest of the breast tissue.

NEUROVASCULATURE

- The breast is innervated by the anterior and lateral cutaneous branches of the thoracic intercostal nerves (T4–T6). Sensory fibres provide innervation to the skin; autonomic fibres provide innervation to vessels and the smooth muscles of the nipple and areola.
- Arterial supply to the breast:
  - Internal mammary (thoracic) artery (60%).
  - Branches of axillary artery—lateral thoracic and thoraco-acromial arteries.
  - Terminal branches of the intercostal arteries.
- The superficial veins of the breast drain into the internal thoracic vein, while the deep veins drain into the internal thoracic, intercostal, and axillary veins.

- 75% of the lymphatic drainage of the breast is into the axillary lymph nodes, with the rest to the internal mammary lymph nodes. Lymphatic vessels follow the blood supply.

PATHOLOGY

- Carcinoma in situ is a premalignant breast condition and typically found on imaging.
  - Ductal carcinoma in situ (the most common subtype) is often managed with WLE, but if widespread or multifocal, mastectomy is the treatment of choice.
  - Lobular carcinoma in situ carries a higher risk of transforming into an invasive breast malignancy. If an invasive component is identified, and the individual possesses the BRCA1/2 gene, bilateral prophylactic mastectomy is considered.
- Invasive carcinoma of the breast can be classified into invasive ductal carcinoma (80%), invasive lobular carcinoma (10%), and rarer subtypes such as medullary/colloid carcinoma.
  - Medullary carcinoma presents typically as a well-defined tumour mass often easily mistaken for a fibroadenoma.
  - Colloid carcinoma (also known as gelatinous carcinoma), like tubular carcinomas, are very rare but carry a good prognosis. They are more common in elderly/postmenopausal woman.
  - Size, grade, node involvement, and receptor status influence prognosis.

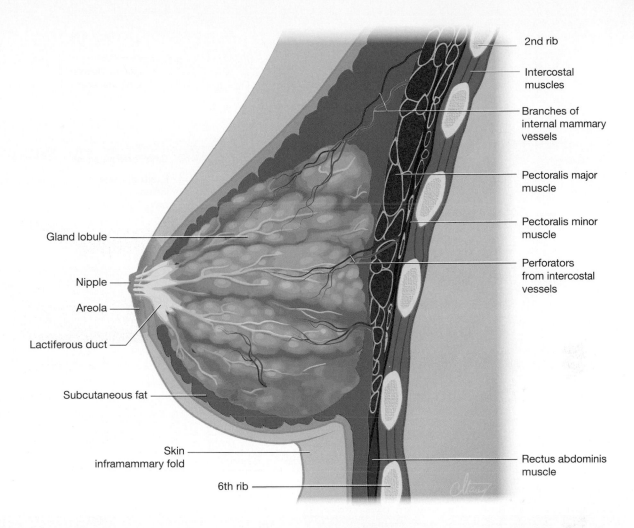

Gross anatomy of the breast.

2nd rib

Intercostal muscles

Branches of internal mammary vessels

Pectoralis major muscle

Pectoralis minor muscle

Perforators from intercostal vessels

Gland lobule

Nipple

Areola

Lactiferous duct

Subcutaneous fat

Skin inframammary fold

6th rib

Rectus abdominis muscle

123 STEP-BY-STEP OPERATION

Anaesthesia: general, but can be performed under local anaesthetic with sedation.

Position: supine with the ipsilateral arm abducted ≤90 degrees on padded arm boards away from the breast.

Considerations: Preoperatively, whilst the patient is awake and upright, the breast lump is palpated and the incision marked with a marker pen. For nonpalpable tumours, a breast radiologist will localise the tumour via guidewire insertion (the tip of the flexible wire is positioned into the centre of the tumour).

Steps:

1. An incision is made using oncoplastic principles (ensuring cancer clearance whilst preserving breast cosmesis), for example, using peri-areolar, inframammary, or round block technique incisions. Incisions should try and include any previous open biopsy site scar.

2. The incision is then deepened into the subcutaneous tissue.

3. The palpable tumour is excised using diathermy scissors or bipolar, with a 1–1.5 cm margin of surrounding macroscopically normal breast tissue (if a re-excision, a margin of similar thickness around the cavity of the previous excision is made).

4. For nonpalpable tumours, the surgeon dissects along the guide wire and resects a 2–3-cm margin around the wire tip.

5. The removed tissue is oriented for the histopathologist with sutures or surgical clips. Usually, a short suture marks the superior border, a long suture marks the lateral border, and the inferior/ductal margins are marked with double knots.

6. Once the specimen is removed, an intraoperative radiograph of the specimen is obtained to assess for adequate margins (calcifications within the specimen indicate the site of malignancy; if calcifications are too close to a margin, further cavity shavings are performed).

7. Haemostasis is achieved using diathermy.

8. Surgical metal clips are left in the site where the lump has been removed (this assists in locating the site on later mammograms for administration of adjuvant radiotherapy and if re-excision of margins are required).

9. The cavity edges are closed with an absorbable suture, then the skin is closed with an absorbable subcuticular suture.

10. Steri-Strips can be applied across the wound edges, followed by a compression dressing with gauze and tape over the wound.

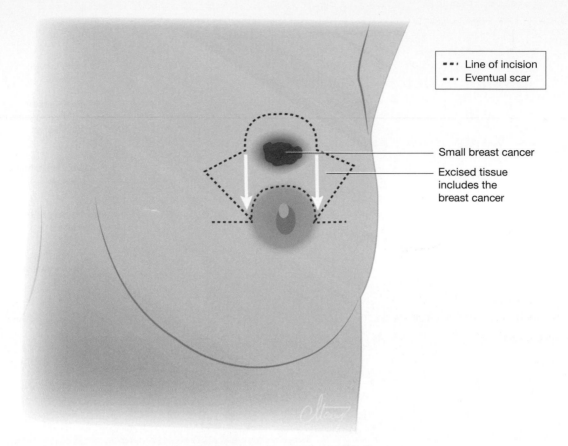

	- - · Line of incision
	- - · Eventual scar

Small breast cancer

Excised tissue includes the breast cancer

Wide local excision lines of incision and closure.

Complications

EARLY
- Haematoma.

INTERMEDIATE AND LATE
- Infection.
- Inadequate surgical margins requiring either further WLE or mastectomy.
- Seroma—typically after drains removed.
- Breast asymmetry and alteration of body image.

Postoperative Care

INPATIENT
- WLE is usually a day case surgery with discharge home the same day.

OUTPATIENT
- Review by the breast clinical nurse specialist (CNS) within a week of discharge to assess wound healing and monitor for seroma formation.
- Consultant-led follow-up clinic in 2 weeks after multidisciplinary team (MDT) review.
- Annual mammography for at least 5 years or until the patient reaches NHS screening age. Frequency of further screening is in line with patient risk category.
- If the patient is known to have a faulty *TP53* gene, they may be offered yearly MRI scans between ages of 20 and 69.

Surgeon's Favourite Question

What are the types of breast cancer, and which is the most common?

Breast cancers can be divided into 'invasive' or 'in situ'. 'In situ' carcinomas are the earliest form of cancer and are completely contained within the duct (DCIS) or lobule (LCIS—lobular carcinoma in situ) and have not invaded into surrounding tissues.

Invasive cancers have several histological subtypes:
- Infiltrating ductal (75%).
- Invasive lobular (8%).
- Ductal/lobular (7%).
- Mucinous, tubular, medullary, papillary (all <2%).

Sentinel Lymph Node Biopsy (SLNB)

30

Katie Nightingale

Definition

Removal of sentinel nodes (first cancer-draining axillary lymph nodes) to identify local lymph node spread of breast cancer in order to stage disease.

Indications and Contraindications

INDICATIONS

- Early invasive breast cancer with no evidence of lymph node involvement on preoperative ultrasound or following a negative ultrasound-guided needle biopsy. Axillary node spread is the most significant prognostic indicator and one of the major determinants of appropriate systemic adjuvant therapy.
- All patients having mastectomy for ductal carcinoma in situ (DCIS).
- Patients having breast conserving surgery for:
  - High-grade DCIS.
  - DCIS + microinvasion seen on core biopsy.
- DCIS + mammography or ultrasound suggesting invasive disease.

CONTRAINDICATIONS
Relative
- Allergy to radio-colloid or blue dye (an alternative is to have single technique—e.g. blue dye or radio isotope only).

Absolute
- Axillary lymph node positive at presentation—confirmed by core biopsy. These patients should have axillary lymph node clearance as first-line, without an SLNB.
- Inflammatory breast cancer.
- Previous axillary surgery or radiotherapy.

Anatomy

GROSS ANATOMY
- The axilla is a quadrangular space with the following boundaries:
  - Superiorly—posterior border of clavicle, outer border of first rib and superior scapular border.
  - Medially—serratus anterior and the chest wall.
  - Laterally—intertubercular sulcus of the humerus.
  - Anteriorly—pectoralis major and minor.
  - Posteriorly—latissimus dorsi, teres major, and subscapularis.
  - Inferiorly—axillary skin.
- The axillary lymph nodes are divided into three surgical levels, corresponding to their anatomical location and path of drainage:
  - Level 1—up to the lateral border of the pectoralis minor.
  - Level 2—up to the medial border of the pectoralis minor.
  - Level 3—extend up to the apex of the axilla.

NEUROVASCULATURE
- The axillary artery arises from the subclavian artery and runs from the lateral border of the first rib to the inferior border of the axilla.
- The axillary vein courses through the axilla and drains the upper limb. Major contributes include the cephalic and basilic veins.
- The brachial plexus forms the nerves of the upper limb.
- The thoracodorsal nerve is approximately 2 cm medial to where the axillary vein crosses the latissimus dorsi and takes an inferior course along with the thoracodorsal vessels.
- The long thoracic nerve follows a similar course, but is more medially positioned, descending inferiorly close to serratus anterior, which it supplies.
- Axillary lymph nodes drain the upper limb and pectoral region. Enlargement is a nonspecific indication of a breast malignancy.

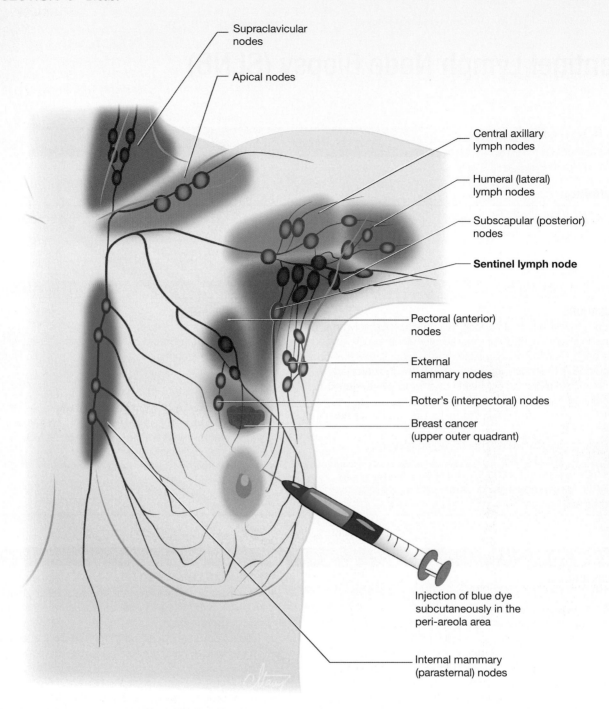

Supraclavicular nodes

Apical nodes

Central axillary lymph nodes

Humeral (lateral) lymph nodes

Subscapular (posterior) nodes

Sentinel lymph node

Pectoral (anterior) nodes

External mammary nodes

Rotter's (interpectoral) nodes

Breast cancer (upper outer quadrant)

Injection of blue dye subcutaneously in the peri-areola area

Internal mammary (parasternal) nodes

Periareolar subcutaneous injection of blue dye into the same quadrant as the breast cancer in order to identify the sentinel lymph node.

1,2,3 STEP-BY-STEP OPERATION

Anaesthesia: general; can also be done under local anaesthetic.

Position: supine with arm abducted 90–110 degrees on an arm board away from the breast.

Considerations: The day prior to, or morning of surgery, a peri-areolar injection of radioactive isotope is given.

Steps:

1. Once the patient is under anaesthesia, a blue dye is injected subcutaneously next to the areola (both the radioactive isotope and blue dye travel through the lymphatic system of the breast and will be taken up by the sentinel node to allow for both visual (blue) and Geiger counter (radioactive) detection of the node, a 'dual technique').

2. A Geiger counter is used to detect the location of the sentinel node in axilla.

3. A small incision, approximately 2–3 cm in length, is made over the location of the sentinel lymph node.

4. Using forceps, scissors, or blunt dissection, the subcutaneous and axillary fat is dissected to visualise the sentinel lymph node.

5. The sentinel node will be identifiable due to the blue colour.

6. Once visualised, the sentinel node is dissected away and removed.
7. The axilla is then explored for further radioactive or blue nodes. If identified, these are removed and sent for analysis. The specific count on the Geiger counter is recorded on the histology form for each node (radioactive nodes are referred to as 'hot' nodes and, if dyed, they are labelled as 'blue'. Nodes can be both, either, or none of these categories).

8. If available, one-step nucleic amplification testing (OSNA) is used to confirm malignancy in approximately 30 minutes. If OSNA shows the node(s) to be positive, then axillary node clearance can be performed whilst the patient is still anaesthetised (and has appropriately consented).
9. The wound is then closed with subcuticular sutures.
10. A simple Steri-Strip dressing is applied to the skin.

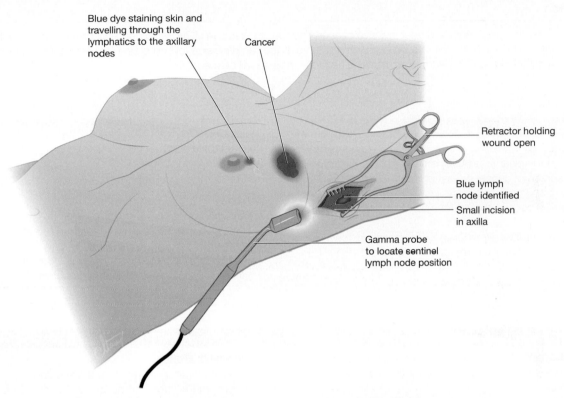

Use of gamma probe to detect a 'hot' sentinel node, which is also blue.

 Complications

EARLY

- Anaphylaxis or allergic reaction to blue dye.
- Blue-green discolouration of urine—resolves after a few days.
- Pain.
- Haematoma.
- Blue discolouration of the skin of the breast, which can last for months to years.

INTERMEDIATE AND LATE

- Infection.
- Seroma.

Postoperative Care

INPATIENT

- SLNB is usually day-case surgery with discharge home the same day.

OUTPATIENT

- Node analysis takes approximately 1 week if OSNA is not available.
- Consultant-led clinic after multidisciplinary team (MDT) review in 4–6 weeks.

? Surgeon's Favourite Question

Briefly outline the lymphatic drainage of the breast.

Seventy-five percent of lymphatic drainage is facilitated by the axillary nodes. The remainder occurs via the internal mammary/thoracic nodes. There are three axillary lymph node 'levels': 1, 2, and 3.

31

Axillary Node Clearance (ANC)

Katie Nightingale

Definition

Removal of axillary lymph nodes to treat invasive cancer. The aim is to remove all gross evidence of disease and should in general contain at least 10 nodes. It can be performed through the same incision following simple mastectomy, but when skin-sparing mastectomy (SSM) is performed, usually a separate incision will be made.

Indications and Contraindications

INDICATIONS

- Axillary node clearance (ANC) is used to treat local lymph node spread of cancer (breast or malignant melanoma) as proven by:
  - Sentinel node(s) positive for macro- or micro-metastases OR
  - A preoperative ultrasound-guided needle biopsy with histologically proven metastatic cancer.

CONTRAINDICATIONS

Relative
- Pre-existing arm lymphoedema.

Absolute
- Known distant metastasis.
- Unknown lymph node status—should be offered sentinel lymph node biopsy (SLNB) first.
- Only isolated tumour cells in sentinel node biopsy samples (these patients are regarded as lymph node-negative).

Anatomy

GROSS ANATOMY

- The axilla is a quadrangular space with the following boundaries:
  - Superiorly—posterior border of clavicle, lateral border of first rib and superior scapular border.
  - Medially—serratus anterior and the thoracic wall
  - Laterally—intertubercular sulcus of the humerus
  - Anteriorly—pectoralis major and minor
  - Posteriorly—latissimus dorsi, teres major, and subscapularis
  - Inferiorly—axillary skin.
- The axillary lymph nodes are divided into three surgical levels, corresponding to their anatomical location and path of drainage:
  - Level 1—up to the lateral border of the pectoralis minor.
  - Level 2—up to the medial border of the pectoralis minor.
  - Level 3—extend up to the apex of the axilla.

NEUROVASCULATURE

- The axillary artery arises from the subclavian artery and runs from the lateral border of the first rib to the inferior border of the axilla.
- The axillary vein courses through the axilla and drains the upper limb. Major contributes include the cephalic and basilic veins.
- The brachial plexus forms the nerves of the upper limb.
  - The thoracodorsal nerve is approximately 2 cm medial to where the axillary vein crosses the latissimus dorsi and takes an inferior course along with the thoracodorsal vessels.
  - The long thoracic nerve follows a similar course but is more medially positioned, descending inferiorly close to serratus anterior, which it supplies.
- Axillary lymph nodes drain the upper limb and pectoral region. Enlargement is a nonspecific indication of a breast malignancy.

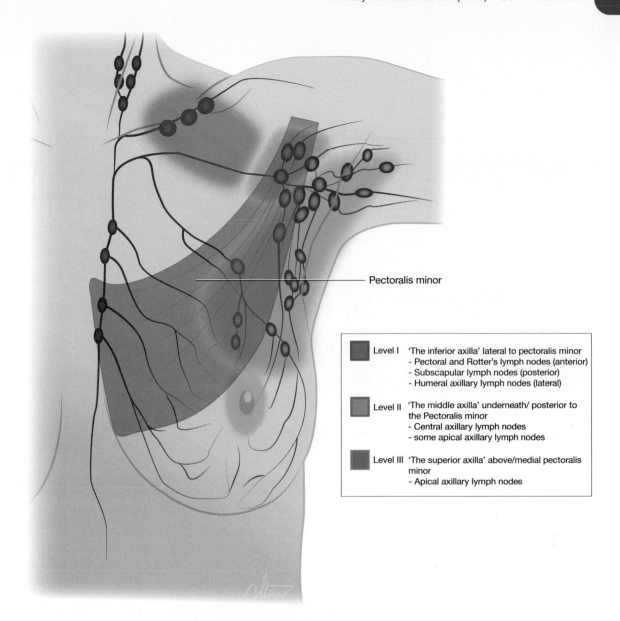

Level I   'The inferior axilla' lateral to pectoralis minor
- Pectoral and Rotter's lymph nodes (anterior)
- Subscapular lymph nodes (posterior)
- Humeral axillary lymph nodes (lateral)

Level II   'The middle axilla' underneath/ posterior to the Pectoralis minor
- Central axillary lymph nodes
- some apical axillary lymph nodes

Level III   'The superior axilla' above/medial pectoralis minor
- Apical axillary lymph nodes

Pectoralis minor

Breast and axillary lymph nodes.

STEP-BY-STEP OPERATION

Anaesthesia: general.

Position: supine with arm abducted 90–110 degrees on an arm board away from the breast

Considerations: To facilitate nerve dissection, paralytic agents are often avoided so that nerve function can be tested.

Steps:

1. A 4–5-cm incision is made along the skin crease of the axilla between the borders of pectoralis major and latissimus dorsi.

2. Dissection is made into the axilla using a combination of diathermy, scissors, and blunt dissection (e.g. 'peanut' swabs held in forceps).

3. The contents of the axilla are visualised through the retraction of the pectoralis major and minor anteriorly and the latissimus dorsi posteriorly (as the axilla is deep and dark, a head-light and retractors with lights attached are often required).

4. This axillary vein is dissected out and acts as the superior border of the axillary lymph node dissection (ALND).

5. Inferior branches of the axillary vein are either clipped or ligated and then cut.

6. The thoracodorsal pedicles are then identified and preserved via dissection inferior to the axillary vein following the posterior wall of the axilla.

7. The long thoracic nerve is dissected free from the contents of the axilla and preserved.

8. The axillary fat pad (containing level 1 lymph nodes) is retracted and removed.

9. Level 2 nodes are removed by medial retraction of the pectoralis minor and the removal of fatty nodal tissues. Level 3 nodes are sometimes also removed. These are then sent to the laboratory.

10. A drain is inserted, and closure is performed with interrupted deep dermal sutures followed by a continuous subcuticular stitch.

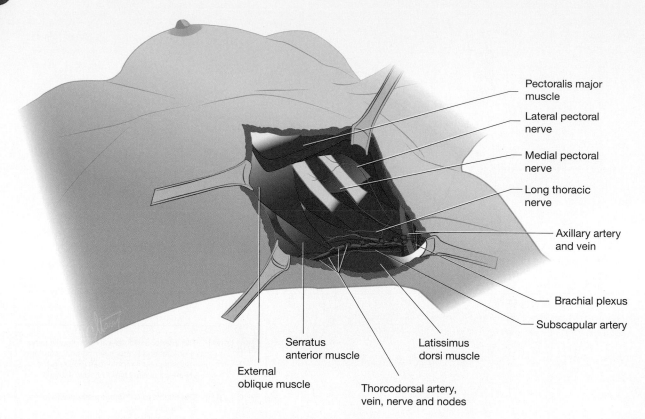

Pectoralis major
muscle

Lateral pectoral
nerve

Medial pectoral
nerve

Long thoracic
nerve

Axillary artery
and vein

Brachial plexus

Subscapular artery

Serratus
anterior muscle

Latissimus
dorsi muscle

External
oblique muscle

Thorcodorsal artery,
vein, nerve and nodes

Visualisation of lymph nodes within the axilla.

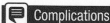

Complications

EARLY
- Bleeding/haematoma.
- Nerve injuries causing:
  - Numbness or paraesthesia of upper arm (medial cutaneous nerve and intercostobrachial nerve).
  - Postmastectomy pain syndrome (intercostobrachial nerve).
- Winged scapula (long thoracic nerve injury affecting serratus anterior)
- Immobility and loss of stabilisation of the shoulder (thoracodorsal and medial pectoral nerve).

INTERMEDIATE AND LATE
- Infection.
- Seroma.
- Temporary shoulder stiffness.
- Lymphoedema of the arm, likelihood increased if level 3 nodes cleared.

Postoperative Care

INPATIENT
- Drains removed at surgeon's discretion, usually when output <30 mL/24 hours after mobilisation.
- Physiotherapy to reduce risk of lymphoedema and shoulder stiffness.

OUTPATIENT
- Review by the breast clinical nurse specialist (CNS) within a week of discharge to assess wound healing and monitor for seroma formation.
- Consultant-led follow-up clinic in 4–6 weeks after multidisciplinary team (MDT) review.

Surgeon's Favourite Question

What complication is likely to have happened if a patient is found to have winged scapula after a mastectomy?

Injury and damage to the long thoracic nerve, which supplies the serratus anterior.

Latissimus Dorsi Flap Reconstruction of the Breast

32

Katie Nightingale

Definition

Reconstruction of the breast using a pedicled latissimus dorsi (LD) flap.

Indications and Contraindications

INDICATIONS
- Breast cancer reconstruction following mastectomy or wide local excision (with significant defect) can be done in conjunction with implant reconstruction.
- An alternative to other autologous tissue-based reconstruction (e.g. deep inferior epigastric perforator (DIEP) flap) if these donor sites are unsuitable.

CONTRAINDICATIONS
Relative
- Active radiotherapy—should be completed before reconstructive surgery.
- Patient occupation requiring excessive use of the latissimus muscle (e.g. climbers and swimmers).

Absolute
- Previous surgery that has damaged the donor site or compromised its vascular supply.
- Extensive local and metastatic disease.

Anatomy

- The LD is a muscle that originates at the spinous processes of T7–L5, the posterior iliac crest, and the thoracolumbar fascia and inserts on to the humerus at the intertubercular groove.
- It is responsible for extension, adduction, and internal rotation of the shoulder joint and has a synergistic role in lateral flexion and extension of the lumbar spine.
- In LD flap reconstruction, it is essential to preserve the thoracodorsal pedicle, which comprises of the thoracodorsal artery, vein, and nerve.

- The thoracodorsal artery branches from the subscapular artery, which originates at the axillary artery. It travels inferiorly after branching, entering the muscle in the posterior axilla. The vein is closely associated with the artery.
- The thoracodorsal nerve supplies the LD and is a branch of the posterior cord of the brachial plexus, from nerve roots C6–C8. It follows a similar inferior course to the artery.

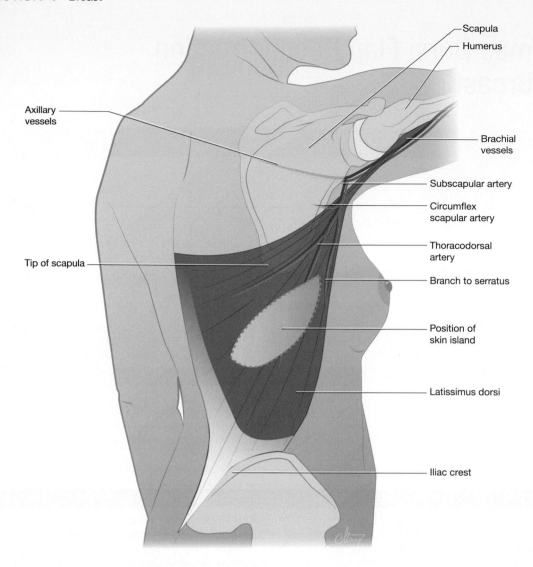

The attachments and neurovasculature of latissimus dorsi.

🔢 STEP-BY-STEP OPERATION

Anaesthesia: general.

Position: lateral decubitus position with the arm abducted; the patient lies on the contralateral side of the LD flap harvest and reconstruction site.

Considerations: LD flap reconstruction can be either immediate, at the same time as the mastectomy, or delayed once adjuvant therapy has been completed. An LD flap is usually pedicled but can be a 'free flap' (lifted from the donor site and moved to a different anatomical location). When pedicled, the donor site is always ipsilateral to the recipient site.

Steps:

1. The LD flap is marked out elliptically to give an 'island' of skin and underlying muscle that is going to be positioned below the bra strap line.
2. The recipient site is then cleared and its incision extended laterally, towards the axilla (if a delayed procedure, the old mastectomy is reopened).
3. The marked donor unit is then incised, and the underlying LD muscle is reflected by separating it from the serratus and the teres major, leaving an exposed thoracodorsal pedicle (nerve, artery, and vein).
4. A 'tunnel' is dissected through the subcutaneous tissues from the pedicle to the chest to allow the flap to be transferred to the anterior chest wall.
5. Minor branches of the thoracodorsal artery are clipped.
6. The thoracodorsal nerve is cut to stop nervous supply to the muscle.
7. The LD flap is then pulled anteriorly via the axillary tunnel to rest over the chest, creating a new breast mound or filling a breast defect (implants can be inserted at this point if it is a combined reconstructive procedure).
8. The LD flap is sutured to the chest wall with absorbable sutures and the skin island closed in two layers (deep and superficial) with buried sutures to distribute tension. The donor site is also closed.
9. Surgical drains are left in situ at both sites—usually two donor site drains and one to two breast drains.
10. Simple dressings are applied to the wound; however, the skin of the LD flap must be accessible and visible for essential 'flap observations' postoperatively.

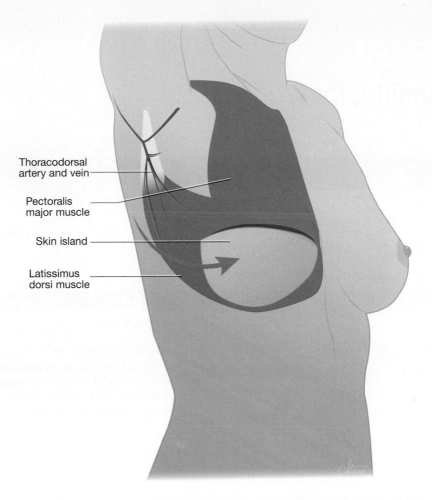

Thoracodorsal
artery and vein

Pectoralis
major muscle

Skin island

Latissimus
dorsi muscle

Relocation of a latissimus dorsi flap through a subcutaneous tunnel onto anterior chest wall.

Complications

EARLY
- Haematoma.
- Flap failure.

INTERMEDIATE AND LATE
- Necrosis of adipose tissue requiring further treatment.
- Seroma (of donor or harvest site).
- Infection.
- Asymmetry and alteration of body image.
- Reduced donor site function, particularly weakness of the LD muscles.

Postoperative Care

INPATIENT
- Hourly 'flap observations' postoperatively, including blood pressure, urine output, and flap checks to assess for warmth, congestion, and turgor, all signs of vascular compromise of the flap. These are less important for pedicled versus 'free' LD flaps but are still common practice.
- Surgical drains removed at the surgeon's discretion, usually when output <30 mL/24 hours after mobilisation.

OUTPATIENT
- Review by the breast clinical nurse specialist (CNS) within a week of discharge to assess wound healing and monitor for seroma formation.
- Consultant-led follow-up clinic in 4–6 weeks.

Surgeon's Favourite Question

What is the difference between a flap and a graft?

A graft has no transferred blood supply and relies on the donor site, whilst a flap has an intact vascular supply.

33 Tonsillectomy

Katrina Mason

Definition

Surgical removal of the palatine tonsils from their fossae in the pharynx.

Indications and Contraindications

INDICATIONS
- Recurrent tonsillitis.
- Scottish Intercollegiate Guidelines Network (SIGN) criteria:
  - Seven episodes in 1 year.
  - Five episodes per year over 2 years.
  - Three episodes per year over 3 years.
- Severely enlarged tonsils causing obstructive sleep apnoea (OSA) or dysphagia.
- Suspected malignancy.
- Peritonsillar abscess (quinsy).

CONTRAINDICATIONS
Relative
- Severe bleeding diathesis.
- Acute tonsillitis—surgery should ideally be delayed.
- Patients at risk of atlanto-axial subluxation (e.g. Down's syndrome, achondroplasia)—often, modified positioning and spine stabilization techniques can be employed.

Anatomy

GROSS ANATOMY
- Tonsils are glands of dense lymphoid tissue on the posterolateral walls of the oropharynx.
- Anatomical boundaries of the tonsils are:
  - Anterior—palatoglossus muscle.
  - Posterior—palatopharyngeus muscle.
  - Deep—superior constrictor muscle.
  - Superior—soft palate.
  - Inferior—lingual tonsil and tongue edge.
- Fibres of the palatopharyngeus and palatoglossus are found in the tonsil bed and attach to the capsule.

NEUROVASCULATURE
- Nerve supply is by the lesser palatine nerve (branch of maxillary division of the trigeminal nerve) and the glossopharyngeal nerve.

- Arterial supply:
  - Superior pole—tonsillar branches of the ascending pharyngeal artery, lesser palatine artery.
  - Inferior pole—branches of facial artery, dorsal lingual artery, and ascending palatine artery.
- Venous drainage is via the peritonsillar plexus, which drains into the lingual and pharyngeal veins, which then drain into the internal jugular vein.
- Lymphatic drainage is to the jugulodigastric nodes and deep cervical lymph nodes.

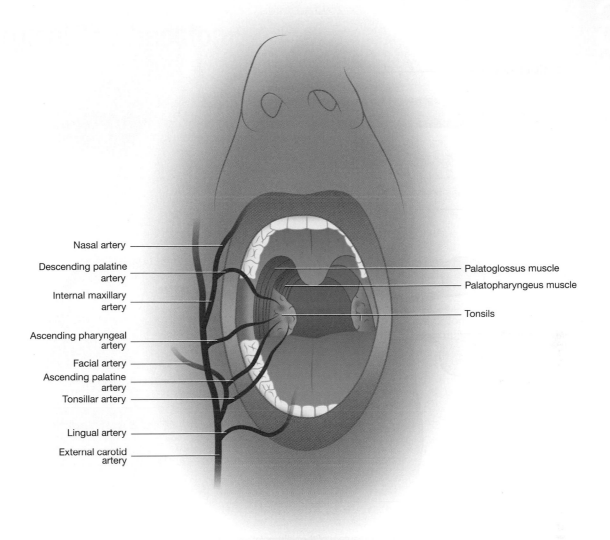

Nasal artery

Descending palatine artery

Internal maxillary artery

Ascending pharyngeal artery

Facial artery

Ascending palatine artery

Tonsillar artery

Lingual artery

External carotid artery

Palatoglossus muscle

Palatopharyngeus muscle

Tonsils

Blood supply to the tonsils.

1 2 3 STEP-BY-STEP OPERATION

Anaesthesia: general; patients are often intubated to secure the 'shared airway'/protect from aspiration of blood. However, a laryngeal mask may be used.

Position: supine with a shoulder roll/sandbag under the shoulder blades to extend the neck and head.

Steps:

1. A Boyle-Davis mouth gag with a mounted mouth guard is used to open the mouth, protect the teeth, and expose the tonsils.

2. Forceps are used to grab hold of the tonsil, and traction is applied medially in order to assist dissection.

3. The following methods may be used to dissect the tonsils:
   a. 'Cold steel' (dissectors and scissors).
   b. Monopolar or bipolar cautery.
   c. Radiofrequency ablation.
   d. Coblation—where radiofrequency energy and saline are combined to create a plasma field at a relatively low temperature (preferred in young children, low weight, and complex comorbidities).

4. The tonsillar capsule is used as a plane of dissection, thereby 'shelling' the tonsil out from its fossa in a cranial-to-caudal direction.

5. Methods used in haemostasis include:
   a. Pressure with gauze (can be soaked with adrenaline).
   b. Silk ties around the bleeding vessel.
   c. Bipolar diathermy cautery.

6. Once the tonsil has been dissected to the base of the tongue, it is often tied with silk ties and the remaining attachment cut with scissors.

7. The postnasal space is suctioned for clots using a soft suction catheter passed through the nostril until it is seen in the oropharynx.

8. The mouth gag is released, and the endotracheal tube is then held in place by the surgeon in one hand as the gag is removed from the mouth with the other in order to prevent accidental extubation.

9. The lips and teeth are inspected for accidental damage and the temporomandibular joint is checked to ensure it has not been dislocated.

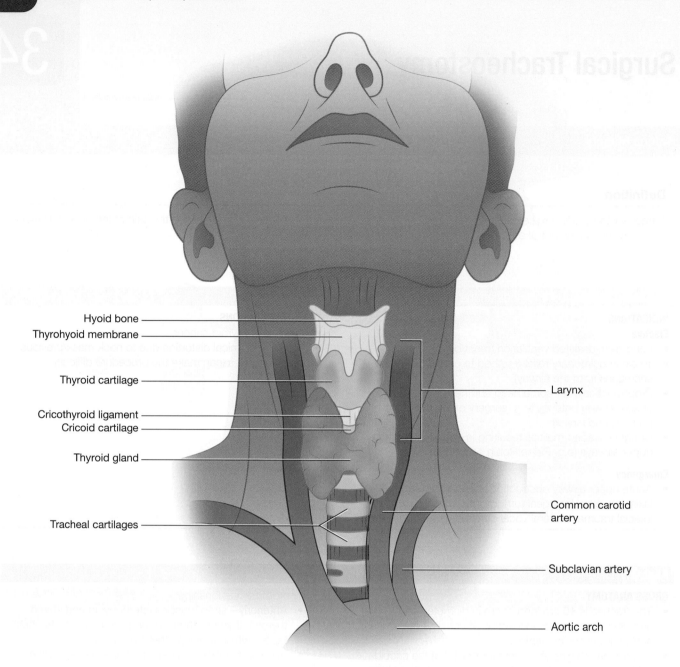

Hyoid bone

Thyrohyoid membrane

Thyroid cartilage

Cricothyroid ligament
Cricoid cartilage

Thyroid gland

Tracheal cartilages

Larynx

Common carotid artery

Subclavian artery

Aortic arch

Anatomical relations of the trachea.

STEP-BY-STEP OPERATION

Anaesthesia: general or local if unable to intubate.

Position: supine with head and neck extended using shoulder roll and head secured with a ring.

Considerations: Tracheostomies can be either percutaneous, using the Seldinger technique with progressive dilatation, or via traditional open surgery. Percutaneous tracheostomies are frequently performed in intensive treatment unit (ITU) by anaesthetists, whereas open techniques are performed by surgeons either as emergencies or electively. The surgical technique is described here.

Steps:

1. A 2–3-cm horizontal incision is made midway between the cricoid and the sternal notch. Vertical incisions can be done in emergencies. The horizontal incision confers superior cosmesis, whereas vertical incisions allow for a more bloodless field.

2. Subcutaneous fat is dissected, and the platysma muscle is divided in the same plane as the incision, revealing the midline raphe.

3. The investing fascia is divided in the midline, allowing the strap muscles to be retracted laterally. The thyroid gland is revealed. Anterior jugular vessels can cross the midline and need to be ligated if encountered.

4. The thyroid gland is retracted superiorly, and the thyroid isthmus is divided in the midline and closed with locking sutures to both stumps to prevent further bleeding. This exposes the trachea situated behind the thyroid gland.

5. Further local anaesthetic can be injected into the tracheal rings and the tracheal lumen itself. Either a vertical incision (always in paediatrics), a window, or a flap can be created through cartilage rings 2–4 (never ring 1).
6. The anaesthetist is always informed prior to cutting into the trachea. They should also retract the endotracheal (ET) tube to prevent bursting the ET balloon. Diathermy is not used in order to decrease the risk of airway fire.
7. After the incision has been performed, the ET tube cuff is deflated and pulled back until the tip can be seen above the tracheostomy opening. 'Stay sutures', nonabsorbable sutures secured to the lateral aspects of the tracheal opening, can be inserted and brought out to be secured with tapes to the neck skin. In an emergency, these can be pulled and the tracheal opening will be brought to the wound surface. In children, the trachea is sutured to the skin with absorbable sutures.
8. The tracheostomy tube is inserted, and the cuff of the tracheostomy tube is inflated. The tube is secured around the neck with collar ties or ribbon gauze.

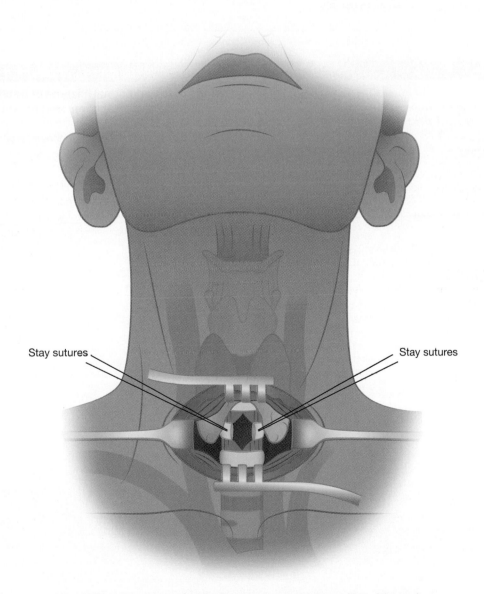

Stay sutures   Stay sutures

Use of 'stay sutures' in surgical tracheostomy to secure the position of the trachea.

Complications

EARLY
- Bleeding.
- Damage to surrounding structures:
  - Oesophagus—can lead to mediastinitis.
  - Recurrent laryngeal nerve paresis or palsy (hoarse/weak voice) or external branch of superior laryngeal nerve paresis or palsy (loss of high pitch) <1%.
  - If recurrent laryngeal nerve injury is bilateral, a permanent tracheostomy will be required due to airway obstruction from closed vocal cords.
  - Pleura-pneumothorax.
- Air embolus.
- Creation of false passage and resultant surgical emphysema.

INTERMEDIATE AND LATE
- Accidental extubation—may result in loss of airway and death.
- Swallowing difficulty.
- Crusting or blockage.
- Local site infection or tracheitis.
- Tracheoesophageal fistula.
- Persistent tracheo-cutaneous fistula after decannulation.
- Tracheal necrosis—may lead to tracheal stenosis.
- Tracheal ulceration.
- Tracheo-innominate artery fistula—can result in massive bleeding.

Postoperative Care

INPATIENT
- Usually first night on ITU/high-dependency unit (HDU), then stepped down to a ward capable of managing tracheostomies.

OUTPATIENT
- Patient education on how to care for their tube and recognise emergency situations (e.g. blockage/displacement).
- The first tube change should be postoperative day 7 on the ward.
- Further tube changes are required every 2–3 months.
- Permanently removing a tracheostomy tube in a patient who can safely ventilate orally/nasally must be done by experienced staff. An occlusive dressing is applied, and the tracheal stoma will close completely by secondary intention.

? Surgeon's Favourite Question

What are the additional hazards of tracheostomy in the paediatric population compared to adults?

Mostly, this is due to the differences in anatomy:
- Trachea is less rigid and therefore difficult to palpate and highly mobile.
- Neck is short, limiting the surgical field.
- Closer proximity to the domes of the pleura extending into the neck, which are vulnerable to injury.
- The innominate vein sits higher in children and is susceptible to injury.

Septoplasty

Katrina Mason

Definition

Surgical straightening of a deviated nasal septum.

Indications and Contraindications

INDICATIONS

- Nasal obstruction due to a deviated nasal septum.
- May be performed as a part of other procedures:
  - A septorhinoplasty procedure.
  - To allow access for functional endoscopic sinus surgery or endoscopic skull base procedures.
  - As part of surgical management of epistaxis.
  - Obtaining septal cartilage for use in an autograft.

CONTRAINDICATIONS

- Extensive autoimmune disease affecting the nasal septum—e.g. granulomatosis with polyangiitis (GPA).

Anatomy

GROSS ANATOMY

- The nasal septum consists of:
  - Anterior part: septal cartilage and maxillary crest.
  - Posterior part: perpendicular plate of the ethmoid, vomer, and palatine bone.
- Deviation of the nasal septum from the midline is common and may be asymptomatic. Localised areas of marked deviation are known as spurs. The septum may even deviate in different directions along its length.

NEUROVASCULATURE

- Innervation:
  - Superiorly: olfactory nerve.
  - Anteriorly: anterior ethmoidal nerve.
  - Posteriorly: medial posterior superior nasal and naso-palatine nerves.
- Arterial supply:
  - Mainly via the sphenopalatine artery (SPA), as per the rest of the nasal cavity. The SPA supplies, in particular, the posterior septum.
- The SPA anastomoses with:
  - Superior labial artery (septal branch).
  - Greater palatine artery (ascending branch).
  - Anterior and posterior ethmoid arteries.
- This anastomosis forms Kiesselbach's plexus, located on the antero-inferior aspect of the cartilaginous septum in an area known as Little's area.
- Venous drainage:
  - The veins accompany the arteries.
  - Veins drain to the pterygoid plexus, facial vein, and ophthalmic veins.
  - Importantly, the veins may carry infection to the cavernous sinus, which can result in a cavernous sinus thrombosis, carrying a 50% mortality.

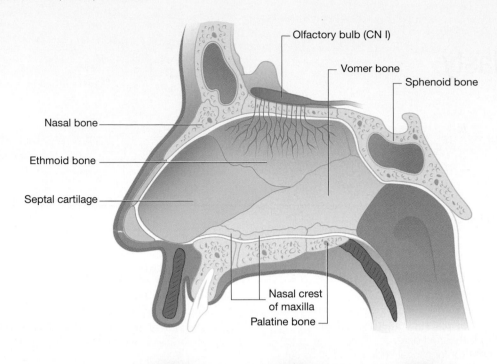

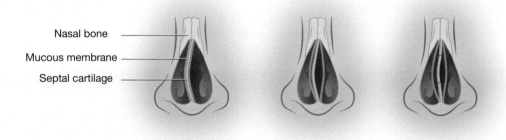

The nasal septum and realignment of septal cartilage.

STEP-BY-STEP OPERATION

Anaesthesia: general; topical Moffet's solution (cocaine, adrenaline, saline, sodium bicarbonate) may be given locally in the nose preoperatively to vaso-constrict and anaesthetise the nose. Variations of this topical solution can be used depending on surgeon preference.

Position: supine with the head secured with a head ring.

Steps:

1. Nasal specula (Killian's or Cottle's) are used to inspect the nasal cavity. Both sides of the septum are infil-trated with lidocaine and adrenaline or saline.
2. The mucoperichondrium is incised down to cartilage with a vertical incision at the anterior septal edge. Inci-sion can be placed on left or right depending on the direction and nature of deformity.
3. A Freer's elevator is inserted into the subperichondrial plane and used to raise a subperichondrial flap, with care being taken not to tear the flap.
4. A contralateral flap may need to be elevated using the technique described earlier in severe deviations. The cartilaginous septum can be dislocated off the bony vomer/perpendicular plate of the ethmoid.

5. The areas of cartilaginous and/or bony septal deviation are resected. Care is taken to avoid twisting of the perpendicular plate of the ethmoid (connects to cribriform plate; fractures may cause cerebrospinal fluid (CSF) leaks). Resected cartilage can then be re-aligned and replaced. Care is also taken not to remove excess cartilage and compromise nasal tip support.
6. Removed septal cartilage can have the deviation corrected through scoring. It can then be replaced, or it can be removed completely.
7. The maxillary crest can be fractured or removed with a gouge to remove any further nasal obstruction.
8. The flaps can be closed with absorbable mattress sutures used to 'quilt' the septum, and the incision with an absorbable suture. This reduces the risk of septal haematoma.
9. Silastic nasal splints may be inserted in both nasal cavities and secured to the septum with an anterior stitch to support the septum and prevent scar tissue forming, or nasal packs may be inserted to prevent flap movement and further reduce haematoma risk.

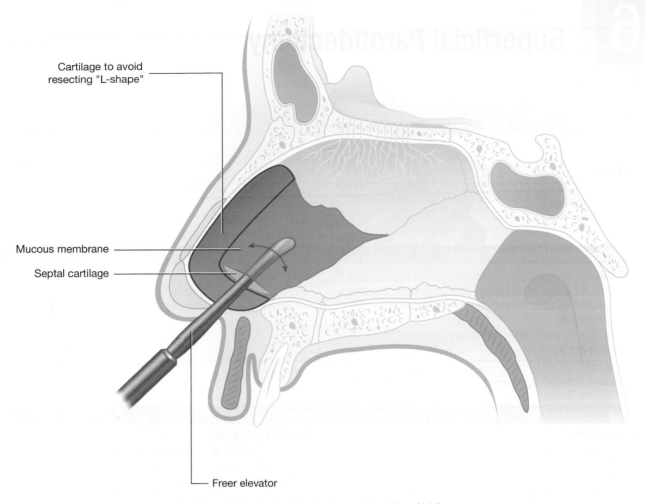

Cartilage to avoid resecting "L-shape"

Mucous membrane

Septal cartilage

Freer elevator

Use of a Freer's elevator to raise a subperichondrial flap.

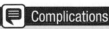

Complications

EARLY
- Bleeding.

INTERMEDIATE AND LATE
- Infection.
- Septal haematoma.
- Septal perforation.
- Cosmetic changes—e.g. collapse of the nasal bridge from reduced septal support ('saddle nose' deformity).
- Failure to resolve symptoms.
- Teeth or upper lip numbness.
- Reduction in sense of smell/anosmia resulting from fracture of the cribriform plate.

Postoperative Care

INPATIENT
- The operation is typically day-case surgery, or patients are discharged after an overnight stay. Nasal packing, if used, can be removed prior to discharge, or dissolvable packing washed out with saline rinses.

OUTPATIENT
- Nasal splints, if used, can be removed after 1 week in the outpatient setting.
- Outpatient review in 6–8 weeks to assess functional outcome.

Surgeon's Favourite Question

Why might patients get a 'saddle nose' deformity after a septoplasty?

A loss of anterior cartilaginous support of the nose can lead to a sagging of the nose, the classical 'saddle nose' deformity. This can be due to either overresection or necrosis of cartilage.

36   Superficial Parotid

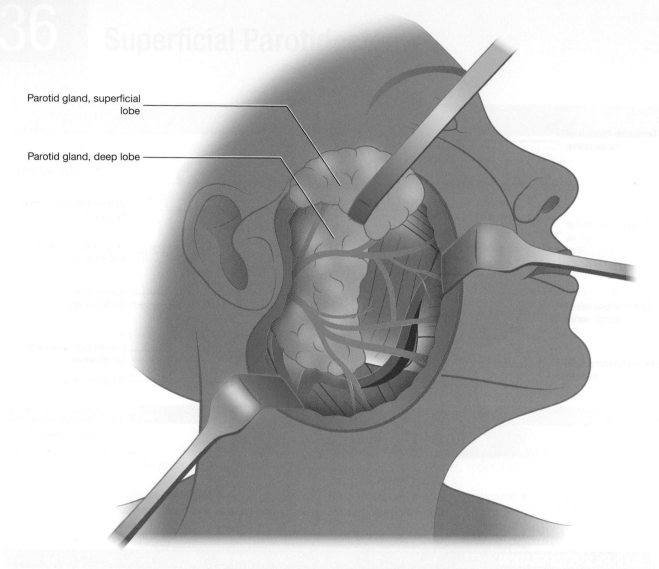

Parotid gland, superficial lobe

Parotid gland, deep lobe

Careful excision of the superficial lobe of the parotid gland.

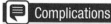 Complications

EARLY
- Bleeding and haematoma formation.
- Facial nerve palsy causing unilateral facial muscle weakness—can be temporary or permanent.
- Loss of sensation of the lower pinna due to greater auricular nerve injury/division—extremely common.

INTERMEDIATE AND LATE
- Infection.
- Facial asymmetry.
- Tumour recurrence.
- Sialocele and salivary fistula.
- Gustatory sweating, also known as Frey's syndrome.

Postoperative Care

INPATIENT
- Drain removed after 24–48 hours or when <30 mL in 24 hours.

OUTPATIENT
- Sutures can be removed at 5–7 days.
- Follow-up appointment to review histology and monitor for side effects. This is within 2 weeks for possible malignant lesions, or 4–6 weeks for benign lesions.

? Surgeon's Favourite Question

In a postparotidectomy follow-up appointment, a patient mentions that he/she sweats on the side of the surgery when he/she eats or even thinks of food. What is this condition called, and why does it occur?

Frey's syndrome—This is due to aberrant reinnervation of the exposed secreto-motor (parasympathetic) nerves to the skin's sweat glands (instead of to the parotid). This can result in 'gustatory sweating', whereby when you eat, the skin overlying the parotid gland sweats. It can be treated with botulinum toxin injection.

Katrina Mason

Definition

FESS encompasses a group of diagnostic and therapeutic operations to improve the function of the para-nasal sinuses and nasal cavity and/or provide access to the skull base, orbit, or brain.

Indications and Contraindications

INDICATIONS

- Chronic rhinosinusitis (CRS) refractory to medical treatment.
- Recurrent acute sinusitis or acute sinusitis with complications (e.g. intracranial collection, orbital abscess).
- Mucoceles.
- Sinonasal tumours (e.g. squamous cell carcinoma, adenocarcinoma, adenoid cystic carcinoma, olfactory neuroblastoma, antrochoanal polyp, inverted papilloma).
- Nasal polyposis—inflammatory, benign.
- Refractory epistaxis—FESS provides access for cautery ± sphenopalatine artery ligation.
- Performed in conjunction with other procedures:
  - Eye: orbital decompression, tear duct surgery (dacryocystorhinostomy).
  - Brain: transsphenoidal pituitary tumour removal, cerebrospinal fluid (CSF) leak repair in anterior skull base defects or fractures.

CONTRAINDICATIONS

- Where an open approach to the nose, skull base, or eye would be more appropriate.

Anatomy

- The nasal vestibule is the most anterior part of the nasal cavity and is lined by stratified squamous epithelium.
- The remainder of the nasal cavity is lined by respiratory epithelium, a ciliated pseudostratified columnar epithelium that warms and moistens the air.
- The upper third of the nasal mucosa is innervated by the olfactory bulb (cranial nerve 1) and is responsible for olfaction.
- Turbinates are bony protrusions from the lateral nasal wall covered by respiratory epithelium.
- There are three turbinates in each nasal cavity:
  - Superior.
  - Middle.
  - Inferior.
- The space below each turbinate is called the meatus and is responsible for draining sinuses and air cells.
  - Superior meatus—drains the posterior ethmoid air cells.
- Middle meatus—drains the maxillary sinus, anterior ethmoid air cells, and the frontal sinus.
- Inferior meatus—drains the nasolacrimal duct.
- The sphenoid sinus drains through an ostium on the posterior wall to the superior turbinate.
- The frontal sinus drains via the frontal recess.
- There are four paired sinuses (air spaces within the skull lined by respiratory epithelium):
  - Maxillary—positioned inferolateral, lies beneath the orbit and above the alveolar process of maxilla.
  - Frontal—positioned superiorly, lies anterior to the frontal lobe and anterior cranial fossa.
  - Ethmoid (anterior and posterior)—sit between the orbits, lying below the cribriform plate and anterior cranial fossa.
  - Sphenoid—the most posteriorly positioned sinus, lies anterior to the hypophyseal fossa (containing the pituitary gland) and the middle cranial fossa. The optic nerve runs within the roof of the sinus.

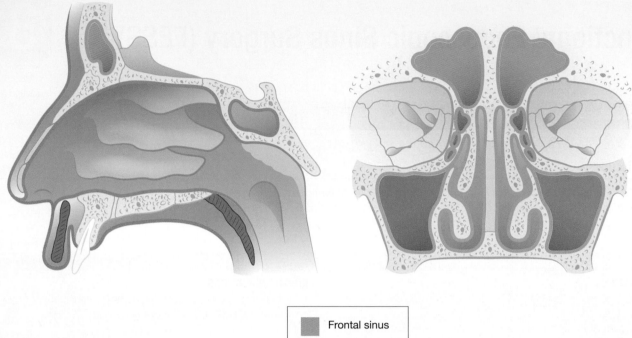

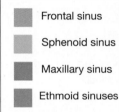

Frontal sinus

Sphenoid sinus

Maxillary sinus

Ethmoid sinuses

Paired sinuses.

1̅2̅3̅ STEP-BY-STEP OPERATION

Anaesthesia: general.

Position: supine, on a head ring; the eyes must not be covered by surgical drapes in order to visualise orbital bleeding, orbital intrusion, or traction on the eye.

Considerations: All patients require a preoperative CT scan of the sinuses for anatomical planning and safety.

Steps:

1. Local anaesthetic and vasoconstrictor are applied to the nasal mucosa (commonly 'Moffett's solution' of sodium bicarbonate, adrenaline, and cocaine) to reduce intraoperative bleeding.

2. A rigid endoscope with a camera attached is passed into the nasal cavity—usually 0 degrees, but 30- or 40-degree scopes can be used to visualise hidden areas. The surgeon watches on a video screen, illuminating the nasal cavity by holding the endoscope in the nondominant hand whilst using a variety of FESS instruments in the dominant hand.

3. Nasal polyps can be removed if present.

4. The uncinate process can be removed to expose the maxillary ostium. The ostium can be enlarged with a microdebrider instrument or curved sucker.

5. Depending on the extent of disease, the anterior ethmoid, posterior ethmoid, sphenoid, and frontal sinuses can be opened to improve sinus drainage. The microdebrider or various FESS instruments can be used.

6. Any mucopus can be suctioned out of the sinus with a curved sucker (and sent for microbiology culture) and saline flushing performed if required.

7. The eyes can also be balloted during the operation whilst observing the lateral nasal wall endoscopically for movement (suggesting lamina papyracea dehiscence).

8. Adrenaline-soaked neuropatties (small squares of dressings on long strings) can be inserted to provide vasoconstriction and to stop bleeding.

9. Absorbable nasal packing can be used to reduce bleeding.

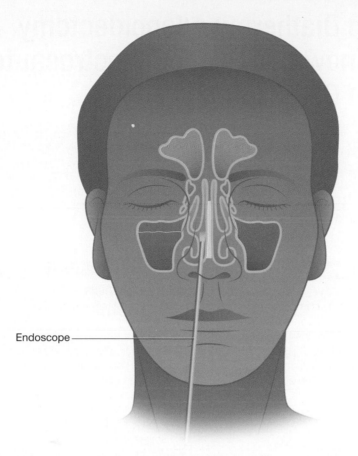

Endoscope

Passage of a rigid endoscope into the nasal cavity to visually assess air sinuses.

Complications

EARLY
- Epistaxis.
- Orbital penetration with ocular complications (e.g. diplopia with damage to the extraocular muscles, orbital haematoma, and, rarely, blindness if the optic nerve is affected).
- Injury to skull base, causing CSF leak.

INTERMEDIATE AND LATE
- Infection within the sinuses or extending to the cranial cavity (e.g. meningitis).
- Synechia or adhesions between mucosal nasal surfaces.
- Epiphora (teary eyes) due to injury to the nasolacrimal duct.
- Failure to improve patient symptoms.

Postoperative Care

INPATIENT
- The patient is discharged from hospital either on the same day or the day after the operation, ensuring no complications such as CSF leak or orbital damage.
- If absorbable nasal packing is used, it will need to be flushed out with saline rinses.

OUTPATIENT
- Upon discharge, the patient usually commences nasal douching (salty water rinses of the nasal cavity) for a few weeks to prevent crusting and adhesions. Steroid nasal drops for CRS can then be recommenced.
- 1–2 weeks off work is recommended. The patient should be advised to avoid excessive activity, blowing their nose, swimming, and contact sports for at least a month.
- Routine outpatient appointment in 4–6 weeks postoperatively.

? Surgeon's Favourite Question

How do you define CRS?

This is a group of disorders characterised by inflammation of the nose and sinuses. It is defined by:
- Two or more of the following four symptoms, of which one must be either obstruction or rhinorrhoea:
  - Nasal obstruction
  - Rhinorrhoea
  - Facial pain/pressure
  - Smell loss/reduction
- And symptoms lasting for more than 12 weeks.
- And objective evidence of inflammation from:
  - CT scan
  - Nasendoscopy.

38

Suction Diathermy Adenoidectomy (Also Known as Suction Electrocautery or Suction Coagulation)

Katrina Mason

Definition

Surgical removal of the adenoids using suction and diathermy under direct vision.

 ## Indications and Contraindications

INDICATIONS

- Nasal obstruction due to adenoidal hypertrophy causing obstructive sleep apnoea (OSA), often performed in conjunction with tonsillectomy ('adenotonsillectomy').
- Chronic otitis media with effusion (OME), 'glue ear'.
- Recurrent acute otitis media (the adenoids may harbour chronic infection or physically obstruct the eustachian tube from draining the middle ear cavity).
- Recurrent or chronic adenitis and/or rhinosinusitis refractory to medical treatment.

CONTRAINDICATIONS

- Children at increased risk of velopharyngeal insufficiency (VPI)—improper closing of the soft palate against the posterior pharyngeal wall during speech and swallowing, leading to regurgitation of food/air and hypo-nasal speech. At-risk groups include those with:
  - Cleft palate.
  - Muscle weakness or neurological disorders with hypotonic conditions.
  - Short palate.
- Severe uncorrected bleeding disorders.
- Patients at risk of atlanto-axial subluxation (e.g. Down's syndrome, achondroplasia)—often, modified positioning and spine stabilisation techniques can be employed.

Anatomy

GROSS ANATOMY

- The adenoids are glands of dense lymphoid tissue. They are large in young children and atrophy by adulthood.
- The adenoids sit on the medioposterior wall of the nasopharynx slightly above the level of the soft palate.
- They form part of Waldeyer's ring of lymphoid tissue in the pharynx.
- Anatomical boundaries of the adenoids are:
  - Anterior—nasal cavity and nasal choanae (the posterior nasal apertures).
  - Posterior—superior pharyngeal constrictor muscle.
  - Lateral—eustachian tube openings.
  - Superior—skull base.
  - Inferior—oropharynx.

NEUROVASCULATURE

- Nerve supply is by the glossopharyngeal nerve (CN IX).
- Arterial supply:
  - Ascending palatine artery, a branch of the facial artery responsible for supplying the soft palate and palatine glands.
  - Ascending pharyngeal, a branch of the maxillary artery that also supplies the pharynx.
  - Tonsillar branch of the facial artery supplying the palatine tonsil.
- Venous drainage is via the pharyngeal and pterygoid plexus, which ultimately drain to the internal jugular vein.
- Lymphatic drainage is to the retropharyngeal and parapharyngeal lymph nodes, which drain to the upper jugular nodes.

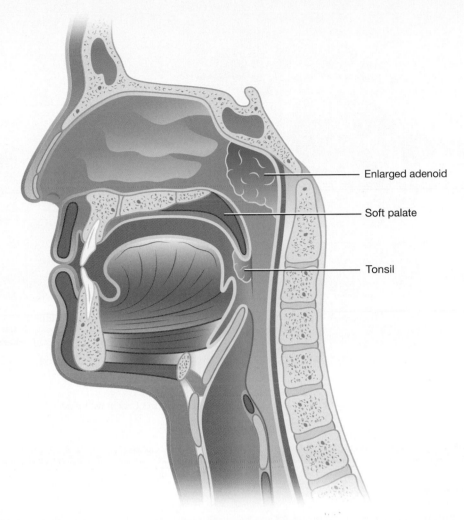

Anatomic relations of the adenoids.

- Enlarged adenoid
- Soft palate
- Tonsil

¹²₃ STEP-BY-STEP OPERATION

Anaesthesia: general; patients are often intubated to secure the 'shared airway'/protect from aspiration of blood.

Position: supine with a shoulder roll/sandbag under the shoulder blades to extend the neck and head.

Considerations: Indirect visualisation using a mirror is the traditional technique, but endoscopic visualisation can be used. If using indirect visualisation, the surgeon wears a head-mounted light.

Steps:

1. A Boyle-Davis mouth gag with a mounted mouth guard is used to open the mouth, protect the teeth, and expose the oropharynx.

2. One or two flexible suction catheters are passed through the nose into the oral cavity and pulled out of the mouth, then secured with a clamp. This 'loop' of catheter pulls the palate and uvula out of the field of vision.

3. A small circular dental mirror is inserted into the mouth and is used to visualise the adenoidal tissue behind the palate throughout the surgery.

4. The suction diathermy probe (a long, thin instrument that combines diathermy and integrated suction) is bent at a slight (20 degrees) angle to allow for the cauterisation of adenoidal tissue in the posterior nasopharynx.

5. Working along the midline, the adenoidal tissue is simultaneously burnt/coagulated with the diathermy and suctioned out into a vacuum system.

6. Gentle, controlled movements are repeated along the length of the adenoids, removing the bulk of the tissue whilst being careful not to cauterise the eustachian tube cushions laterally. Often, a small inferior rim of adenoid tissue is left to prevent VPI.

7. When the choanae are clearly visible and the nasopharynx has a smooth contour, haemostasis is ensured, and the procedure is complete.

8. The mouth gag is released. The endotracheal tube is then held in place by the surgeon in one hand as the gag is removed from the mouth with the other in order to prevent accidental extubation. The teeth and lips are checked for iatrogenic trauma.

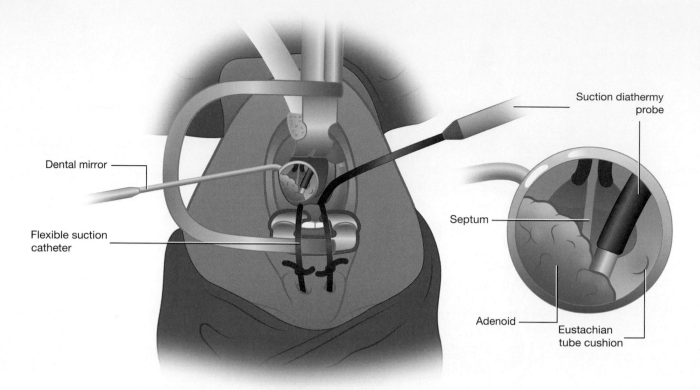

Use of suction diathermy to gently excise adenoid tissue under direct vision with a dental mirror.

Complications

EARLY

- Primary (within 24 hours) or secondary (delayed) haemorrhage.
- Burns to nasopharynx or surrounding structures leading to scarring.
- Temporomandibular joint dislocation.
- Dental injuries (e.g. chipped tooth or loss of tooth—children with loose teeth are at higher risk).
- Velo-palatine insufficiency (VPI).

INTERMEDIATE AND LATE

- Infection.
- Halitosis.
- Neck injury ranging from stiffness to torticollis to, extremely rarely, Grisel's syndrome.
- Adenoid tissue regrowth and recurrence of symptoms.

Postoperative Care

INPATIENT

- Adenoidectomy is usually a day procedure, but patients who have OSA may require overnight stay.
- Postoperative antibiotics and nasal drops may be prescribed.

OUTPATIENT

- One week off school is generally recommended.
- Outpatient follow-up depends upon indication, usually 6 weeks postprocedure.

? Surgeon's Favourite Question

What is Grisel's syndrome?

Subluxation of the atlanto-axial joint not associated with trauma; it may be caused by pathological relaxation of the transverse ligament of the atlanto-axial joint by, for example, pharyngitis, adenotonsillitis, post adenotonsillectomy, or cervical abscess.

Myringotomy and Tympanostomy Tube Grommet Insertion

39

Katrina Mason

Definition

Insertion of a ventilation tube across the tympanic membrane (TM).

Indications and Contraindications

INDICATIONS
- Otitis media with effusion (OME), aka 'glue ear', causing hearing loss that does not resolve over 3 months of observation (can lead to speech and language delay and behaviour problems).
- Atelectatic or retracted TMs, which are at risk of cholesteatoma formation due to chronic negative middle ear pressures (e.g. eustachian tube dysfunction).
- Facilitate use of intratympanic steroids, e.g. for Meniere's disease.
- Acute otitis media (AOM) with complications: sepsis, mastoiditis, meningitis, intracranial abscess, facial nerve palsy.
- Recurrent AOM with middle ear effusion.

CONTRAINDICATIONS
- Suspected intratympanic glomus tumour.

Anatomy

GROSS ANATOMY
- Sections of the ear:
  - External—pinna, external auditory canal.
    - Function—amplifies and transmits sound to middle ear.
  - Middle—ossicles (malleus, incus, stapes).
    - Function: amplifies and transmits sound to inner ear.
  - Inner—semicircular canals, vestibule, cochlea.
    - Function: conducts sound to the brain via conversion of mechanical wave to electrical signals and assists in balance.
- The TM is an oval, transparent membrane separating the middle and external ear and is composed of three layers:
  - Outer epithelial layer (ectoderm)—lined by stratified squamous epithelium continuous with the skin of the ear canal.
  - Middle fibrous layer (mesoderm)—contains outer radiating and inner circular fibres.
  - Inner mucous layer (endoderm)—a single layer of squamous epithelium continuous with the lining of the middle ear cavity.
- The TM is divided into two parts:
  - Pars flaccida—above the malleolar folds.
  - Pars tensa—the rest of the drum.
- The manubrium (handle) of the malleus attaches to the TM, which is held in place by a ring of cartilage (annulus).
- The eustachian tube connects the middle ear to the nasopharynx, allowing for equalisation of atmospheric pressure across the TM.

NEUROVASCULATURE
- The sensory nerve supply to the TM includes:
  - Auriculotemporal nerve (mandibular branch of trigeminal nerve).
  - Auricular branch of vagus nerve (Arnold nerve).
  - Tympanic branch of glossopharyngeal nerve (Jacobson nerve).
- The blood supply is derived from the stylomastoid branch of the posterior auricular, deep auricular, and anterior tympanic branches from the maxillary artery.
- Venous drainage comprises veins on the superficial aspect of the TM draining to the external jugular vein, and veins from the deep surface of the TM draining to the transverse sinus and dural veins.

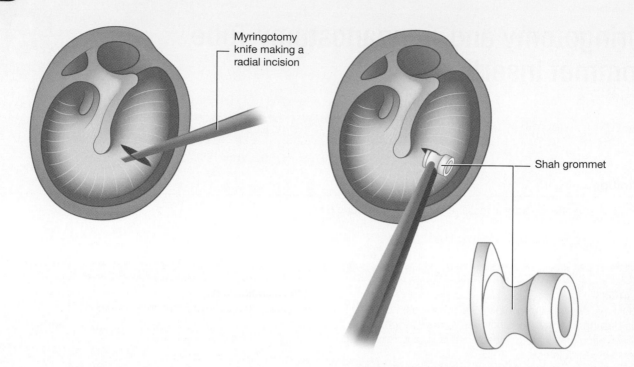

Myringotomy
knife making a
radial incision

Shah grommet

Use of a myringotomy knife to make a small incision in the pars tensa for the insertion of a shah grommet.

1 2 3 STEP-BY-STEP OPERATION

Anaesthesia: general; can be undertaken using local anaesthesia in compliant adults.

Position: supine with a head ring to support the head, and the head tilted slightly away from the surgeon.

Considerations: Prior to surgery, patients should have an up-to-date audiological assessment of hearing—pure tone audiometry and tympanometry.

Steps:

1. Microscope assistance is used to magnify the small operating field. An aural speculum is inserted into the canal and wax removed using suction or fine ear instruments (e.g. a wax hook or crocodile forceps).
2. The entire TM should be visualised for unexpected disease and to identify the location of grommet placement. Most grommets are placed in the antero-inferior portion of the pars tensa but can be placed in any location except the postero-superior quadrant, which overlies the incus and stapes.
3. A myringotome (fine knife) is used to make a small 2-mm incision ('myringotomy') in a radial direction in the TM.
4. Fluid from the middle ear can be suctioned through the incision with a fine suction tip. If infection is present, this can be flushed with saline and suctioned.
5. The grommet is held by the crocodile forceps and placed through the incision under direct vision.
6. Often, a fine needle is needed to push the grommet so that is sits across the TM.
7. Topical antimicrobial eardrops can be dropped into the canal and middle ear through the grommet.

Tympanic Membrane

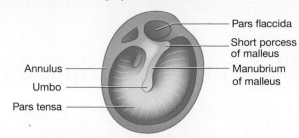

- Pars flaccida
- Short porcess of malleus
- Annulus
- Manubrium of malleus
- Umbo
- Pars tensa

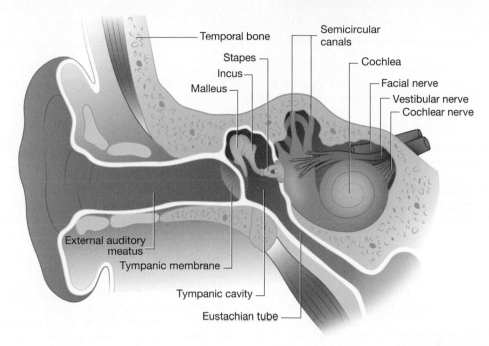

- Temporal bone
- Semicircular canals
- Stapes
- Cochlea
- Incus
- Malleus
- Facial nerve
- Vestibular nerve
- Cochlear nerve
- External auditory meatus
- Tympanic membrane
- Tympanic cavity
- Eustachian tube

Anatomy of the middle and inner ear and components of the tympanic membrane.

 ## Complications

EARLY
- Pain.
- Bleeding.
- Injury to the incudo-stapedial joint (if misplaced in the postero-superior quadrant).
- Grommet accidentally placed within or migrating to the middle ear space.

INTERMEDIATE AND LATE
- Infection.
- Early extrusion or failure to extrude (grommets usually extrude within 6–18 months).
- Persistent TM perforation.
- Tympanosclerosis (scarring of the TM).
- Focal atrophy at the site of insertion—increases risk of retraction pocket and cholesteatoma formation.
- Deterioration in hearing.
- Blocked grommets.

Postoperative Care

INPATIENT
- A day-case surgery.

OUTPATIENT
- Antibiotic ear drops for 3–5 days, water precautions for 2 weeks.
- The first outpatient follow-up is usually 6 weeks after surgery with audiological hearing assessment.
- Regular outpatient review every 6 months with audiological hearing assessment until the grommets have fallen out, the TM has healed, and/or the preoperative condition has resolved.

? Surgeon's Favourite Question

Which groups of children are at increased risk of OME?

Children who are more prone to Eustachian tube dysfunction, such as children with Down's syndrome, and those with craniofacial disorders or cleft palate. Bone-conducting hearing aids are an alternative to surgery for these patients.

40 Bilateral Sagittal Split Osteotomy (BSSO)

Mark Lawrence, Elizabeth Yeung

Definition

Surgical repositioning of mandible to correct congenital and acquired dentofacial deformities. Often combined with a maxillary osteotomy when this becomes a bimaxillary osteotomy ('bimax').

Indications and Contraindications

INDICATIONS

- Correction of mandibular dentofacial deformities:
  - Increased overjet (top teeth too far in front of bottom teeth in occlusion) secondary to mandibular skeletal position.
  - Posttraumatic lateral open bite (from previous mandibular condyle fracture).
- Facial aesthetics.

CONTRAINDICATIONS

Absolute

- Skeletal growth not completed (paediatric patients).
- Patient unwilling to commit to a full course of treatment (average 18–24 months, including preparatory/finishing orthodontics).

Relative

- Peridontal disease.
- Coagulation disorders.
- Previous head and neck radiation.
- Temporomandibular joint (TMJ) dysfunction.
- Mental health conditions.

Anatomy

GROSS ANATOMY

- The mandible consists of a horizontal body (anteriorly) and two vertical rami (posteriorly).
- The mandibular alveolar process contains the mandibular teeth.
- The mandibular body and rami join together on each side at angle of the mandible.
- Anteriorly, the two body regions fuse in the midline at the mandibular symphysis.
- Posteriorly, bilaterally the rami project superiorly to form the condyles. Each condyle articulates with the temporal bone to form the TMJ.

- The mandibular foramen is located on the internal aspect of the ramus and allows the inferior alveolar nerve (IAN) and inferior alveolar artery to pass through the mandible and exit at the mental foramen.
- The muscles of mastication are attached to the mandible—masseter, temporalis, medial, and lateral pterygoid.

NEUROVASCULATURE

- Preoperatively—blood supply to the mandible is primarily via the inferior alveolar artery.
- Postoperatively—blood supply is from a combination of the periosteum and the inferior alveolar artery.

Lateral pterygoid
muscle

Temporalis muscle

Inferior alveolar artery

Inferior alveolar nerve

Lingula

Mandibular foramen

Medial pterygoid
muscle

Lingual nerve

Mylohyoid
muscle

Mentalis
muscle

Masseter muscle

Mental foramen

Buccinator muscle

Mental nerve

Gross anatomy of the mandible.

[123] STEP-BY-STEP OPERATION

Anaesthesia: general anaesthesia with nasal tube.

Position: Supine on head ring/horseshoe. Surgical drapes to allow exposure of the face to allow visual reference to facial midlines during procedure. Throat pack to be placed within the posterior oropharynx so that it doesn't affect the position of the tongue within the oral cavity and thus impact intraoperative occlusion, permissive hypotension, antibiotics, steroids, and tranexamic acid on induction.

Steps:

1. Infiltrate along the external oblique ridge, retromolar trigone, and posterior buccal sulcus bilaterally using local anaesthetic with adrenalin.
2. A full-thickness mucoperiosteal incision is made lateral to the external oblique ridge adjacent the last standing mandibular molar (proximally) to the mandibular second premolar (distally) leaving a cuff of at least 5 mm of unattached mucosa to allow suturing later.
3. The periosteum is reflected to expose the mandible from the mandibular second premolar (distally) to the mandibular ramus (proximally). The inferior fibres of temporalis are stripped from the inferior aspect of the ascending ramus and the dissection continued on the medial aspect of the mandible to identify the lingula and entry point of the associated IAN.
4. A saw is used to perform a stepped osteotomy from just above the level of the lingula (proximally) on the medial surface of the mandible to the inferior border on the buccal surface of the mandible between the first and second molars (distally).
5. Sequential osteotomes and spreaders are used to guide completion of the osteotomy along the underside of the mandible (the 'split').
6. The neurovascular bundle is identified, making sure it is free from the proximal segment and confirming that the two fragments are independent of each other.
7. The mandibular and maxillary teeth are placed into intermaxillary fixation (IMF), using the orthognathic wafer fabricated during surgical planning and secured with elastic chain or wire.
8. Any bony interference between the proximal and distal mandibular fragments is removed with a bur (this may include third molars if present) and the new mandibular position is fixed bilaterally using titanium osteosynthesis plates, ensuring the inferior border of the mandible is aligned.
9. IMF is released checking passive movement of the mandible into the wafer/occlusion.
10. The incisional wounds are closed with resorbable sutures.

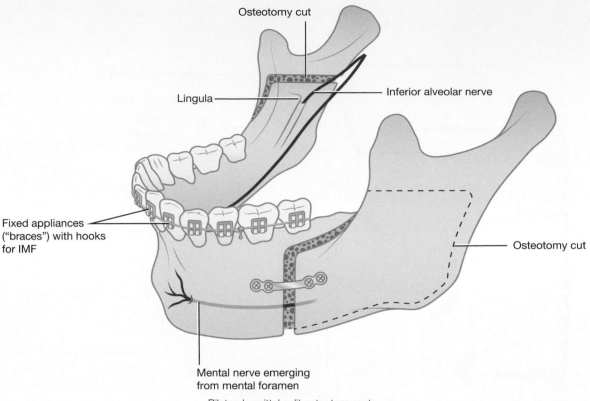

Bilateral sagittal split osteotomy cuts.

 Complications

EARLY
- Unfavourable mandibular splits/fractures (e.g. condyle remains on the dentate fragment).
- Pain/swelling.
- Reduced mouth opening.
- Haemorrhage.
- Numbness of lips.

INTERMEDIATE AND LATE
- Malocclusion.
- Infection.
- Symptomatic metal work necessitating removal.
- Malunion/nonunion.
- Relapse.

Postoperative Care

INPATIENT
- Nurse head up at 45 degrees.
- Encourage use of cooling mask.
- Two postoperative doses of IV antibiotics and dexamethasone.
- Encourage oral intake (fluids/liquid/soft diet) as tolerated.
- Meticulous oral hygiene.
- Aim to discharge patient 24 hours postoperatively.

OUTPATIENT
- Follow up the patient within 2 weeks postoperation to ensure uncomplicated surgical recovery.
- Postoperative review in orthognathic joint clinic for final postsurgical orthodontics.

 Surgeon's Favourite Question

What is the lingula?

A tongue-shaped projection of bone on the medial surface of the mandible that is used as a more visible marker for the entry point of the IAN into the bone.

The Coronal Flap

41

Rebecca Exley, Elizabeth Yeung

Definition

A common trans-midscalp approach to access the cranial vault and upper-midface structures for reconstruction or resection.

Indications and Contraindications

INDICATIONS

Allows access to the following upper and middle facial structures:

- Cranial vault.
- Frontal sinus.
- Nasal dorsum.
- Orbit (medial, lateral, roof).
- Ethmoid.
- Zygoma.
- Infratemporal fossa.
- Temporomandibular joint, condyle and subcondyle.
- Lateral skull base.

CONTRAINDICATIONS

Relative Contraindications

- Male pattern baldness or strong family history (more prominent scarring post procedure)—incision may be placed more posteriorly to accommodate.
- Medically unstable patients (due to length of procedure).
- Uncorrected coagulopathies.
- Previous coronal access or poor quality scalp tissues (poor healing risk).

Anatomy

GROSS ANATOMY

- Coronal suture—between the frontal bone and the parietal bone.
- Sphenofrontal suture—between the frontal bone and sphenoid bone.
- Frontonasal suture—between the frontal bone and nasal bones.
- Frontozygomatic suture—between the frontal bone and zygomatic bone.
- The SCALP consists of Skin, Connective tissue, (galea) Aponeurosis, Loose connective tissue, and Pericranium.

NEUROVASCULATURE

- Temporal branch of the facial nerve (TBFN):
  - The TBFN leaves the parotid gland inferior to the zygomatic arch.
  - The course may be mapped by using a point 0.5 cm below the tragus to a point 1.5 cm above the lateral eyebrow (Pitanguy's line). It crosses the zygomatic arch 0.8–3.5 cm anterior to the external auditory canal.

- Superior to the zygomatic arch, TBFN runs between the temporoparietal fascia and the deep temporal fascia (covering the temporal muscle). As the nerve runs towards the frontalis muscle, it divides into three to four branches. The anterior branches supply the superior portion of the orbicularis oculi muscle and the frontalis muscle.
- Superficial temporal artery (STA):
  - The STA is a terminal division of the external carotid artery and originates in the substance of the parotid gland (posterior to the mandibular condyle).
  - The STA runs a tortuous superior course, crossing over the zygomatic process anterior to the tragus accompanied by the superficial temporal vein and the auriculotemporal nerve.
  - The STA has a frontal (anterior) and a parietal (posterior) branch superficial to the temporal fascia.

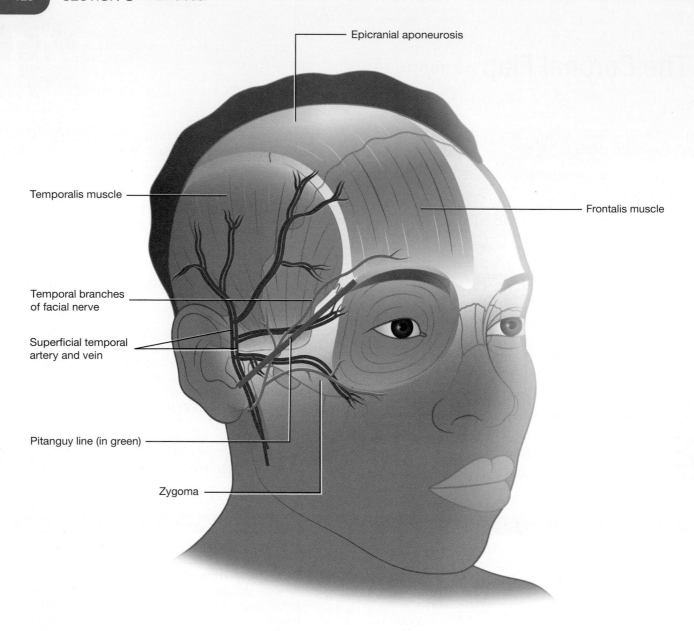

Gross anatomy of the temporal region.

Labels on figure: Epicranial aponeurosis; Temporalis muscle; Frontalis muscle; Temporal branches of facial nerve; Superficial temporal artery and vein; Pitanguy line (in green); Zygoma

⑫₃ STEP-BY-STEP OPERATION

Anaesthesia: general; endotracheal intubation either oral or nasal depending on whether occlusion is required for the reduction of fractures.

Position: Supine and head up.

Considerations: Hair preparation: hair can be parted and a 15–25 mm corridor shaved or the hair completely shaved. Antibiotics at induction.

Steps:

1. The hairline incision is made posterior to the temporal line (preserving the deep branch of the supraorbital nerve avoiding scalp sensory disturbance) to above the root of the helix (this permits access to the upper facial third). Preauricular or postauricular extension is required for access to the middle facial third and or the temporomandibular joint and subcondyle.

2. Compound solution (adrenaline, local anaesthetic, hyalase and steroid in a saline base) may be injected along the planned incision line to provide anaesthesia, control bleeding and provide hydrodissection.

3. The scalp skin incision is made and the dissection begins in the subgaleal plane between the temporal lines. The soft tissue envelope is undermined with curved scissors. Lateral to the temporal line, the temporalis fascia is the inferior limit of the dissection. Preauricular extension continues in this plane.

4. The coronal flap is elevated with sharp and blunt dissection and countertraction. Once sufficiently free, the flap is everted.

5. A pedicled pericranial flap may be required for reconstructive procedures and a rectangular flap of the desired size is created between the temporal lines and elevated from the bone. If no pericranial flap is required

a horizontal incision is made 2–3 cm above the supra-orbital ridges between the temporal lines.

6. An oblique incision from the root of the zygomatic arch to above the frontozygomatic suture is made. Dissection below the superficial layer of temporalis fascia allows for protection of the TBFN during exposure of the zygomatic arch.
7. The supraorbital neurovascular bundle is released to permit access to the orbital roof, medial wall, and nasal bones. Access to the orbital floor is via supplemental transconjunctival or a transcutaneous incision to the lower lid.

EXTENDED ACCESS

8. The infratemporal fossa may be accessed if the temporalis muscle is divided from its bony attachments 1 cm below the superior temporal line. The deep temporal vessels are preserved (the divided temporalis muscle is resuspended later).
9. The temporomandibular joint and subcondylar region may be accessed below the zygomatic arch by stripping the posterior masseter. Alternatively, the zygomatic arch may be segmentally osteotomised, keeping the masseteric attachment undisturbed. The facial nerve trunk remains within the flap.
10. The facial soft tissues must be resuspended and the galea and skin of the scalp definitively closed. Drains may be used to prevent haematoma. A compressive head bandage with padding posterior to the pinna may be applied.

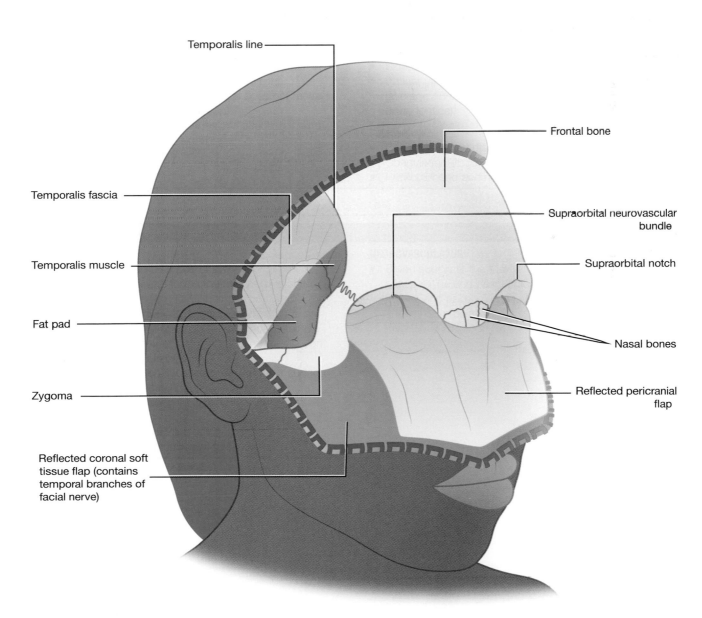

Coronal flap.

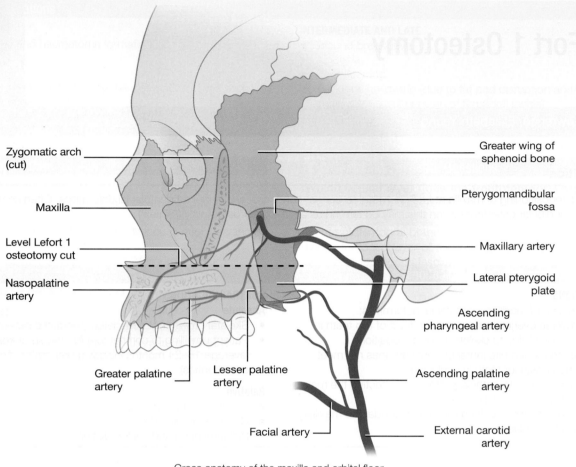

Zygomatic arch (cut)

Maxilla

Level Lefort 1 osteotomy cut

Nasopalatine artery

Greater palatine artery

Lesser palatine artery

Facial artery

Greater wing of sphenoid bone

Pterygomandibular fossa

Maxillary artery

Lateral pterygoid plate

Ascending pharyngeal artery

Ascending palatine artery

External carotid artery

Gross anatomy of the maxilla and orbital floor.

STEP-BY-STEP OPERATION

Anaesthesia: general anaesthesia with nasal tube.

Position: supine.

Considerations: The nasal tube can be sutured to the nose to prevent tube displacement during movement of the maxilla. Throat pack to be placed within the posterior oropharynx so that it does not affect the position of the tongue within the oral cavity and impact the intraoperative occlusion.

Steps:

1. The maxillary buccal sulci are infiltrated bilaterally using local anaesthesia with adrenalin.

2. A full-thickness mucoperiosteal incision is made from upper right first molar to the upper left first molar (leaving at least 5-mm cuff of unattached mucosa for suturing later).

3. The maxillary periosteum is reflected to identify the infraorbital nerves (superiorly), floor, and lateral walls of the bony nasal cavity—pyriform fossae (medially) and zygomatic maxillary buttresses (laterally). The sub-periosteal dissection is extended distally behind the tuberosity, avoiding the buccal fat pads, to access the pterygomaxillary junction. The nasal mucosa is dissected off the lateral nasal walls and nasal floor.

4. A reciprocating saw is used to cut the anterior and lateral walls of the maxilla (avoiding the tooth roots), from the pterygomaxillary junction (laterally) to the lateral walls of the bony nasal cavity (medially). The pterygoid plates are separated from the posterior maxilla (ptery-gomaxillary disjunction) using a curved osteotome. The nasal septum is divided from the maxilla.

5. Using firm digital pressure, the maxilla is down frac-tured so that the tooth-bearing segment is mobile (connected by soft tissue only).

6. The teeth are positioned into the desired relationship (occlusion), guided by the preplanned orthognathic guide (wafer), and secured in position using elastic chain or wires (intermaxillary fixation (IMF)).

7. Any bony interference between the parts of the maxilla is removed with a bur to establish bilateral bony con-tact, and avoiding vascular pedicles posteriorly.

8. The new maxillary position is fixed bilaterally using titanium osteosynthesis plates at the lateral aspects of piriform fossae and the zygomatic maxillary buttresses.

9. IMF is released, ensuring passive movement of the mandible into the wafer/occlusion.

10. Incisional wounds are closed with resorbable sutures.

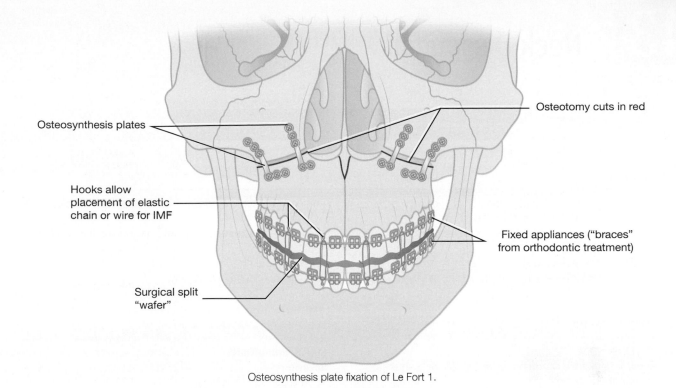

Osteosynthesis plates

Osteotomy cuts in red

Hooks allow placement of elastic chain or wire for IMF

Fixed appliances ("braces" from orthodontic treatment)

Surgical split "wafer"

Osteosynthesis plate fixation of Le Fort 1.

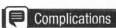 Complications

EARLY
- Pain/swelling.
- Reduced mouth opening.
- Haemorrhage (rare).
- Epistaxis.
- Blocked nose.
- Numbness of lips.

INTERMEDIATE AND LATE
- Infection.
- Symptomatic metal work necessitating removal.
- Malunion/nonunion.
- Deviated nasal septum.
- Unfavourable aesthetic result.

Postoperative Care

INPATIENT
- Nurse head up at 45 degrees.
- Encourage use of cooling mask.
- Two postoperative doses of IV antibiotics and dexamethasone.
- Meticulous oral hygiene with toothbrushing and mouthwash.
- Encourage oral intake (fluids/liquid/soft diet) as tolerated.
- Aim to discharge the patient within 24 hours postoperatively.

OUTPATIENT
- Follow up with the patient within 2 weeks.
- Postoperative review in orthognathic joint clinic for final postsurgical orthodontics.

? Surgeon's Favourite Question

What is the blood supply to the maxilla after surgery?

After orthognathic/Le Fort 1 surgery, blood supply is primarily from the ascending pharyngeal and ascending palatine arteries and the mucosal alveolar anastomotic network.

43 Neck Dissection

Angela Hancock, Elizabeth Yeung

Definition

Surgical excision of the lymph nodes of the neck to eradicate or to prevent metastatic disease in head and neck cancer. Neck dissection can be subdivided into:

- Radical neck dissection—resection of the sternocleidomastoid muscle, accessory nerve and internal jugular vein, and all lymph node levels.
- Modified radical neck dissection—aims to preserve some or all of the above structures.
- Selective neck dissection—lymph nodes and their connective tissue within selected levels only.

Indications and Contraindications

INDICATIONS

- Known metastatic lymph nodes in a previously untreated patient (therapeutic).
- Suspicion of occult metastatic disease (elective).
- Salvage surgery for recurrent disease after failure of radiotherapy, chemotherapy or previous surgery.

CONTRAINDICATIONS

Relative
- Multiple comorbidities.
- Neurocognitive impairment.

Absolute
- Unresectable extensive neck disease on preoperative imaging such as encasement of carotid arteries or deep infiltration into prevertebral space.
- Untreatable primary tumour.
- Distant metastases.

Anatomy

The lymph nodes of the neck are divided into six levels on each side:

- Level Ia—in the submental triangle bounded by the hyoid bone and anterior belly of the digastric muscle bilaterally.
- Level Ib—in the submandibular triangle where the submandibular gland and duct and lingual and hypoglossal nerve are (provides motor innervation to the extrinsic and intrinsic muscles of the tongue).
- Level II—the upper jugular lymph nodes found adjacent to the internal jugular vein which is bounded by the stylohyoid muscle anteriorly and posterior border of the sternocleidomastoid muscle posteriorly, the base of skull superiorly and inferiorly by line drawn from the level of the hyoid bone. Here, the accessory nerve will be encountered (provides motor innervation to the sternocleidomastoid and trapezius muscles).
- Level III and level IV—the mid and lower jugular nodes, respectively, and bordered by the sternohyoid muscle anteriorly and sternocleidomastoid posteriorly. They are divided by a line drawn from the cricoid cartilage.
- Level V—within the triangular space made by the anterior border of the trapezius muscle, posterior border of the sternocleidomastoid, and the clavicle.
- Level VI—lymph nodes lying in the anterior central compartment and is bounded by the hyoid bone and suprasternal notch and carotid sheath.

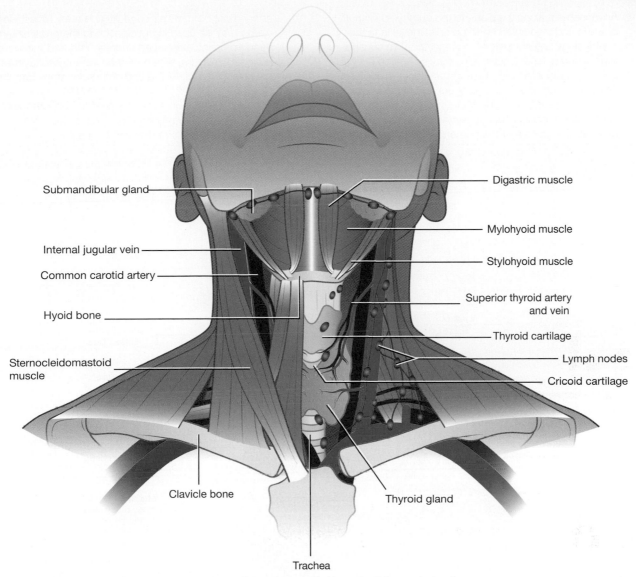

Submandibular gland

Internal jugular vein

Common carotid artery

Hyoid bone

Sternocleidomastoid
muscle

Clavicle bone

Digastric muscle

Mylohyoid muscle

Stylohyoid muscle

Superior thyroid artery
and vein

Thyroid cartilage

Lymph nodes

Cricoid cartilage

Thyroid gland

Trachea

The neurovascular and lymphatic channels of the cervical region.

¹²₃ STEP-BY-STEP OPERATION

Anaesthesia: general.

Position: supine with a head ring ± sand bag at the shoulder, head turned to the contralateral side.

Considerations: Unilateral or bilateral neck dissection depending upon the position of the primary tumour relative to midline and nodal metastases found on staging with CT, MRI, and ultrasound-guided fine needle aspiration cytology. The number of lymph node levels dissected is affected by site of primary tumour and anticipated tumour spread.

Steps:

1. A horizontal neck crease incision is made at least two fingers from the inferior border of the mandible (to avoid the marginal mandibular nerve). This may be extended to allow bilateral neck dissection.

2. A subplatysmal flap is raised superiorly and inferiorly. The great auricular nerve may be seen (it may not be possible to preserve this structure). Care is taken to avoid or to ligate the external jugular vein.

3. The marginal mandibular nerve is identified at the level of the submandibular gland and a fascial flap containing the nerve is raised superiorly.

4. The lower border of the mandible is dissected with control of the facial vessels. A facial lymph node may be found and should be included along with the main specimen.

5. The anterior border of the sternocleidomastoid muscle is found and developed. The accessory nerve is identified (running posterolaterally at level II). The nerve is preserved and the fibrofatty lymph node containing tissue freed and resected.

6. The cervical plexus nerves deep to the sternocleidomastoid muscle are identified to give the plane of dissection for the remaining fibrofatty tissue. Dissection moves anteriorly with care taken to identify and preserve the internal jugular vein and common carotid artery (care should be taken with the branches of the internal jugular vein to avoid tears and haemorrhage). The vagus and phrenic nerves should be seen and the ansa cervicalis may also be identified. The thoracic duct may be visualised on the left side and accessory ducts on the right.

7. Advancement along the plane to the omohyoid inferiorly is made and then anteriorly to complete level Ia to the contralateral anterior belly of the digastric. The superior thyroid and anterior jugular veins may be ligated.

8. Level Ib is resected with the submandibular gland and its duct ligated and cut. The lingual and hypoglossal nerves are preserved. The facial vessels will be re-encountered and ligated. If a microvascular free flap is to be used to reconstruct the primary defect, the facial artery must be handled carefully and a microvascular clamp may be used in anticipation at the proximal end.

9. Vacuum drains are placed and secured and the wound is closed in layers, with one deep interrupted layer at the level of the platysma and sutures or staples to the skin.

10. The neck dissection sample is sent to histopathology in formalin, usually mounted on a card to orientate and indicating the levels of dissection taken.

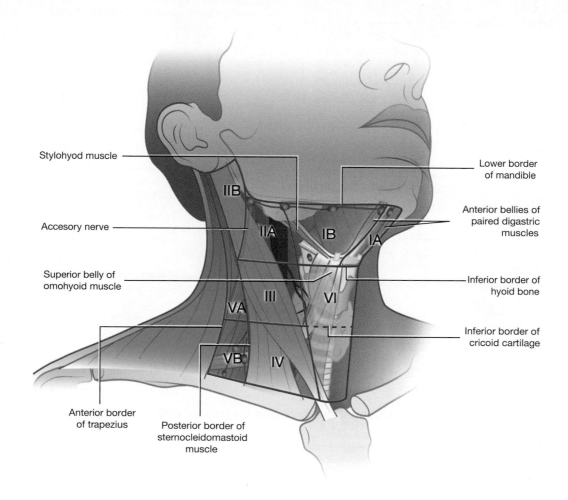

Stylohyod muscle

Accesory nerve

Superior belly of omohyoid muscle

Anterior border of trapezius

Posterior border of sternocleidomastoid muscle

Lower border of mandible

Anterior bellies of paired digastric muscles

Inferior border of hyoid bone

Inferior border of cricoid cartilage

Cervical lymph nodes.

 Complications

EARLY

- Airway compromise—consider use of a temporary tracheostomy in selected cases where significant postoperative swelling may occur, e.g. bilateral neck dissection in previously irradiated patient.
- Bleeding and haematoma—a significant bleed postoperatively may necessitate relook in theatres, washout, and control of the bleeding source.
- Infection.
- Chyle leak—opaque or white exudate in drain bottles may be seen which can be tested for triglycerides.
- Skin flap necrosis—particularly in those with a previously irradiated neck.

INTERMEDIATE AND LATE

- Shoulder weakness, stiffness, and winging of the scapula due to accessory nerve morbidity.
- Scar and paraesthesia to skin of neck.
- Weakness of the lower lip due to damage to the marginal mandibular branch of the facial nerve.
- Morbidity of the tongue due to nerve damage or sacrifice of lingual nerve and hypoglossal nerve affecting speech, mastication, and swallow.
- Ear paraesthesia from greater auricular nerve damage or sacrifice.
- Localised lymphedema of the neck.

Postoperative Care

INPATIENT
- Drains kept in until approximately 20 mL output in 24 hours.
- Speech and language therapy (SALT), dietician review.

OUTPATIENT
- Once pathological TNM staging confirmed, may require radiotherapy or chemotherapy.
- May require ongoing SALT and dietician input if complications relating to hypoglossal or lingual nerve.
- Physiotherapy for accessory nerve morbidity.

 Surgeon's Favourite Question

What are the branches of the internal carotid artery in the neck?

This is a trick question. There are no branches in the neck!

44 Orbital Floor Reconstruction

Rhodri Davies, Elizabeth Yeung

Definition

Open reduction and internal fixation/reconstruction of the floor of the bony orbit (commonly following trauma) using a titanium plate.

Indications and Contraindications

INDICATIONS

- Restricted eye movement or painful entrapment of soft tissue in the fracture.
- Persistent diplopia, after swelling reduction, that impacts the patient's life.
- Macroscopically altered globe position.
- Large defects in which there is an anticipated postinjury increase in orbital volume resulting in enophthalmos or hypoglobus.
- Significant physiological disturbance caused by the oculocardiac reflex (more common in paediatric patients – "trapdoor fracture").

CONTRAINDICATIONS
Absolute

- Asymptomatic patients.
- Small or undisplaced fractures with normal acuity and full range of eye movements.
- Acute binocular diplopia, but with normal acuity and full range of eye movements, should be reassessed once the swelling has reduced.
- Globe rupture (may consider as a delayed procedure when cleared by ophthalmology).

Relative

- Uncontrolled hypertension.
- Anticoagulation.
- Nonseeing eye.

Anatomy

GROSS ANATOMY

- The orbit is created from a coalition of seven bones that come together forming an inverted pyramid with its tip posteriorly (apex) and base anteriorly (orbital rim).
- Extraocular muscles (four recti and two obliques) coordinate the movement of the globe and superior eyelid (levator palpebrae superioris).
- The optic nerve enters the orbit at the apex through the orbital canal (alongside the ophthalmic artery).
- The superior orbital fissure transmits the lacrimal, frontal, trochlear (CN IV), oculomotor (CN III), nasociliary, and abducens (CN VI) nerves alongside the superior ophthalmic vein.
- The inferior orbital fissure transmits the zygomatic branch of the maxillary nerve, the inferior ophthalmic vein, and sympathetic nerves.
- The infraorbital nerve (branch of the maxillary division of the trigeminal nerve—CN V2) travels within the infraorbital canal in the bone of the floor of the orbit and exits onto the anterior surface of the maxilla at the infraorbital foramen. The infraorbital nerve transmits sensory information from the infraorbital and perinasal tissues so injury to the orbital floor results in characteristic paraesthesia of these areas.
- The orbital apparatus are surrounded by fat that cushions and stabilises.

NEUROVASCULATURE

- The orbital contents are supplied by the ophthalmic artery and drained by the superior and inferior ophthalmic veins.
- The optic nerve (CN II) is formed from the convergence of retinal ganglion cell axons and transmits sight information to the primary cortex of the brain.
- Superior rectus, inferior rectus, medial rectus, inferior oblique, and levator palpebrae superioris are innervated by the oculomotor nerve (CN III). A palsy of this nerve results in a characteristic dilated 'down and out' pupil with ptosis of the upper eyelid.
- Superior oblique is innervated by the trochlear nerve (CN IV).
- Lateral rectus is innervated by the abducens nerve (CN VI).
- The corneal blink reflex is controlled by the ophthalmic branch of the trigeminal nerve (CN V1—afferent) and the facial nerve (CN VII—efferent).

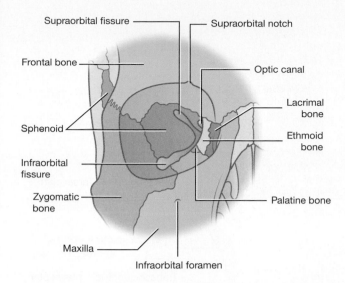

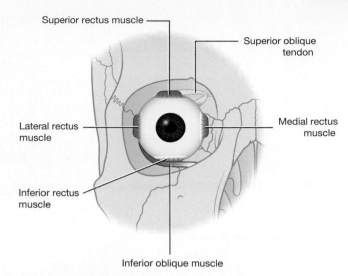

Gross anatomy of the orbit.

¹²₃ STEP-BY-STEP OPERATION

Anaesthesia: General with endotracheal tube or laryngeal mask.

Position: Supine, neck extended, head supported in head ring/horseshoe.

Considerations: Permissive hypotension and tranexamic acid.

Steps:

1. A lateral canthotomy may be performed by making a small incision through skin at the lateral canthus. The subcutaneous tissue is then crushed or cauterised. The tip of the scissors is 'strummed' across the tissue to feel the inferior crus of the canthal tendon. The tendon is then cut (cantholysis) and the lower lid is retracted away from the orbit.

2. The lower lid is everted over a Desmarres retractor, and monopolar diathermy is used to dissect through the conjunctiva and septum just inferior to the tarsal plate and onto the orbicularis oculi muscle. The conjunctiva and septum are pulled up and towards the globe and a predominantly avascular plane becomes apparent. The dissection is continued down until the infraorbital rim is palpable.

3. Traction sutures are placed in the conjunctival/septal flap. These may be used to pull the flap over the globe for protection (alternatively a plastic eye shield may be used).

4. Dissection continues subperiosteally to expose the orbital rim anteriorly, and then posteriorly into the orbit.

The infraorbital canal and inferior orbital fissure are used as landmarks.

5. The intraorbital anatomy (periosteum, fat, muscle, etc.) is gently released from the defect in the floor of the orbit. Traction on the orbital contents may trigger the oculocardiac reflex, inducing bradycardia, so caution and close communication with the anaesthetic team are vital.

6. The deep orbital extent of the defect must be determined by palpating the posterior ledge (the orbital plate of the palatine bone).

7. A preformed titanium plate is trimmed to size and slid under the periosteum to reconstruct the orbital floor.

8. The titanium plate is then secured with one to two screws anteriorly (either inside the orbit or over the rim, to avoid them being palpable).

9. A fixed duction test is performed to ensure there is no entrapment. This is done by grasping the inferior conjunctiva and ensuring smooth unrestricted elevation of the globe.

10. The periosteum or the muscle is tacked together to cover the plate. The conjunctiva may also be closed. The lateral canthus is sutured to the periosteum of the lateral rim of the orbit with a permanent or long-lasting suture and the canthotomy is sutured closed at the grey line (lash root line) with a resorbable suture.

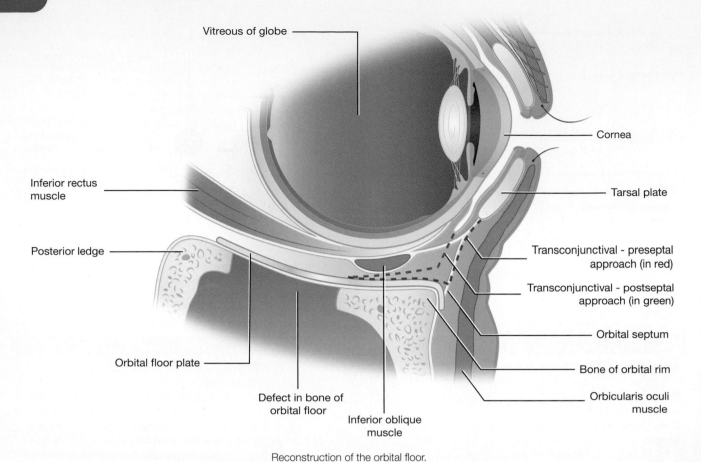

Vitreous of globe

Cornea

Inferior rectus muscle

Tarsal plate

Posterior ledge

Transconjunctival - preseptal approach (in red)

Transconjunctival - postseptal approach (in green)

Orbital septum

Orbital floor plate

Bone of orbital rim

Orbicularis oculi muscle

Defect in bone of orbital floor

Inferior oblique muscle

Reconstruction of the orbital floor.

💬 Complications

EARLY

- Retrobulbar haemorrhage.
- Painful restriction in eye movement/entrapment.
- Reduced acuity or blindness.
- Chemosis/subconjunctival haemorrhage.
- Postoperative mydriasis.

INTERMEDIATE/LATE

- Diplopia.
- Suboptimal eye position.
- Enopthalmos/hypoglobus.
- Ectropion.
- Infraorbital nerve paraesthesia.
- Lateral canthal dystopia.

Postoperative Care

INPATIENT

- Eye observations (usually at increasing intervals from 15 minutes until 6–8 hours postoperatively—includes pain, pupil size and response, acuity, colour vision, and motility).
- Eye drops/ointment—chloramphenicol drops/ointment for 7 days.
- Two postoperative doses of steroids.

OUTPATIENT

- Clinic review within 1–2 weeks postoperatively.
- Postoperative imaging (if not done as inpatient—usually CT).
- Appearance, acuity, and motility assessments.

❓ Surgeon's Favourite Question

What are the bones that make up the orbit?

Maxilla, zygoma, frontal, nasal, lacrimal, ethmoid, palatine, and sphenoid.

Open Reduction and Internal Fixation of Mandibular Fractures (Tooth-Bearing Regions)

Chrysavgi Oikonomou, Elizabeth Yeung

Definition

Operative fixation of mandibular fractures using osteosynthesis plates and/or screws.

Indications and Contraindications

INDICATIONS

- Displaced fracture with abnormal occlusion.
- Unresolving pain from an undisplaced fracture.
- Lateral extracapsular displacement of the mandibular condyle.
- Displacement of the mandibular condyle into the middle cranial fossa.
- Foreign body in the temporomandibular joint (TMJ).
- Unsuccessful reduction with intermaxillary fixation (IMF).
- Undisplaced fracture with poor patient compliance of conservative management (elastic traction),
- Systemic conditions contraindicating IMF (e.g. seizures).

CONTRAINDICATIONS

Relative

- Undisplaced/minimally displaced single fracture without malocclusion.
- Edentulous patient.

Absolute

- Patient not expected to survive other injuries.

Anatomy

GROSS ANATOMY

- Each half of the mandible consists of a horizontal body (anteriorly) and a vertical ramus (posteriorly). The transition region between the body and ramus is called the angle.
- The mandibular alveolar process contains the mandibular teeth.
- Anteriorly, the two body regions fuse in the midline at the mandibular symphysis. Posteriorly, the rami project superiorly to form the condyles on each side. Each condyle articulates with the temporal bone to form the TMJ.
- The mandibular foramen is located on the internal aspect of the ramus and allows the inferior alveolar nerve and inferior alveolar artery to pass through the mandible and exit at the mental foramen. The posterior margin of the mandibular foramen coincides with a tongue-like projection of bone (the lingula) that is used as a key operative landmark for the neurovascular bundle.
- The muscles of mastication are attached to the mandible—masseter, temporalis, medial, and lateral pterygoid.

NEUROVASCULATURE

- Blood supply to the mandible is primarily via the inferior alveolar artery and enters the mandible via the mandibular foramen with the inferior alveolar nerve.
- The muscles of mastication are supplied by the mandibular branch of the trigeminal nerve (CNV3).

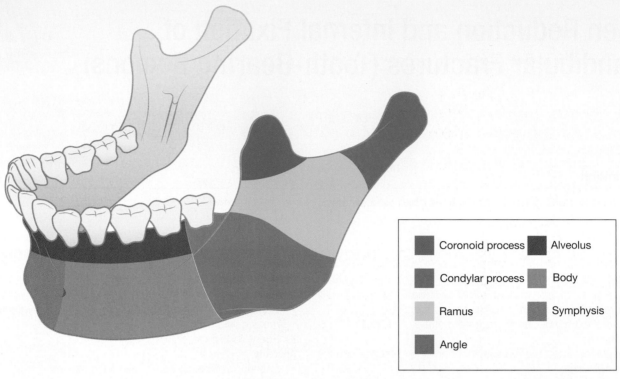

Coronoid process	Alveolus
Condylar process	Body
Ramus	Symphysis
Angle	

Subdivisions of the mandible.

🅱 STEP-BY-STEP OPERATION

Anaesthesia: General with nasopharyngeal intubation (must be able to check occlusion).

Position: Supine on head ring or horseshoe.

Considerations: The transoral approach is most commonly the access for simple fractures of the symphysis, body, and angle regions. Extraoral approach via submandibular and/or submental incisions may be used for complex fractures. Direct access to the fracture site can also be given by existing skin lacerations.

Steps:

1. The incision area is infiltrated with a local anaesthetic with adrenalin.
2. For an intraoral approach, an incision is made through the mucosa 10–15 mm away from the attached gingivae for access of the symphysis and body, and 5 mm for the angle region.
3. The dissection is carried through the underlying muscle and periosteum (protecting the neurovascular structures of the region) until fracture ends are fully exposed.
4. The exposed bone ends are debrided of soft tissue and fracture haematoma.
5. The fracture is anatomically reduced and the patient is placed in occlusion either manually (hand held) or via IMF (can be achieved with IMF screws, IMF plating systems, interdentally wired arch bars, or interdentally wired IMF buttons).
6. In the case of an angle fracture with a third molar in the fracture site, the tooth may be removed (if interfering with reduction). This may take place after step 7 if the tooth is not interfering with reduction (by removing the anterior screws to make space, extracting the tooth and then replacing the screws with the fracture re-reduced).
7. Fixation of the fracture is achieved by placement of long screws across the fracture fragments or osteosynthesis plates and screws.
8. IMF is removed and occlusion is checked. If there is need to reestablish the occlusion or support the occlusion, the IMF may be maintained for 4 to 6 weeks with the use of elastics to allow some function.
9. The wound is thoroughly irrigated.
10. Closure is achieved in layers with resorbable sutures.

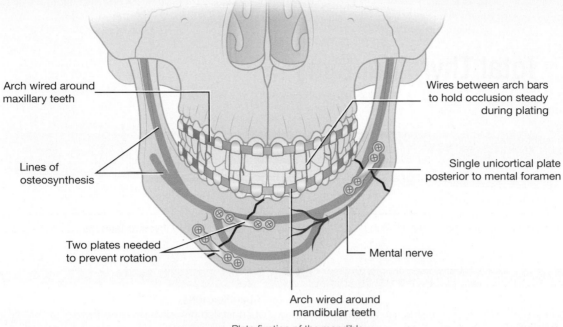

Arch wired around
maxillary teeth

Lines of
osteosynthesis

Two plates needed
to prevent rotation

Arch wired around
mandibular teeth

Wires between arch bars
to hold occlusion steady
during plating

Single unicortical plate
posterior to mental foramen

Mental nerve

Plate fixation of the mandible.

Complications

EARLY
- Inferior alveolar nerve injury resulting in altered sensation/ numb lip and chin.
- Facial nerve injury (most commonly the marginal mandibular branch of the facial nerve).
- Occlusal changes.
- Wound breakdown.

INTERMEDIATE/LATE
- Metal work mobility/fracture.
- Nonunion/malunion.
- Reduced range of mouth opening.
- Periprosthetic fracture (metal work introduces new stress points).

Postoperative Care

INPATIENT
- Soft diet in order to avoid full masticatory force for 4–6 weeks.
- Excellent oral hygiene.
- Postoperative imaging (usually dental panoramic and PA mandible X-rays).

OUTPATIENT
- Follow-up is tailored to the patient. Stability of occlusion or the need for occlusal adjustment postoperatively (change elastic position), range of mandibular movement, and patient's oral hygiene and compliance.
- Mouth-stretching exercises (initially passive, active once bony union).

Surgeon's Favourite Question

What are Champy's lines of osteosynthesis?

They are normal areas of tension and compression that act through the mandibular bone during function. We can exploit these in simple fractures (only) by placing unicortical plates that restore the disrupted tension line and share mechanical force through the bone during healing ('load-sharing').

46 Total Thyroidectomy

Roberta Bullingham

Definition

Complete removal of the entire thyroid gland. Can be performed using open or minimally invasive techniques (video assisted).

Indications and Contraindications

INDICATIONS

- Compressive symptoms—airway obstruction and dysphagia, most commonly from a multinodular goitre.
- Total thyroidectomy for thyroid malignancy is indicated in:
  - Papillary or follicular cancer with a primary tumour >4 cm, extrathyroidal extension, or metastases to lymph nodes or distant sites.
  - Papillary or follicular cancer with a tumour <4 cm with abnormalities in the contralateral lobe or when postoperative radioiodine is indicated.
  - Multifocal papillary microcarcinoma (more than five foci).
  - Medullary carcinoma.
  - Metastasis in the thyroid—usually from renal cell carcinoma or melanoma (very rare).
- Hyperthyroidism refractory to medical therapy, or patients with contraindications to radioiodine treatment, e.g. pregnant women.
- Moderate to severe Graves' ophthalmopathy. Surgery is preferred over radioiodine since radioiodine may exacerbate Graves' ophthalmopathy.
- Cosmetic—where the goitre is very large and unsightly

CONTRAINDICATIONS

- Uncontrolled preoperative hyperthyroidism (risk of 'thyroid storm').
- Locally advanced anaplastic carcinoma.
- Hemithyroidectomy/unilateral lobectomy is preferred in small tumours <4 cm or indeterminate or suspicious nodules.

Anatomy

GROSS ANATOMY

- The thyroid is a butterfly-shaped endocrine gland that sits in the midline of the neck.
- Components of the adult thyroid gland:
  - Central 'isthmus'—overlying the second and third cartilaginous tracheal rings.
  - Two lateral lobes—projecting laterally from the isthmus down to the sixth tracheal ring (the superior and inferior parts of which are called the 'poles').
- A superior pyramidal lobe, an embryological remnant, may also be present.
- The adult thyroid is invested in the pretracheal fascia, blending superiorly with the larynx. The gland therefore moves cranially with tongue protrusion and on swallowing.

NEUROVASCULATURE

- On either side of the thyroid, within the tracheaoesophageal grooves, lies the recurrent laryngeal nerve (RLN). This nerve supplies the intrinsic muscles of the larynx. Deep to the upper pole of the thyroid sits the external branch of the superior laryngeal nerve, which supplies the cricothyroid muscle and contributes to vocal strength and pitch.
- The superior thyroid arteries (a branch of the external carotid artery) supply the superior thyroid poles.
- The inferior thyroid arteries (a branch of the thyrocervical trunk of the subclavian artery) supply the inferior thyroid poles.
- The superior, middle, and inferior thyroid veins drain the thyroid gland.
- The thyroid lymph fluid drains to the lateral deep cervical nodes and pre- and paratracheal lymph nodes.

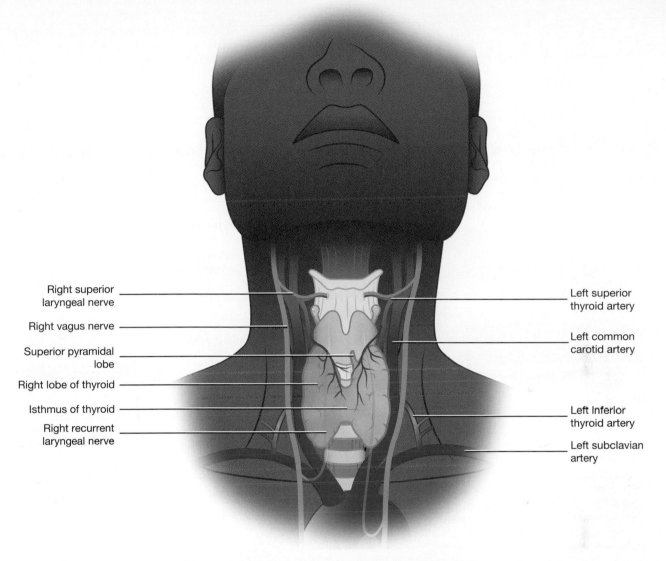

Right superior laryngeal nerve

Right vagus nerve

Superior pyramidal lobe

Right lobe of thyroid

Isthmus of thyroid

Right recurrent laryngeal nerve

Left superior thyroid artery

Left common carotid artery

Left inferior thyroid artery

Left subclavian artery

Neurovasculature innervations and relations of the thyroid gland.

¹²₃ STEP-BY-STEP OPERATION

Anaesthesia: general.

Position: reverse Trendelenburg with a shoulder roll and head ring to extend and expose the neck.

Considerations: A neural integrity monitor electromyogram endotracheal tube is used to detect vocal fold movement from laryngeal nerve stimulation during the procedure.

Steps:

1. A transverse 'collar' incision is made two finger-breadths above the sternal notch and extending to the medial border of the sternocleidomastoid on either side.

2. The skin and platysma are divided. Superior and inferior subplatysmal flaps are raised.

3. The strap muscles are exposed and separated with dissection down through the pale midline raphe onto the thyroid. Lateral substrap dissection is then performed until the common carotid is encountered the lateral extent of dissection.

4. The middle thyroid vein (if present) is ligated and divided. The upper pole is mobilised, and the superior vessels are isolated, ligated, and divided.

5. RLN is located in the tracheoesophageal groove and identified and protected (assisted by neurostimulation to confirm the nerve). The neighbouring inferior thyroid artery is secured and double-ligated.

6. The RLN is then traced cranially and dissected off the thyroid until it enters the larynx posterior to the cricothyroid joint.

7. The parathyroid glands (and their vasculature) are identified and preserved if possible.

8. The same steps of lateral substrap dissection, mobilisation and ligation of superior pole, and dissection and preservation of RLN and parathyroids are repeated on the contralateral lobe. The thyroid gland can then be dissected off the trachea.

9. Haemostasis is checked with head down tilt and a Valsalva manoeuvre. One or two drains are placed.

10. The strap muscles and platysma are closed with absorbable sutures and the skin with nonabsorbable sutures or clips.

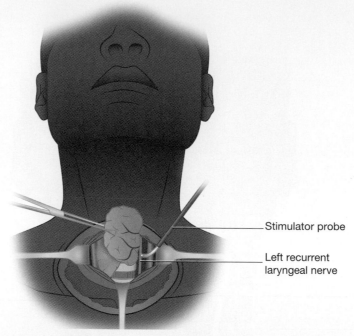

Stimulator probe

Left recurrent
laryngeal nerve

Identification of the left recurrent laryngeal nerve during a total thyroidectomy.

Complications

EARLY

- Haematoma—can cause acute life-threatening airway obstruction from tracheal compression and oedema.
- RLN paresis or palsy (hoarse/weak voice) or external branch of superior laryngeal nerve paresis or palsy (loss of high pitch). If RLN injury is bilateral, a tracheostomy may be required due to airway obstruction from closed vocal cords.
- Thyroid 'storm'—intraoperative hyperpyrexia, sweating, tachycardia, heart failure.
- Pneumothorax.
- Horner's syndrome—miosis, ptosis, anhidrosis, and enophthalmos—due to damage to sympathetic trunk.
- Oesophageal perforation or tracheal injury.
- Hypothyroidism.

INTERMEDIATE AND LATE

- Hypocalcaemia due to hypoparathyroidism caused by inadvertent removal of or damage to the parathyroid glands.
- Seroma.
- Chyle leak due to damage to the thoracic duct.

Postoperative Care

INPATIENT

- Calcium and parathyroid hormone (PTH) levels checked the same day, with calcium and vitamin D replacement as appropriate.
- Patients undergoing surgery for benign disease should be commenced on a weight-appropriate dose of levothyroxine.
- Patients requiring postoperative radioiodine ablation >3 weeks postoperatively are commenced on liothyronine (T3).
- Drains removed when <30 mL in 24 hours.

OUTPATIENT

- Follow-up appointment 4 weeks postoperatively for benign disease or 2 weeks for malignant disease to plan further oncological treatment.
- Levothyroxine dose is titrated to thyroid-stimulating hormone (TSH) level at 6 weeks.

Surgeon's Favourite Question

Describe the embryology of the thyroid gland. Why is it important?

The thyroid bud is a diverticulum (pouch) that projects through the floor of the pharynx. The thyroid tissue descends to its adult locality, leaving the foramen caecum of the tongue and pyramidal lobe of the thyroid in its wake. Thyroid remnants can be found along this tract, such as lingual thyroid, thyroglossal cysts, and ectopic thyroid tissue.

Parathyroidectomy

Roberta Bullingham

Definition

Removal of a single or multiple parathyroid glands. Can be performed using open or minimally invasive techniques (video assisted).

Indications and Contraindications

INDICATIONS

- Symptomatic primary hyperparathyroidism (HPT) or parathyroid crisis caused by a parathyroid adenoma.
- Asymptomatic primary HPT with (a) raised serum calcium levels (variable cut-offs) and (b) objective evidence of end organ damage; reduced glomerular filtration rate or bone density T-score <−2.5.
- Parathyroid cancer.

CONTRAINDICATIONS

Absolute
- Familial hypocalciuric hypercalcaemia: urine calcium <200 mg/day.

Relative
- Known contralateral recurrent laryngeal nerve injury—bilateral recurrent laryngeal nerve palsy results in acute airway obstruction from closed vocal cords and will require a tracheostomy.
- Symptomatic cervical disc spondylopathy.

Anatomy

GROSS ANATOMY

- The parathyroids are very small (5 mm) glands that typically lie in upper and lower pairs. They can vary in number from two to six in total and have a characteristic tan-brown colour.
- The superior parathyroid glands originate from the fourth branchial pouch. They only migrate a short distance, located close to the inferior thyroid artery in the adult, and tend to have a posterior lie.
- The inferior parathyroid glands arise from the third branchial pouch, along with the thymus. Typically, the thymus is said to 'point' to the glands. Whilst the thymus descends into the thorax, the inferior parathyroids lie either (a) underneath the lower pole of the thyroid (90%) or (b) along the tract of the inferior thyroid veins (10%). This can be as far inferior as the anterior mediastinum.
- Parathyroid adenomas can be identified preoperatively using ultrasound scan, 99-c sestamibi scintigraphy, and CT.

NEUROVASCULATURE

- The inferior thyroid artery (from the thyrocervical trunk of the subclavian artery) supplies the superior parathyroid glands. The inferior parathyroids receive their blood supply from either the inferior thyroid artery or the variable thyroid ima artery.
- Small veins from the parathyroid glands drain into neighbouring superior, middle, and inferior thyroid veins.
- Lymph from the parathyroid drains to the lateral deep cervical nodes and paratracheal lymph nodes.

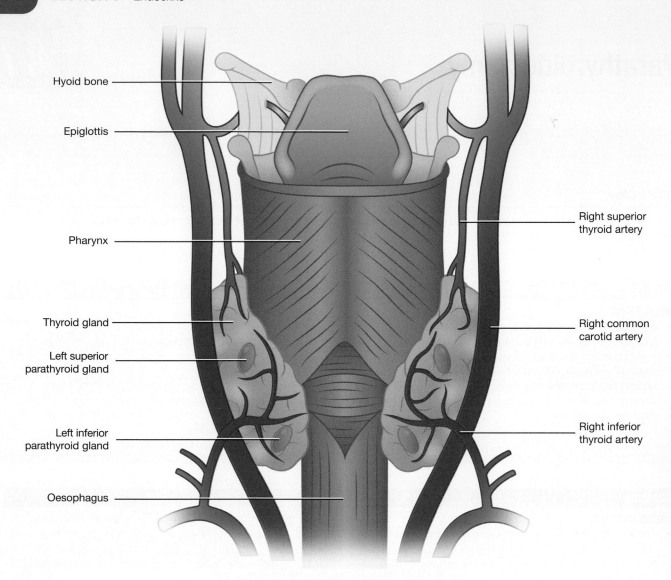

Hyoid bone

Epiglottis

Pharynx

Thyroid gland

Left superior parathyroid gland

Left inferior parathyroid gland

Oesophagus

Right superior thyroid artery

Right common carotid artery

Right inferior thyroid artery

Vasculature and anatomical location of the parathyroid glands.

1 2 3   STEP-BY-STEP OPERATION

Anaesthesia: general; a neural integrity monitor electromyogram endotracheal tube is used to detect vocal fold movement from laryngeal nerve stimulation during the procedure.

Position: reverse Trendelenburg supine with shoulder roll and head ring to extend and expose the neck.

Considerations: An open-neck exploration is the standard approach (described here), but a focused 'minimally invasive' parathyroidectomy may be performed where single gland disease is clearly localised.

Steps:

1. A transverse 'collar' incision is made two finger-breadths above the sternal notch and extending to the medial border of the sternocleidomastoid on either side.
2. The skin and platysma are divided. Superior and inferior subplatysmal flaps are raised.
3. The strap muscles are exposed and separated with dissection down through the pale midline raphe onto the thyroid. Lateral substrap dissection is then performed until the common carotid is encountered.

4. A thyroid lobe is anteromedially displaced to locate the parathyroid gland.
5. The recurrent laryngeal nerve is located in the tracheoesophageal groove and identified and protected. This step is assisted by neurostimulation to confirm the nerve.
6. Once located, single or multiple enlarged glands are removed. If all four are enlarged, at least three are resected, typically leaving half a gland in situ.
7. Intraoperative frozen sections or rapid parathyroid hormone (PTH) assays (intraoperative PTH reduction of >50% from baseline) may be utilised to confirm correct identification of an adenoma.
8. Haemostasis is achieved meticulously, using diathermy cautiously around the recurrent laryngeal nerve. A drain can be placed.
9. The strap muscles and platysma are closed with absorbable sutures and skin with nonabsorbable sutures or clips.

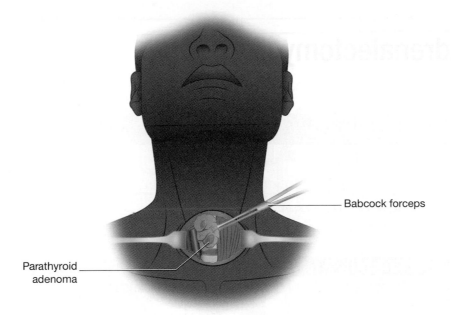

Babcock forceps

Parathyroid adenoma

Identification of abnormal parathyroid gland.

 Complications

EARLY
- Recurrent laryngeal nerve palsy (hoarse/weak voice) or external branch of superior laryngeal nerve palsy (loss of high pitch).
- Haematoma—can cause acute life-threatening airway obstruction from tracheal compression and oedema.

INTERMEDIATE AND LATE
- Transient hyperthyroidism.
- Temporary hypocalcaemia (usually resolves within 6 weeks to 1 year).
- Permanent hypocalcaemia (higher risk with multiglandular resection).
- Prolonged, severe hypocalcaemia or 'hungry bone syndrome'; can develop in the presence of normal or even elevated PTH postoperatively.
- Persistent HPT; commonly due to incomplete excision, supernumerary, or ectopic parathyroid tissue.

Postoperative Care

INPATIENT
- Minimal 6-hour postoperative observation to exclude cervical haematoma prior to discharge if no drain used.
- PTH and serum calcium levels are checked prior to discharge and abnormal calcium levels corrected. Additional vitamin D supplementation may be required.
- Drain (if used) removed when <30 mL output in 24 hours.
- Next-day discharge is common for a routine uncomplicated surgery; however, renal HPT patients often require several days to allow for careful biochemical monitoring and correction.

OUTPATIENT
- Follow-up appointment for wound review and biochemical profiling 4 weeks postoperation.
- A single 6-month follow-up appointment for serum calcium testing and confirmation of cure may be acceptable in those with a single adenoma. More regular, long-term follow-up is recommended in multiglandular disease.

? Surgeon's Favourite Question

With which multiple endocrine neoplasia (MEN) syndrome(s) is primary HPT associated?

Parathyroid hyperplasia is present in 90% of patients with MEN1A (pancreatic tumours, pituitary adenoma, parathyroid hyperplasia). It is also found in 50% of patients with MEN2A (medullary thyroid carcinoma, phaeochromocytoma, parathyroid hyperplasia).

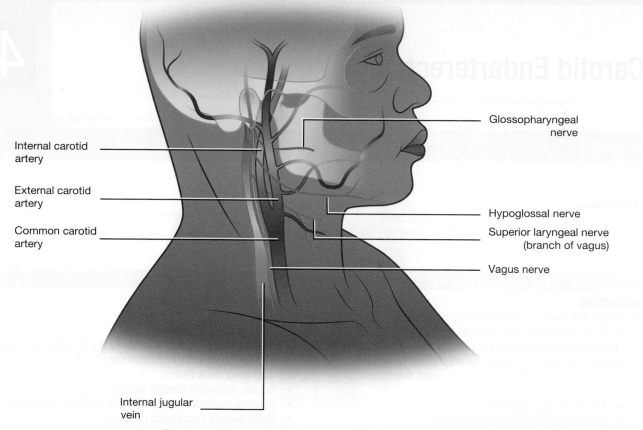

Internal carotid artery

External carotid artery

Common carotid artery

Internal jugular vein

Glossopharyngeal nerve

Hypoglossal nerve

Superior laryngeal nerve (branch of vagus)

Vagus nerve

Branches of the external carotid artery and associated nerves.

🔢 STEP-BY-STEP OPERATION

Anaesthesia: general or local/regional with a superficial cervical plexus block.

Position: supine with the neck extended and face turned to the contralateral side.

Considerations: Patients should be commenced on anti-platelets and statin therapy preoperatively and continued lifelong. In symptomatic bilateral stenosis, a staged procedure is recommended.

Steps:

1. An incision over the bifurcation of the CCA is made along the anterior border of the SCM.
2. The subcutaneous tissues and platysma are divided, and the SCM is reflected postero-laterally. The carotid sheath is exposed.
3. The IJV is identified; the facial vein is identified, ligated, and divided to provide access; the IJV is then retracted laterally or medially.
4. The CCA, ICA, and ECA are dissected free from surrounding tissues and encircled with slings ready for clamping.
5. Immediately prior to the clamping, a bolus of IV heparin is administered. Clamps are then placed on the ICA first (above the plaque preventing embolisation), and then on the CCA (below the plaque) and the ECA.
6. A longitudinal arteriotomy (incision) is made along the full length of the diseased CCA and ICA.
7. If using a general anaesthetic, a shunt may be placed from the common carotid below the level of the clamp to the ICA above the clamp. With local anaesthetic, the patient is monitored for evidence of neurological compromise whilst the ICA is clamped. A shunt can be used to restore blood flow if required.
8. The plaque is removed from the lumen of the artery by dissection in the layers of the deep media. Care is taken to create a smooth and tapered transition between normal artery and the endarterectomized section (to prevent subsequent arterial dissection).
9. The artery is then closed either primarily, or with a patch (commonly either bovine pericardium or synthetic material such as Dacron) to increase vessel diameter.
10. The wound is closed in layers; skin can be closed with either a subcuticular suture or metal clips; a drain can be inserted.

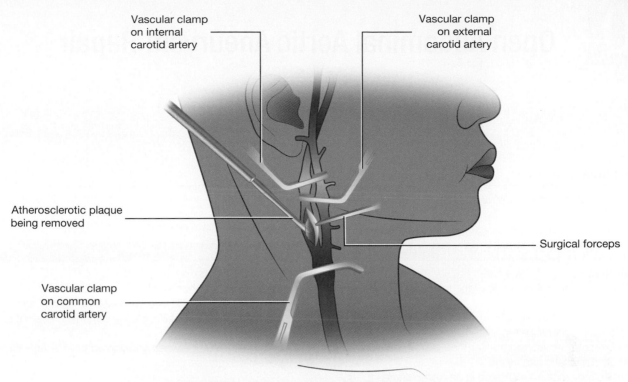

Excision of atherosclerotic plaque at the site of an arterlotomy in the internal carotid artery.

Complications

EARLY
- Intra- and postoperative stroke.
- Myocardial infarction.
- Mortality.
- Bleeding or haematoma—can result in a compressive airway obstruction requiring an emergency haematoma evacuation.
- Infection.
- Nerve damage:
  - Hypoglossal nerve—tongue weakness, deviates towards side of damage—difficulty in speaking and swallowing.
  - Glossopharyngeal nerve—difficulty swallowing.
  - Mandibular branch of the facial nerve— asymmetrical smile.
  - Recurrent laryngeal nerve—vocal cord palsy.
  - Vagus nerve injury – change of voice, difficulty swallowing and loss of gag reflex.

INTERMEDIATE AND LATE
- Hyperperfusion syndrome (rare) as a result of rapid reperfusion of previously hypoxic areas of the brain. Presents with headache, focal motor seizures, and intracerebral haemorrhage.
- Ongoing neurological deficit from perioperative stroke or nerve damage.
- Restenosis of the artery.
- Patch infection.

Postoperative Care

INPATIENT
- Hourly neurological observations in a high dependency unit (HDU) setting are required for 24 hours postoperatively.
- Patients should be monitored with an arterial line to allow for accurate control of blood pressure (commonly labile for the first 12–24 hours).
- Drain (if inserted) removed once <20 mL in 24 hours.

OUTPATIENT
- Routine follow up in 4–8 weeks.

Surgeon's Favourite Questions

What are the branches of the ECA?

Superior thyroid, ascending pharyngeal, lingual, facial, occipital, posterior auricular, maxillary, superficial temporal.

50 Open Abdominal Aortic Aneurysm Repair

Ijaz Ahmad

Definition

Open surgical repair of an infrarenal abdominal aortic aneurysm (AAA).

Indications and Contraindications

INDICATIONS

- Elective repair of AAA if one of the following conditions apply:
  - A diameter of over 5.5 cm—indicates the risk of rupture is higher than repair.
  - Diameter expanding greater than 10 mm per year.
  - Symptomatic aneurysms.
- Emergency repair is indicated in an AAA rupture.
- Some cases of aneurysms caused by microbiological infection (mycotic aneurysms).

CONTRAINDICATIONS

- Elective repair—those unlikely to survive or recover from the operation. The decision is based on comorbidities, life expectancy, quality of life, cardiopulmonary reserve, and exercise tolerance.
- Emergency repair—when considered futile or against the patient's expressed wishes.

Anatomy

- The thoracic aorta transitions into the abdominal aorta as it passes through the diaphragm's aortic hiatus at the level of T12. The abdominal aorta descends along the posterior wall of the abdomen, anterior to the vertebral column.
- The abdominal aorta has nine branches that supply the abdominal viscera:
  1. Right and left phrenic arteries—supply the diaphragm.
  2. Coeliac trunk—supplies the liver, stomach, oesophagus, duodenum, and pancreas (foregut).
  3. Right and left suprarenal arteries—supply the adrenal glands.
  4. Superior mesenteric artery (SMA)—supplies the small bowel from the lower half of the duodenum to the first two-thirds of the transverse colon.
  5. Right and left renal arteries—supply the kidneys (the right renal artery is longer than the left).
  6. Right and left gonadal arteries—supply the testicles in males and the ovaries in females.
  7. Inferior mesenteric artery (IMA)—supplies the large intestine from the splenic flexure to the level of the upper rectum.
  8. Median sacral artery—supplies the sacrum and coccyx.
  9. Lumbar arteries (L1–L4)—supply the lumbar vertebrae.
- At the level of L4, the abdominal aorta bifurcates into the left and right common iliac arteries.
- The common iliac arteries bifurcate into the internal iliac artery (supplying the pelvis) and the external iliac artery (supplying the leg).
- The external iliac artery becomes the common femoral artery as it emerges from under the inguinal ligament. The common femoral artery gives rise to the profunda femoris and the superficial femoral artery (SFA) in the thigh.

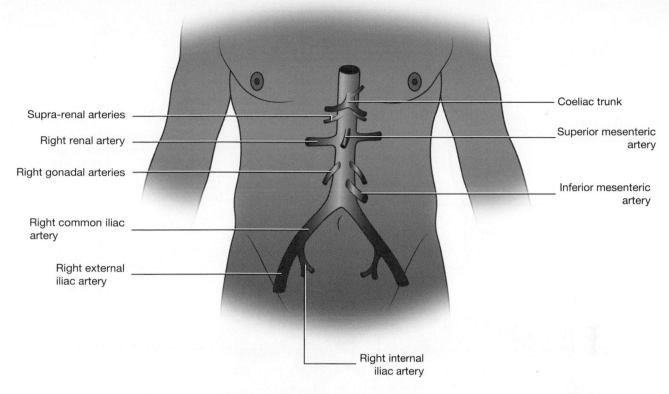

Supra-renal arteries

Right renal artery

Right gonadal arteries

Right common iliac
artery

Right external
iliac artery

Coeliac trunk

Superior mesenteric
artery

Inferior mesenteric
artery

Right internal
iliac artery

Branches and bifurcations of the abdominal aorta.

¹²₃ STEP-BY-STEP OPERATION

Anaesthesia: general anaesthesia, often with an epidural for postoperative pain relief.

Position: supine.

Considerations: Patients require a cross-match of several units of packed red cells preoperatively.

Steps:

1. A transverse or midline laparotomy incision is made and the abdominal cavity accessed.
2. The small bowel and omentum are covered in damp swabs and are then retracted to one side.
3. The retroperitoneal cavity is exposed, and the retroperitoneal duodenum is mobilised towards the patient's right side.
4. The aorta is visualised, and the neck of the aneurysm and the iliac vessels are dissected to gain full proximal and distal exposure. A bolus of IV heparin is administered.
5. Proximal control is obtained by clamping the aorta above the level of the aneurysm. Distal control is obtained by the clamping of both iliac arteries.
6. A longitudinal incision is made along the anterior surface of the aneurysm and the aneurysm sac is opened. Special care is taken to avoid the origin of the IMA. Once incised, thrombus and debris from within the sac are removed. Back-bleeding is controlled from the lumbar arteries by over-sewing.
7. The prosthetic (Dacron) graft is sutured in from the proximal normal aorta to either the normal postaneurysmal aorta (using a straight tube graft) or into the normal iliac arteries (using a bifurcated graft).
8. The proximal clamp is briefly removed, and the graft is flushed with heparin (this removes any thrombus and prevents more thrombus developing). This is repeated just before finishing the distal anastomosis to remove any further thrombus from the graft.
9. The distal limb pulses are assessed using Doppler, and the feet are checked for perfusion.
10. The aneurysm sac and retroperitoneum are closed over the graft, and the bowel is checked for evidence of ischaemia. The abdominal cavity is then closed in layers.

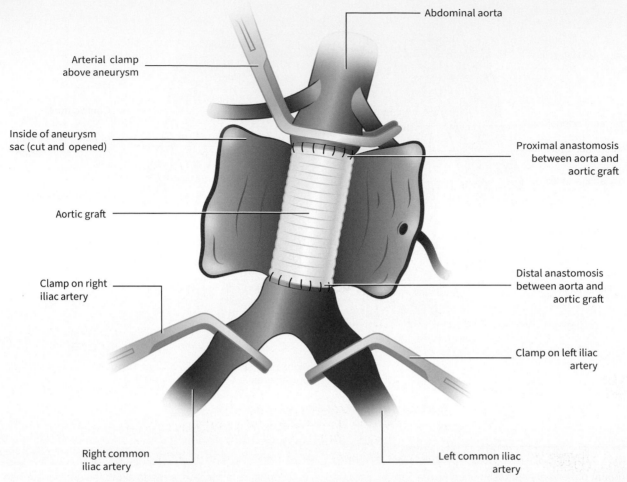

Abdominal aorta

Arterial clamp
above aneurysm

Inside of aneurysm
sac (cut and opened)

Proximal anastomosis
between aorta and
aortic graft

Aortic graft

Clamp on right
iliac artery

Distal anastomosis
between aorta and
aortic graft

Clamp on left iliac
artery

Right common
iliac artery

Left common iliac
artery

The anastomosis of a straight tubed Dacron graft at the site of an abdominal aortic aneurysm.

💬 Complications

EARLY
- Myocardial infarction—a major complication of the aortic surgery, particularly related to sudden periods of hypotension when clamps are removed and distal perfusion is restored.
- Bleeding.
- Lower limb ischaemia due to distal embolisation or thrombosis (trash foot).
- Renal, bowel, and spinal ischaemia.
- Damage to ureters or bowel.
- Paralytic ileus.

INTERMEDIATE AND LATE
- Graft infection.
- Incisional hernia.
- Aorto-enteric fistula.
- 30-day mortality for elective repair.
- 30-day mortality for emergency repair.
- Sexual dysfunction due to pelvic nerve damage.

Postoperative Care

INPATIENT
- Initially, patients should be cared for on either intensive care unit (ICU)/high dependency unit (HDU).
- A clear diet is started day 1 postoperatively and built up as tolerated.

OUTPATIENT
- Patients attend vascular clinic 6 weeks postoperatively.
- Unlike endovascular aneurysmal repair (EVAR), patients who have undergone an open abdominal AAA repair do not require routine long-term follow-up or repeat imaging; however, guidelines do suggest CT imaging after 4–5 years to assess for pseudoaneurysm formation at the site of anastomosis.

❓ Surgeon's Favourite Question

Which major vein crosses the aorta near the renal arteries?

Left renal artery.

Endovascular Aneurysm Repair (EVAR)

Ijaz Ahmad

Definition

Repair of an abdominal aortic aneurysm (AAA) using a minimally invasive endovascular technique.

Indications and Contraindications

INDICATIONS

- Elective repair of AAA if one of the following conditions apply:
  - A diameter of over 5.5 cm indicates the risk of rupture is higher than repair.
  - Diameter expanding greater than 10 mm per year.
  - Urgent repair is indicated in symptomatic aneurysms.
- Immediate repair is indicated in an AAA rupture.
- Emergency cases of aneurysms caused by microbiological infection (mycotic aneurysms).

CONTRAINDICATIONS

- Unsuitable aortic anatomy (as identified on CT angiogram—e.g. tortuous aorta, iliac arteries too small).
- Estimated glomerular filtration rate (eGFR) <30 mL/min—however, CO_2 angiography or small doses of iodinated contrast and the use of fusion imaging techniques can negate this contraindication.

Anatomy

- The thoracic aorta transitions into the abdominal aorta as it passes through the diaphragm's aortic hiatus at the level of T12. The abdominal aorta descends along the posterior wall of the abdomen, anterior to the vertebral column.
- The abdominal aorta has nine branches that supply the abdominal viscera:
  1. Right and left phrenic artery—supply the diaphragm.
  2. Coeliac trunk—supplies the liver, stomach, oesophagus, duodenum, and pancreas (foregut).
  3. Right and left suprarenal arteries—supply the adrenal glands.
  4. Superior mesenteric artery (SMA)—supplies the small bowel from the lower half of the duodenum to the first two-thirds of the transverse colon.
  5. Right and left renal arteries—supply the kidneys (the right renal artery is longer than the left).
  6. Right and left gonadal arteries—supply the testicles in males and the ovaries in females.
  7. Inferior mesenteric artery (IMA)—supplies the large intestine from the splenic flexure to the level of the upper rectum.
  8. Median sacral artery—supplies the sacrum and coccyx.
  9. Lumbar arteries (L1–L4)—supply the lumbar vertebrae.
- At the level of L4, the abdominal aorta bifurcates into the left and right common iliac arteries.
- The common iliac arteries bifurcate into the internal iliac artery (supplying the pelvis) and the external iliac artery (supplying the leg).
- The external iliac artery becomes the common femoral artery as it emerges from under the inguinal ligament. The common femoral artery gives rise to the profunda femoris and the superficial femoral artery (SFA) in the thigh.
- The common femoral arteries are routinely used for endovascular access. Each femoral artery is located at the midinguinal point (medially halfway between the anterior superior iliac spine (ASIS) and the pubic symphysis).
- The deep inguinal ring lies on the midpoint of the inguinal ligament (halfway between the ASIS and the pubic tubercle). The femoral artery lies at the midinguinal point.
- The femoral artery runs medial to the femoral nerve and lateral to the femoral vein (NAVY—nerve, artery, vein, Y fronts from lateral to medial).

Supra-renal arteries

Right renal artery

Right gonadal arteries

Right common iliac artery

Right external iliac artery

Right internal iliac artery

Coeliac trunk

Superior mesenteric artery

Inferior mesenteric artery

Branches and bifurcations of the abdominal aorta.

123 STEP-BY-STEP OPERATION

Anaesthesia: general, regional or local.
Position: supine.
Considerations: EVAR is conducted in an interventional suite or hybrid theatre (a surgical theatre equipped with image intensifier).
Steps:

1. Femoral arteries are accessed through specific percutaneous devices or through cutdowns (incisions in both groins with dissection of the surrounding tissues to expose and control both femoral arteries).
2. Once exposed, the arteries are cannulated and a catheter and guide wire combination is advanced through the femoral arteries via the right femoral artery. A stiff wire is positioned with its tip in the descending thoracic aorta above the AAA. Via the left femoral artery, a diagnostic catheter is inserted to a level just above the AAA. Through this, contrast dye is injected into the aorta and radiographs are taken to demonstrate the anatomy of the aorta and the aneurysm (contrast runs).
3. The main body of the graft is then inserted over the stiff guide wire with the proximal end of the graft being deployed into the infrarenal landing zone (hooks anchor the graft to the aortic wall). Once the proximal portion of the graft is anchored, the remaining graft is deployed.
4. A contrast run is performed in the right iliac artery, and measurements of the vessel are taken in order to select a stent with the correct length landing just proximal to the internal iliac artery orifice.
5. An appropriately sized right iliac limb is deployed so that the proximal portion anchors into the aortic graft whilst the distal end lies within the right common iliac artery. The left iliac limb is then deployed via the left femoral artery.
6. The proximal and distal ends of the graft system and all junctions are gently ballooned (a catheter-deployed balloon is briefly expanded across the junction to fully seal the graft to the artery wall).
7. Further contrast runs are performed to assess the seal of the graft.
8. The femoral artery sheaths and all wires are removed.
9. The defects in the femoral arteries are then repaired with prolene sutures.
10. The incisions are then closed in layers.

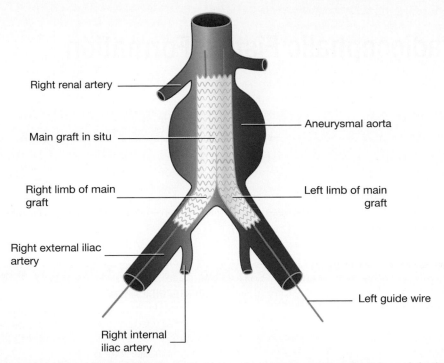

Right renal artery

Main graft in situ

Right limb of main graft

Right external iliac artery

Right internal iliac artery

Aneurysmal aorta

Left limb of main graft

Left guide wire

Positioning of the main body and the right and left limbs of an endovascular aneurysm repair graft within an abdominal aortic aneurysm.

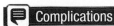 Complications

EARLY
- Renal, bowel, and spinal ischaemia.
- Leg ischaemia due to distal embolisation or thrombosis (may require embolectomy, thrombectomy, bypass, or, rarely, amputation).
- Contrast-induced nephropathy.
- Complications of femoral access—pseudoaneurysm, haematoma, distal embolisation.

INTERMEDIATE AND LATE
- Infection of either the wound or graft.
- Graft migration.
- Renal damage due to multiple contrast CT scans required for follow-up.
- Aorto-enteric fistula.
- Endoleaks:
  - Ia—failure of seal between graft and aneurysm neck.
  - Ib—failure of seal between graft and iliac vessels at the distal end of the graft.
  - II—flow of blood into the aneurysm sac from back-bleeding vessels (typically lumbar vessels).
  - III—failure of a seal between components of the graft device.
  - IV—leaking through the graft material.
  - V—growth of the aneurysm sac with no identifiable (types I–IV) leak.

Postoperative Care

INPATIENT
- Ruptured AAA patients should initially be cared for in intensive care unit (ICU)/high-dependency unit (HDU).
- Elective patients are suitable for ward-level care.
- It is important to ensure that adequate maintenance fluids are prescribed to limit renal damage following CT contrast.

OUTPATIENT
- Stent surveillance—to monitor for signs of the AAA increasing in size or signs of metal fatigue. Most commonly, CT angiogram is used for 1 year, and then a combination of ultrasound and plain radiographs is used to assess for leaks and stent fractures and to measure sac size.

 Surgeon's Favourite Question

What is the difference between a 'true' aneurysm and a pseudoaneurysm?

A true aneurysm is a focal dilatation of all three layers of the arterial wall. A pseudoaneurysm is formed by blood collecting between the tunica media and tunica adventitia of the artery wall, frequently caused by injury to the vessel.

52 Radiocephalic Fistula Formation

Ijaz Ahmad

Definition

Surgical formation of an abnormal connection between an artery and a vein—an arteriovenous (AV) fistula, used for vascular access in haemodialysis treatment.

Indications and Contraindications

INDICATIONS
- Patients requiring long-term vascular access for haemodialysis.

CONTRAINDICATIONS
- Vascular anatomy unsuitable for fistula formation—e.g. small vascular diameter or atherosclerotic disease of the artery. A vein luminal diameter of ≤2.5 mm and an arterial luminal diameter of ≤2 mm.
- Damaged veins from cannulation and blood sampling— patients approaching the need for dialysis should have their veins protected, and blood samples should be taken from the back of the hands.

Anatomy

- Cephalic vein:
  - The cephalic vein is a superficial vein of the anterolateral arm that drains the dorsal network of the hand.
  - Within the anterior cubital fossa, the cephalic vein communicates with the basilic vein via the median cubital vein.
  - The cephalic vein drains into the axillary vein at the deltopectoral groove.
- Radial artery:
  - The radial artery is a branch of the brachial artery. The brachial artery bifurcates into the radial and ulnar arteries just distal to the antecubital fossa.
- The radial artery runs along the anterolateral aspect of the forearm, supplying the posterior forearm and radial border of the hand.
- Within the hand, the radial artery anastomoses with the ulnar artery to form the superficial and deep palmar arches.
- The superficial branch of the radial nerve lies lateral to the radial artery, and care must be taken to avoid injury during the formation of a radiocephalic fistula.

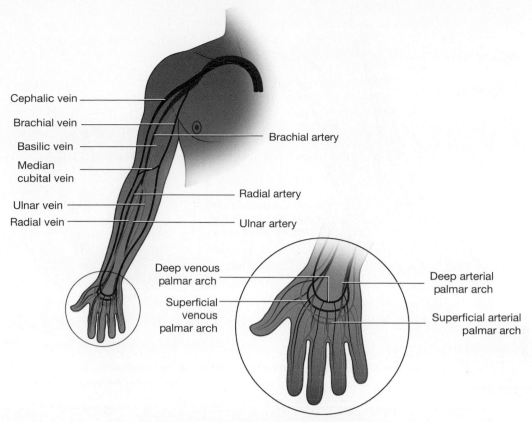

Cephalic vein

Brachial vein

Basilic vein

Median
cubital vein

Ulnar vein

Radial vein

Brachial artery

Radial artery

Ulnar artery

Deep venous
palmar arch

Superficial
venous
palmar arch

Deep arterial
palmar arch

Superficial arterial
palmar arch

Arterial supply and venous drainage of the upper limb.

¹²₃ STEP-BY-STEP OPERATION

Anaesthesia: general, local, or a regional nerve (brachial plexus) block.

Position: supine, with the arm supine on an arm board.

Considerations: Prior to surgery, patients undergo duplex imaging to assess the suitability of their vasculature for a fistula. Within theatre, ultrasound-guided preoperative markings may be performed.

Steps:

1. A 5–7-cm incision is made running over and longitudinal to the cephalic vein, 2–3 cm proximal to the wrist.
2. Through this incision, both the cephalic vein and the radial artery are visualised and accessed.
3. The cephalic vein is mobilised, and branches are ligated.
4. The cephalic vein is divided distally at the wrist. The distal end is left tied off, and a clamp is left on the proximal end. The vein is then flushed with heparinised saline (causing dilation).

5. The radial artery is exposed and dissected from surrounding tissue; care is taken to preserve the superficial branch of the radial nerve.
6. Clamps are applied to the radial artery, one proximal and one distal to the site where the cephalic vein will be anastomosed.
7. A longitudinal arteriotomy is performed on the radial artery.
8. An end (end of vein) to side (side of artery) anastomosis is performed using nonabsorbable monofilament sutures.
9. The arterial clamps are removed, and blood flow is restored.
10. Adequate flow through the fistula is confirmed (a palpable thrill), and the wound is closed in layers.

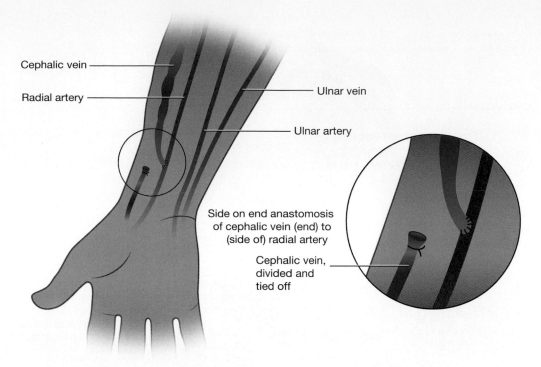

Cephalic vein

Radial artery

Ulnar vein

Ulnar artery

Side on end anastomosis of cephalic vein (end) to (side of) radial artery

Cephalic vein, divided and tied off

End of vein to side of artery anastomosis for the formation of a radiocephalic fistula.

 Complications

EARLY
- Bleeding and haematoma formation.
- Damage to surrounding structures, specifically the superficial branch of the radial nerve.
- Thrombosis of fistula resulting in failure.
- Early and severe steal syndrome (rarely).

INTERMEDIATE AND LATE
- Wound infection.
- Failure of fistula to mature (early fistula failure).
- Excessive vein dilation.
- Stenosis within the vein reducing blood flow and ultimately causing thrombosis.
- Failure of an established fistula due to thrombosis (late fistula failure).
- Steal syndrome—whereby blood is shunted away from the distal circulation and up the AV fistula, causing ischaemic symptoms within the hand.
- Congestive cardiac failure if blood flow through the fistula is very high.

Postoperative Care

INPATIENT
- Patients are discharged on the day of surgery.

OUTPATIENT
- Arterialization of the vein will take approximately 6 weeks. Patients are seen in clinic prior to the AV fistula being used for haemodialysis.
- Patients are warned that tourniquets and blood pressure cuffs, as well as cannulation and venepuncture, should be avoided on the arm with the fistula.
- If there is any concern about the fistula, such as thrombosis, aneurysm, or stenosis, it can be investigated with duplex ultrasound.

Surgeon's Favourite Question

Why do we make a first attempt at forming a fistula as distally as possible down the arm?

Fistulas have a high failure rate with time, and thus, if the first fistula is formed as distally as possible, subsequent attempts can be made, each time moving more proximally.

Below-Knee Amputation (BKA)

53

Ijaz Ahmad

Definition

Amputation of the lower limb below the level of the knee.

Indications and Contraindications

INDICATIONS

Summarised as
- 'Dead':
  - Potentially life-threatening lower limb ischaemia or necrosis with no safe options for revascularisation.
  - Nonsalvageable limb following trauma.
- 'Dying':
  - Potentially life-threatening Infection of the lower limb despite optimal antimicrobial therapy.
  - Malignant tumour of the lower limb (e.g. osteosarcoma).
- 'Damn nuisance':
  - A lower limb that hampers the functionality of the patient.

CONTRAINDICATIONS
- Patients who are not expected to be independently mobile postoperatively. In these patients, an above-knee amputation is more suitable, as the likelihood of successful stump healing is significantly higher for above knee amputation compared to below-knee (BK) amputation.
- Amputations requested by patients with body dysmorphic syndrome.

Anatomy

- The leg has four compartments: anterior, lateral, superficial posterior, and deep posterior.
- The compartments are separated by four fascial layers: the interosseous membrane, the transverse intermuscular septum, the anterior intermuscular septum, and the posterior intermuscular septum.
- Superficial posterior compartment:
  - The superficial posterior compartment is separated from the lateral compartment by the posterior intermuscular septum and from the deep posterior compartment by a transverse intermuscular septum.
  - The superficial posterior compartment contains the soleus, gastrocnemius, and plantaris muscles.
  - There are no major neurovascular structures in this compartment.
- Deep posterior compartment:
  - The deep posterior compartment is separated from the superficial posterior compartment by the transverse intermuscular septum and from the anterior compartment by the interosseous membrane.
  - The deep posterior compartment contains the tibialis posterior, popliteus, flexor hallucis longus, and flexor digitorum longus.

- Importantly, the tibial nerve and the posterior tibial artery descend in the posterior compartment.
- The lateral compartment:
  - The lateral compartment is bounded by the anterior intermuscular septum (anteriorly), the posterior intermuscular septum (posteriorly), and the fibula (medially).
  - It is supplied by the superficial peroneal nerve, which arises from the bifurcation of the common peroneal nerve as it winds around the head of the fibula.
- The anterior compartment:
  - The anterior compartment is bounded medially by the lateral surface of the tibia and laterally by the extensor surface of the fibular and anterior intermuscular septum. It is separated from the deep posterior compartment by the interosseus membrane.
  - It contains the deep peroneal nerve and the anterior tibial artery as it descends the lower legs before transitioning into the dorsalis pedis artery on the dorsal surface of the foot.

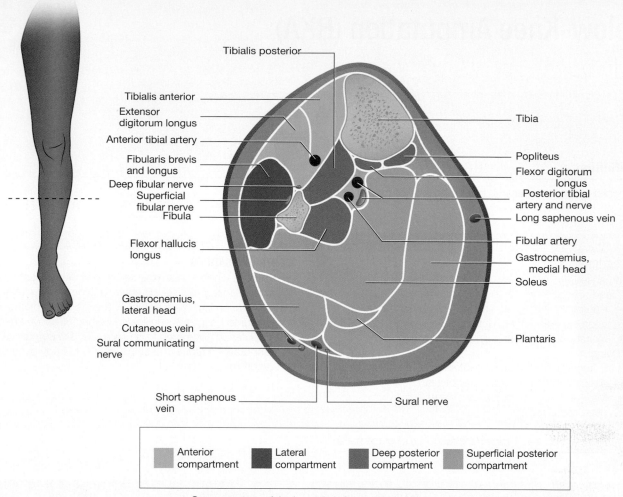

Tibialis posterior

Tibialis anterior

Extensor
digitorum longus

Anterior tibial artery

Fibularis brevis
and longus

Deep fibular nerve
Superficial
fibular nerve
Fibula

Flexor hallucis
longus

Tibia

Popliteus

Flexor digitorum
longus
Posterior tibial
artery and nerve

Long saphenous vein

Fibular artery

Gastrocnemius,
medial head

Soleus

Gastrocnemius,
lateral head

Cutaneous vein

Sural communicating
nerve

Plantaris

Short saphenous
vein

Sural nerve

▨ Anterior compartment	▨ Lateral compartment	▨ Deep posterior compartment	▨ Superficial posterior compartment

Compartments of the lower limb (below the knee).

¹²₃ STEP-BY-STEP OPERATION

Anaesthesia: general or regional.

Position: supine.

Considerations: Use of a tourniquet—e.g. in patients with bleeding diatheses, patients who are unable to receive blood transfusion (e.g. Jehovah's Witness), and young trauma patients (well-vascularised muscle tissue). Stumps can be fashioned in a variety of ways: Burgess flap (long posterior flap), skew flap, or equal anterior-posterior fish-mouth flap. The Burgess flap (most commonly used flap) is described in the following.

Steps:

1. The Burgess flap is marked 10–12 cm distal to the tibial tuberosity. The anterior incision extends across the anterior two-thirds of the leg, and the posterior incision is made more distally and comprises the remaining one-third of the circumference of the leg. It is made long enough so that this posterior flap can wrap over the stump. The transition between the anterior and posterior flaps is gently curved to reduce redundant skin.

2. Muscle and soft tissues of the anterior and lateral compartments are divided.

3. The vascular bundles (anterior tibial and peroneal) are suture-ligated. The long saphenous vein is identified and ligated.

4. The tibial and peroneal nerve are sharply divided and allowed to retract into the soft tissues. The sural nerve is sharply divided 5 cm proximal to the skin edge.

5. The tibia is skeletonised using a periosteal elevator and divided using an oscillating bone saw two fingers' breadth proximal to the skin incision. The cut end is rasped and smoothed over.

6. The fibula is cut 2 cm proximal to the tibia.

7. Muscles of the deep posterior compartment are divided at the same level as the tibia. The posterior flap is created using gastrocnemius, superficial tissues, and skin. If it is too bulky, soleus can be excised to allow tension-free closure.

8. The tourniquet is released, and haemostasis is obtained with sutures and/or cautery. A drain can be inserted between the stump and the flaps.

9. The posterior flap is brought up over the end of the stump to meet the anterior flap, and the muscle fascia is sutured to the tibial periosteum. The fascia and skin are closed in layers.

10. The stump is then dressed simply for protection during healing. Constrictive circumferential dressings should be avoided. The knee is immobilised in a splint or dressing to prevent postoperative knee contracture.

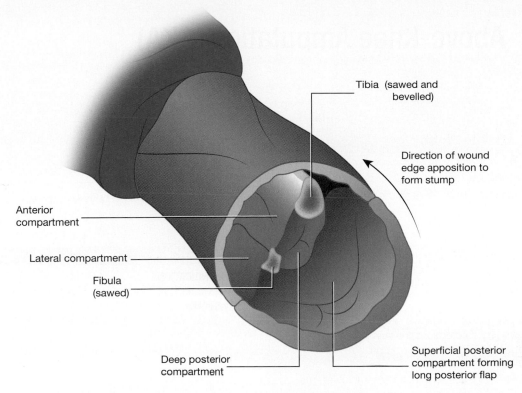

Tibia (sawed and bevelled)

Direction of wound edge apposition to form stump

Anterior compartment

Lateral compartment

Fibula (sawed)

Deep posterior compartment

Superficial posterior compartment forming long posterior flap

Cut surfaces of the tibia, fibula, and anterior and posterior compartments in a below-knee amputation.

Complications

EARLY
- Bleeding and haematoma formation.

INTERMEDIATE AND LATE
- Flap necrosis.
- Mortality—most commonly due to cardiovascular events.
- Infection of the wound or surrounding soft tissues.
- Stump pain.
- Deep vein thrombosis (DVT)/pulmonary embolism (PE).
- Wound dehiscence and nonhealing stump wound.
- Phantom limb pain.
- Flexion contracture of the knee.
- Neuromas.
- Pressure sores from immobility or prosthesis.

Postoperative Care

INPATIENT
- The drain is removed when output has fallen to <30 mL/24 hours.
- Adequate pain control is critical to aid stump healing—patients often require patient-controlled analgesia following amputation and are started early on neuropathic analgesia.
- Postoperative physiotherapy and occupational therapy services provide vital support and rehabilitation for patients undergoing lower limb amputations.

OUTPATIENT
- Specialist rehabilitation services should be engaged to optimise the opportunity of mobilisation with a prosthesis. A special moulding elastic sock ('Juzo' sock) can be applied from 1 week to help shape the stump ahead of fitting for prostheses. Prostheses can be fitted once the stump has fully healed (usually a minimum of 6 weeks).

Surgeon's Favourite Question

What factors must be considered when deciding upon an amputation level?

1) Likelihood of postoperative ambulation with a below knee stump (patient physiology, preexisting contractures).
2) Likelihood of stump healing (depends on extent of disease/trauma).

54

Above-Knee Amputation (AKA)

Ijaz Ahmad

Definition

Amputation of the lower limb between the hip and the knee (transfemoral amputation).

 ## Indications and Contraindications

INDICATIONS
Summarised as
- 'Dead':
  - Potentially life-threatening lower limb ischaemia or necrosis with no safe options for revascularisation.
  - Nonsalvageable limb following trauma.
- 'Dying':
  - Potentially life-threatening infection of the lower limb despite optimal antimicrobial therapy.
  - Malignant tumour of the lower limb (e.g. osteosarcoma).
- 'Damn nuisance':
  - A lower limb that hampers the functionality of the patient.

CONTRAINDICATIONS
- Amputations requested by patients with body dysmorphic syndrome.

Anatomy

GROSS ANATOMY
- The upper portion of the lower limb is divided into three compartments.
- Anterior compartment—contains the sartorius and quadriceps femoris muscles (comprising the three vastus muscles and rectus femoris), pectineus, iliopsoas, and iliacus. These muscles act to extend the knee.
- Medial compartment—contains the adductor muscles (gracilis, obturator externus, adductor brevis, adductor longus, and adductor magnus).
- Posterior compartment—contains the hamstrings (biceps femoris, semitendinosus, and semimembranosus).

NEUROVASCULATURE
- The sciatic nerve innervates the posterior compartment and is found posterior to the femur.
- The obturator nerve innervates the medial compartment of the thigh.
- The femoral nerve innervates the anterior compartment of the thigh.
- The superficial femoral artery (SFA) and vein (SFV) run in the adductor canal between the anterior and medial compartments.
- The profunda femoris artery and vein run close to the femur in the medial compartment, with branches supplying the muscles of the thigh.
- The great saphenous vein (GSV) runs along the medial aspect of the thigh.

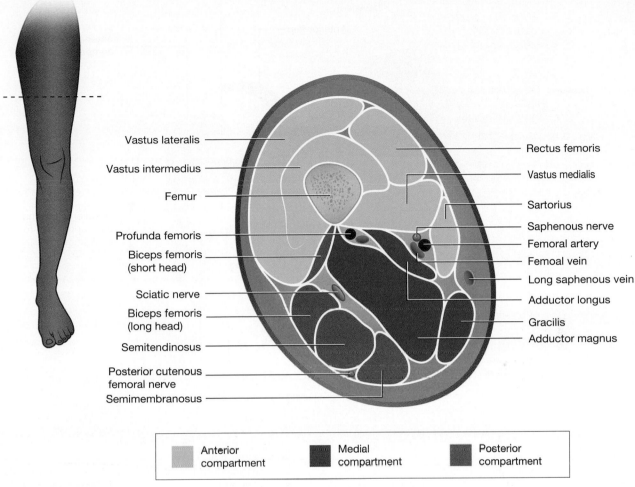

Compartments of the lower limb (above the knee).

1 2 3 STEP-BY-STEP OPERATION

Anaesthesia: general or regional.

Position: supine with bolster placed under ipsilateral buttock.

Considerations: Use of a tourniquet—e.g. in patients with bleeding diatheses, patients who are unable to receive blood transfusion (Jehovah's Witness), and young trauma patients (well-vascularised muscle tissue).

Steps:

1. A transversely oriented 'fish-mouth' incision is made proximal to the knee. The anterior and posterior flaps are generally of equal length with the level of bone division 12–15 cm above the superior margin of the knee joint (to ensure adequate soft tissue coverage of the bone cut).

2. The fascia and muscles of the anterior and medial compartment are divided with a 'raking' incision; special attention is paid to identifying the GSV (encountered early) and the SFA/SFV bundle (encountered late) so that they can be ligated securely.

3. The femur is skeletonised using a periosteal elevator and divided using an oscillating bone saw two fingers' breadth proximal to the skin incision (ensuring adequate soft tissue cover).

4. The remaining muscles of the posterior compartment are divided.

5. Special attention is paid to identifying the sciatic nerve, which is then sharply cut and allowed to retract naturally.

6. A sciatic nerve catheter may be inserted to deliver local anaesthetic to the divided sciatic nerve.

7. If used, the tourniquet is then released, and any additional bleeding points are identified and dealt with by either ligation or cautery; a drain can be inserted between the anterior and posterior muscle flaps.

8. The hip is flexed prior to closing the wound; if tension on the wound is seen, the femur should be shortened.

9. The fascia and skin are then closed in layers, with special attention paid to not create 'dog ears' (out-pouchings of tissue) where the anterior and posterior flaps meet.

10. The stump is then dressed simply for protection during healing. Constrictive circumferential dressings should be avoided.

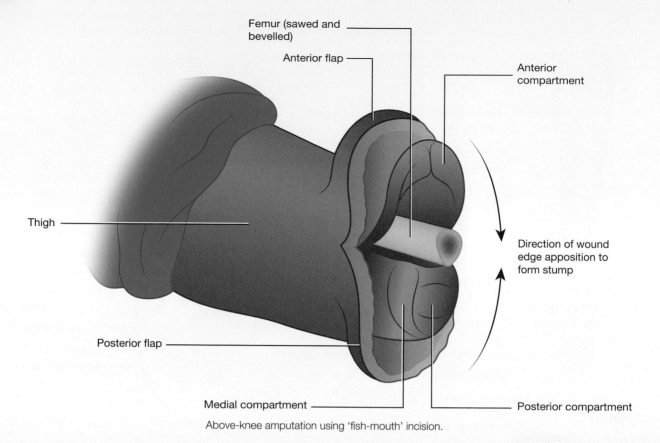

Femur (sawed and bevelled)

Anterior flap

Anterior compartment

Thigh

Direction of wound edge apposition to form stump

Posterior flap

Medial compartment

Posterior compartment

Above-knee amputation using 'fish-mouth' incision.

 Complications

EARLY
- Bleeding and haematoma formation.

INTERMEDIATE AND LATE
- Deep vein thrombosis (DVT)/pulmonary embolism (PE).
- Infection of the wound or surrounding soft tissues.
- Flap necrosis.
- Mortality—most commonly due to cardiovascular events.
- Stump pain.
- Phantom limb pain.
- Wound dehiscence and a nonhealing stump wound.
- Neuroma formation.
- Pressure sores from immobility.

Postoperative Care

INPATIENT
- If inserted, the drain is removed when output has fallen to <30 mL/24 hours.
- Adequate pain control is critical to aid stump healing— This can be achieved with the Sciatic nerve catheter if placed during the operation. Patients often require patient-controlled analgesia following amputation and are started early on neuropathic analgesia.
- Postoperative physiotherapy and occupational therapy services provide vital support and rehabilitation for patients undergoing lower limb amputations.

OUTPATIENT
- Specialist rehabilitation services should be engaged to optimise the opportunity of mobilisation with a prosthetic (if the patient is likely to mobilise).
- Some centres encourage air-cushioned prosthetic mobilisation for selected individuals within 2 weeks of the above-knee amputation (AKA).

 Surgeon's Favourite Question

What percentage of patients are able to mobilise with a prosthetic following an above knee amputation (AKA) compared to a below knee-amputation (BKA)?

Approximately one-third for AKA and two-thirds for BKA.

Femoral-Popliteal Bypass Graft

55

Ijaz Ahmad

Definition

The use of a graft to bypass a section of symptomatic occlusive femoral-popliteal artery disease.

Indications and Contraindications

INDICATIONS
- Patients with critical limb ischaemia or lower limb claudication following failure of medical management who have a diseased superficial femoral artery (SFA) or proximal popliteal artery.

CONTRAINDICATIONS
- Inadequate inflow (insufficient blood flow into the area of stenosis).
- Inadequate outflow (a poor quality distal popliteal artery supplying distal vessels).
- Advanced ischaemic disease requiring amputation.

Anatomy

- The abdominal aorta bifurcates into the common iliac arteries at the level of L4.
- The common iliac arteries bifurcate into the internal and external iliac arteries, which are responsible for supplying the pelvis and legs, respectively.
- As the external iliac artery passes deep to the inguinal ligament, it transitions to become the common femoral artery (CFA).
- The CFA bifurcates into the profunda femoral artery (PFA) and the SFA.
- The SFA supplies the leg; as it descends through the adductor hiatus, it becomes the popliteal artery, which then passes into the popliteal fossa.

- Within the popliteal fossa, the popliteal artery bifurcates into the anterior tibial artery and the tibioperoneal trunk.
- The tibioperoneal trunk then divides into the posterior tibial and peroneal arteries, which descend the remainder of the leg through the posterior compartment.
- The anterior tibial artery passes through a hiatus in the interosseous membrane between the tibia and fibula and then descends in the anterior compartment of the leg alongside the deep peroneal nerve before becoming the dorsalis pedis artery.
- The dorsalis pedis artery, together with the lateral and medial plantar arteries (branches of the posterior tibial artery), supplies blood to the foot.

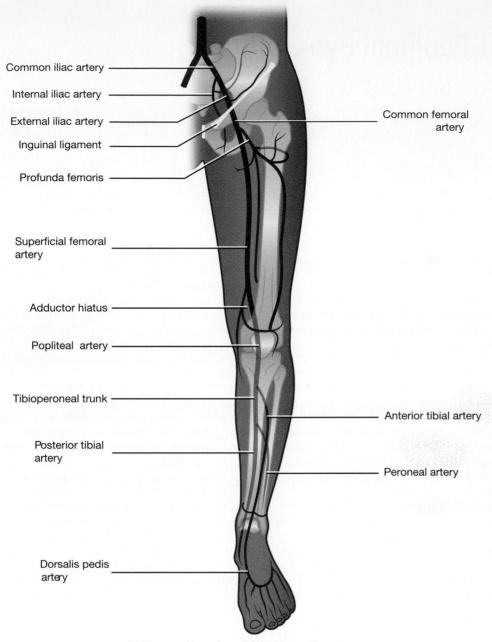

Common iliac artery

Internal iliac artery

External iliac artery

Inguinal ligament

Profunda femoris

Common femoral artery

Superficial femoral artery

Adductor hiatus

Popliteal artery

Tibioperoneal trunk

Anterior tibial artery

Posterior tibial artery

Peroneal artery

Dorsalis pedis artery

Divisions and branches of the common iliac artery.

123 STEP-BY-STEP OPERATION

Anaesthesia: general
Position: supine
Steps:

1. The CFA is identified by palpation, and a groin incision is made longitudinally to expose the CFA, SFA, and PFA, which are then dissected from the surrounding tissues.

2. Sloops are placed around the proximal segment of the CFA and around the SFA and PFA to prepare them for clamping later.

3. An incision is made at the site of distal anastomosis:

   a. For an above-knee popliteal artery bypass—the incision is made over the medial aspect of the distal thigh, anterior to the sartorius, exposing the popliteal artery just below the adductor magnus.

   b. For a below-knee popliteal artery bypass—the incision is made along the posterior border of the medial aspect of the tibia.

4. The popliteal artery is then dissected, and, using sloops, proximal and distal control is obtained.

5. An incision is made along the length of the great saphenous vein, which is then dissected out from the underlying subcutaneous tissue. The proximal and distal ends of the vein are then clamped, and the branches are ligated.

6. The vein graft can either be left in its natural position (in situ) or be tunnelled more deeply beneath the sartorius muscle in the thigh, then between the two heads of gastrocnemius behind the knee to reach the popliteal artery below the knee. If it is tunnelled, the vein is usually reversed so that the valves do not impede the flow of blood. If the graft is to be left in situ or, if tunnelled, not reversed, then a valvulotome instrument is used to obliterate the valves (if using a prosthetic graft, then steps 5 and 6 are omitted). During a fem-pop bypass, most

surgeons will reverse the vein and tunnel deeply. Using an in situ vein bypass is more advantageous when the bypass is being extended down to the calf arteries (e.g. the posterior tibial artery), as the vein needs less preparation and this avoids any discrepancy in vessel size that can occur when a reversed vein is used.

7. A bolus of IV heparin is administered.
8. Clamps are applied proximally and distally to the site of anastomosis of the CFA/SFA, a arteriotomy is made in the artery and the graft is anastomosed to the arteriotomy made. The graft is run to ensure good flow and to check for any leaks.
9. The vein (or prosthetic graft) is then tunnelled deeply or left in situ, and the distal anastomosis onto the popliteal artery is performed.
10. The clamps are removed, allowing blood to flow through the graft. Distal pulses and foot temperature are checked. The wounds are then closed in layers.

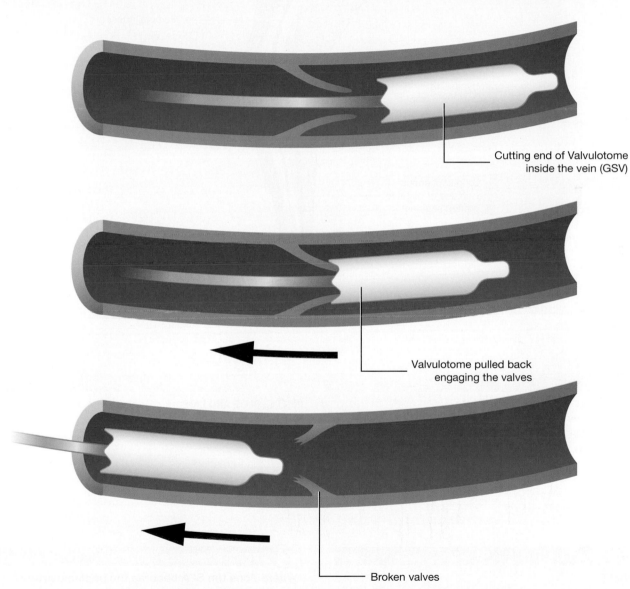

Cutting end of Valvulotome inside the vein (GSV)

Valvulotome pulled back engaging the valves

Broken valves

Use of a valvulotome to prepare the great saphenous vein for anastomosis as a bypass graft.

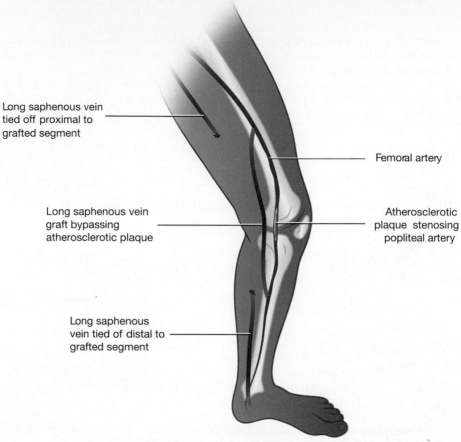

Long saphenous vein tied off proximal to grafted segment

Long saphenous vein graft bypassing atherosclerotic plaque

Long saphenous vein tied of distal to grafted segment

Femoral artery

Atherosclerotic plaque stenosing popliteal artery

Femoral-popliteal bypass graft using the great saphenous vein.

Complications

EARLY

- Bleeding.
- Haematoma.
- Graft failure.
- Nerve damage.

INTERMEDIATE AND LATE

- Graft infection.
- Graft stenosis and/or occlusion.
- Wound infection.
- Seroma formation.
- False aneurysm formation.
- Graft occlusion.

Postoperative Care

INPATIENT

- Patients are encouraged to mobilise day 1 postoperatively.
- Patients are discharged 2–4 days postoperatively with antiplatelet agents (typically aspirin or clopidogrel lifelong).

OUTPATIENT

- Outpatient review at 6 weeks to assess clinical response and to perform duplex ultrasound surveillance of the graft.
- All efforts must be made to modify lifestyle and vascular risk factors in order to maximise long-term benefit and graft longevity.

Surgeon's Favourite Question

Where does the SFA become the popliteal artery?

When it passes through the adductor magnus hiatus.

Embolectomy

Ijaz Ahmad

56

Definition

Removal of embolus from a blood conduit, most commonly an artery.

 Indications and Contraindications

INDICATIONS
- Emergency:
  - Acute upper limb ischaemia caused by brachial artery occlusion (less likely limb threatening but often causes limb claudication).
  - Acute lower limb ischaemia caused by the blockage of an artery (aorta, iliac, femoral, or popllteal) by an embolism.

CONTRAINDICATIONS
- Acute arterial thrombosis in a patient with chronic peripheral arterial disease—these cases should be considered for alternative techniques (e.g. bypass, endarterectomy, or balloon angioplasty with or without stenting).
- Nonviable limb—in these cases, an amputation should be performed or end-of-life care provided.

Anatomy

GROSS ANATOMY
- The abdominal aorta bifurcates into the common iliac arteries at the level of L4.
- The common iliac arteries bifurcate into the internal and external iliac arteries, which are responsible for supplying the pelvis and legs, respectively.
- As the external iliac artery passes deep to the inguinal ligament, it transitions to become the common femoral artery (CFA).
- The CFA bifurcates into the profunda femoral artery (PFA) and superficial femoral artery (SFA).
- The SFA supplies the leg; as it descends through the adductor hiatus, it becomes the popliteal artery, which then passes into the popliteal fossa.
- Within the popliteal fossa, the popliteal artery bifurcates into the anterior tibial artery and the tibioperoneal trunk.

- The tibioperoneal trunk then divides into the posterior tibial and peroneal arteries, which descend the remainder of the leg through the posterior compartment.
- The anterior tibial artery passes through a hiatus in the interosseous membrane between the tibia and fibular and then descends in the anterior compartment of the leg before becoming the dorsalis pedis artery.
- The dorsalis pedis artery, together with the lateral and medial plantar arteries (branches of the posterior tibial artery), supply blood to the foot.

PATHOLOGY
- Limb arterial emboli may originate from any proximal arterial flow location—from the left atrium to the segment of artery immediately proximal to the embolism.

175

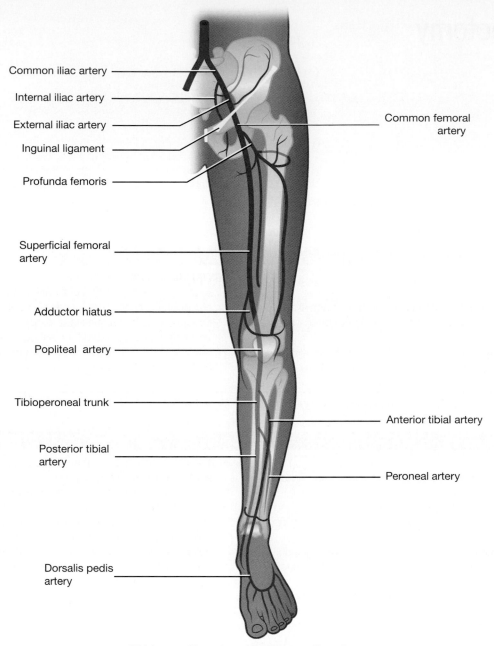

Common iliac artery

Internal iliac artery

External iliac artery

Inguinal ligament

Profunda femoris

Common femoral artery

Superficial femoral artery

Adductor hiatus

Popliteal artery

Tibioperoneal trunk

Anterior tibial artery

Posterior tibial artery

Peroneal artery

Dorsalis pedis artery

Divisions and branches of the common iliac artery.

¹²₃ STEP-BY-STEP OPERATION

Anaesthesia: general or local.
Position: supine.
Steps:

1. The artery through which the embolectomy will be performed is exposed (most commonly the CFA and, more rarely, the below-knee popliteal artery in cases of lower limb emboli or the brachial artery in upper limb emboli).

2. Proximal and distal arterial control is established by applying vascular slings to the artery on either side of the intended arteriotomy site. The slings are held under tension.

3. IV heparin is given if the patient has not been heparinised preoperatively.

4. An arteriotomy is performed proximal to the site of the embolism (longitudinal arteriotomies are used in severely diseased arteries, but in arteries with little disease, a transverse incision is preferred, as a longitudinal incision requires a patch for closure to prevent stenosis).

5. A Fogarty catheter (2–4 French) is passed into the distal arterial segment and guided past the site of anticipated occlusion.

6. The balloon is inflated beyond the embolism, then the catheter is gently withdrawn in a continuous fashion, adjusting the balloon pressure en route as required (the clot will be captured by the balloon and is pulled out of the arteriotomy).

7. This process is then repeated, both distally and proximally, until no further clots remain.
8. A heparin saline flush is then administered into the artery.
9. Proximal inflow is checked by releasing tension on the proximal vascular sling or clamp, and steps 6–8 are repeated as required. An on-table angiogram may be performed to confirm the degree of arterial patency. If the risk of compartment syndrome is high, prophylactic fasciotomies are performed.
10. The artery is once again flushed with heparin and the arteriotomy closed (primary closure or using patch). An intravenous heparin infusion is then continued postoperatively.

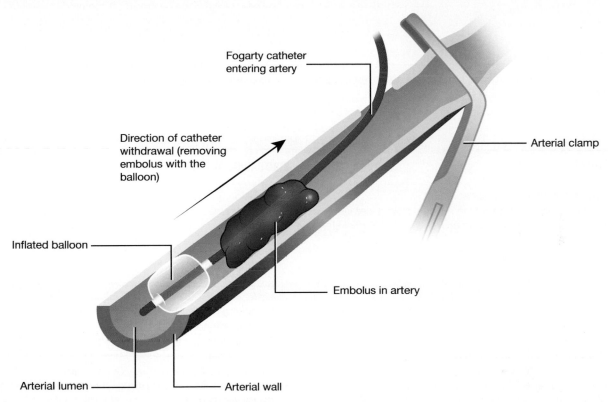

Fogarty catheter entering artery

Direction of catheter withdrawal (removing embolus with the balloon)

Arterial clamp

Inflated balloon

Embolus in artery

Arterial lumen

Arterial wall

Passing of a Fogarty catheter to clear a distal embolus.

Complications

EARLY
• Reperfusion injury causing compartment syndrome.
• Bleeding—can range from a small haematoma to active bleeding from the wound requiring a return to theatre.
• Haematoma.
• Nerve injury.
• Recurrent embolisation.

INTERMEDIATE AND LATE
• Wound infection.
• Lymph leak.
• Reocclusion.

Postoperative Care

INPATIENT
• Patients should be continued on an anticoagulant postoperatively (usually heparin) and then be commenced on anticoagulation therapy prior to discharge.
• To determine the duration of anticoagulation, the source/cause for the thromboembolism should be investigated prior to discharge (echocardiogram, 24-hour ECG tape, CT/MR angiogram of the proximal arterial tree, and thrombophilia screening).

OUTPATIENT
• Follow-up in vascular clinic is not routinely required unless further disease amenable to intervention has been identified.

? Surgeon's Favourite Question

What is the purpose of commencing anticoagulation preoperatively?

The aim of anticoagulation is to reduce the chance of further emboli and to prevent thrombus forming around the occluding embolus, making the ischaemia worse and making it more difficult to treat.

57 Femoral Endarterectomy

Ijaz Ahmad

Definition

Removal of an atherosclerotic plaque from a stenosed or occluded femoral artery. It may be undertaken in isolation or be undertaken to facilitate a bypass procedure.

Indications and Contraindications

INDICATIONS
- Intermittent claudication causing intolerable symptoms despite a trial of medical management.
- Patients with critical limb ischaemia (rest pain, ulceration, gangrene, and tissue loss) and proven femoral arterial stenosis or occlusion.

CONTRAINDICATIONS
- Patients with multilevel disease not amenable to revascularisation. In this situation, the improvement in perfusion would be inadequate for the underlying problem or the patient is not considered fit enough to tolerate the procedure with an acceptable risk of complications.

Anatomy

- The external iliac artery becomes the common femoral artery (CFA) at the midinguinal point (halfway between the pubic symphysis and the anterior superior iliac spine (ASIS) within the femoral triangle).
- The femoral triangle contains, from lateral to medial, the femoral nerve, artery, and vein (NAV-Y fronts). The iliopsoas, pectineus, and adductor longus muscles form the floor of the femoral triangle; the roof is formed by the fascia lata. Its lateral border is the medial border of sartorius, medial border of adductor longus, and superior border of the inguinal ligament.
- The CFA then bifurcates into the profunda femoral artery (PFA) and the superficial femoral artery (SFA).
- The SFA supplies the leg; as it descends through the adductor hiatus, it becomes the popliteal artery, which then passes into the popliteal fossa.
- Within the popliteal fossa, the popliteal artery bifurcates into the anterior tibial artery and the tibioperoneal trunk.
- The tibioperoneal trunk then divides into the posterior tibial and peroneal arteries, which descend the remainder of the leg through the posterior compartment.
- The anterior tibial artery passes through a hiatus in the interosseous membrane between the tibia and fibula and then descends in the anterior compartment of the leg alongside the deep peroneal nerve (deep to tibialis anterior) before becoming the dorsalis pedis artery.
- The dorsalis pedis artery, together with the lateral and medial plantar arteries (branches of the posterior tibial artery), supplies blood to the foot.

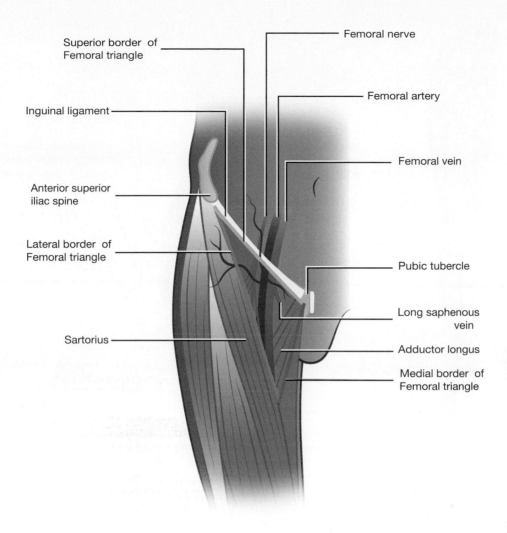

Superior border of Femoral triangle

Inguinal ligament

Anterior superior iliac spine

Lateral border of Femoral triangle

Sartorius

Femoral nerve

Femoral artery

Femoral vein

Pubic tubercle

Long saphenous vein

Adductor longus

Medial border of Femoral triangle

Borders and contents of the femoral triangle.

¹²₃ STEP-BY-STEP OPERATION

Anaesthesia: general or neuraxial (epidural or spinal).
Position: supine.
Steps:

1. The femoral artery is located by palpating the femoral pulse. The pulse may not be palpable in a heavily calcified artery; in this instance, the incision is guided by anatomical landmarks and/or ultrasound.
2. A longitudinal incision is made over the CFA, which is then dissected from the surrounding tissues.
3. The dissection is continued inferiorly to expose the PFA and SFA. Once exposed, they are slooped for later clamping.
4. Side branches of the CFA are dissected and controlled with slings to prevent back-bleeding during the endarterectomy.
5. The patient is administered a bolus of IV heparin and the slooped CFA, PFA, and SFA are clamped.

6. An incision is made along the length of the diseased artery (a longitudinal arteriotomy) to reveal any atherosclerotic plaque surrounding the lumen.
7. The plaque is then removed from the inside of the arterial wall using blunt dissection.
8. The artery is closed by either primary intention (rarely) or by using a patch (autologous vein patch, bovine pericardium, Dacron, or Gore-Tex) to prevent a stenosis and to slightly increase the vessel diameter.
9. Just before the completion of the arterial closure, the clamps are removed and reapplied sequentially to ensure any clot is flushed out of the arteriotomy.
10. The arterial clamps are removed, the distal pulses are checked, and the foot is assessed for perfusion. The wound is then closed in layers.

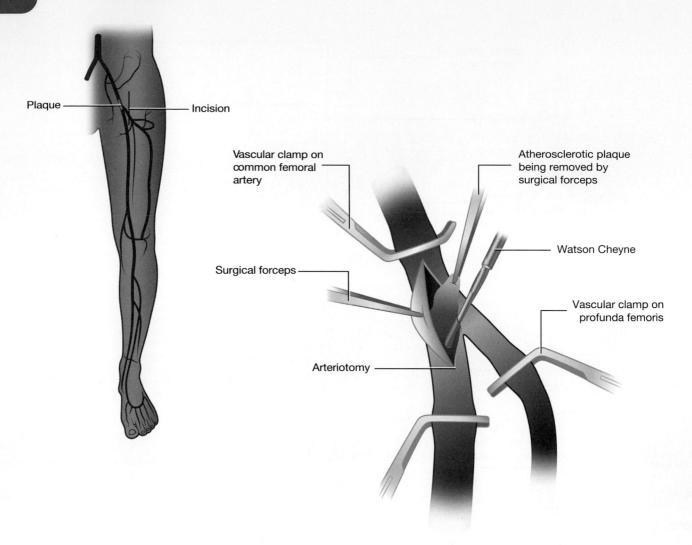

Removal of an atherosclerotic plaque via a longitudinal arteriotomy of the common femoral artery.

Complications

EARLY
- Bleeding.
- Haematoma.
- Arterial thrombosis.
- Distal embolisation/trash foot.

INTERMEDIATE AND LATE
- Leak of lymphatic fluid.
- Wound infection.
- Patch infection.
- Reocclusion.
- Pseudoaneurysm.

Postoperative Care

INPATIENT
- Patients typically discharged after 1–2 days.
- Anticoagulant medication (clopidogrel) and high-dose statins are commenced prior to discharge.

OUTPATIENT
- Patients are followed up in vascular clinic at 6 weeks.

Surgeon's Favourite Questions

What is the difference between the midinguinal point and the midpoint of the inguinal ligament?

The midinguinal point is halfway between the pubic symphysis and the ASIS and is the location of the femoral artery. The midpoint of the inguinal ligament, between the ASIS and the pubic tubercle, marks the deep ring.

Endovenous Thermal Ablation for Varicose Veins

Ijaz Ahmad

DEFINITION

Thermal ablation of the great saphenous and short saphenous veins with endovenous radiofrequency or laser treatment (EVRF, EVLT).

Indications and Contraindications

INDICATIONS

- Symptomatic varicose veins (venous skins changes, leg ulcers, thrombophlebitis, bleeding, pain) with:
  - Documented reflux (seen on duplex ultrasound) within the truncal superficial veins—i.e. great saphenous vein (GSV) or short saphenous vein (SSV).

CONTRAINDICATIONS
Relative Contraindications

- Pre-existing cellulitis over the puncture site(s).
- Previously failed EVRF/EVLT.
- Previous deep vein thrombosis.

Absolute Contraindications

- Previous phlebitis (indicating the vein for treatment is occluded).
- Acute deep vein thrombosis.
- Pregnancy.

Anatomy

- The superficial venous system of the leg comprises the GSV and the SSV.
- The GSV arises from the dorsal venous arch of the foot and the dorsal vein of the great toe.
- The GSV ascends along the medial aspect of the lower leg, anterior to the medial malleolus and across the posterior border of the medial condyle of the femur, before then running along the medial border of sartorius to anastomose with the common femoral (deep) vein at the saphenofemoral junction (SFJ) in the femoral triangle.
- The long saphenous nerve runs adjacent to the GSV and transmits sensation from the antero-medial leg and knee.

- The SSV arises from the dorsal venous arch of the foot and the dorsal vein of the little toe and passes posterior to the lateral malleolus and ascends the posterior aspect of the calf. It then passes between the two heads of gastrocnemius and drains into the popliteal (deep) vein in the popliteal fossa.
- The sural nerve runs adjacent to the SSV in the distal calf and transmits sensation from the lateral foot and fifth toe.
- Named perforating veins run between the deep and superficial systems. They are Hunter's, Dodd's, Boyd's, and Cockett's.

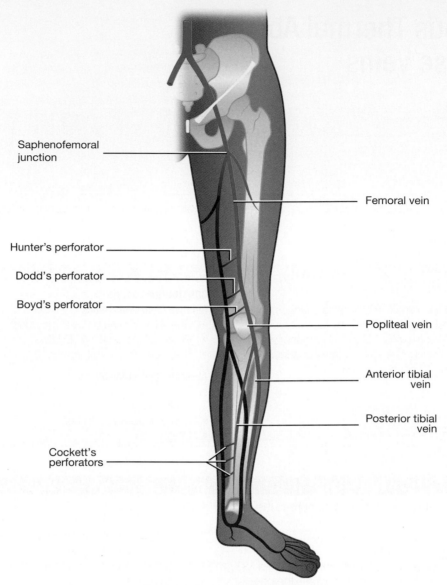

Saphenofemoral junction

Femoral vein

Hunter's perforator

Dodd's perforator

Boyd's perforator

Popliteal vein

Anterior tibial vein

Posterior tibial vein

Cockett's perforators

Venous drainage of the lower limb.

¹²₃ STEP-BY-STEP OPERATION

Anaesthesia: local anaesthetic infiltration around the puncture site.

Position: prone for SSV and supine for GSV treatment.

Considerations: For the purposes of this chapter, endovenous laser treatment is described.

Steps:

1. Ultrasound is used to map the course of the vein and identify an appropriate segment for treatment.
2. Dilute local anaesthetic is injected into and around the puncture site (most commonly the most distal straight section of vein available).
3. A needle is passed into either the GSV or SSV, through which a guide wire is passed up into the vein. The needle is then removed.
4. A sheath is then passed over the guide wire, and the wire is removed, leaving the sheath in situ. The laser fibre is passed through the sheath (a red light can be seen through the skin above where the tip of the probe lies).

5. The position of the tip of the probe is checked with ultrasound (at least 2 cm distal to the SFJ within the GSV).
6. To compress the wall of the vein against the laser probe and to protect tissues, dilute local anaesthetic (typically 250 mL) is injected under ultrasound guidance around the entire length of the vein.
7. The laser fibre is switched on and is then progressively withdrawn down the length of the vein at a rate of 10 seconds per 1 cm.
8. Foam sclerotherapy injections or direct avulsion of tortuous tributaries not treated by the laser can be performed subsequently.
9. Direct pressure is applied to the puncture sites to control bleeding.
10. Compression bandaging should be applied and left in place for 48 hours, to then be replaced by thigh-length compression stockings.

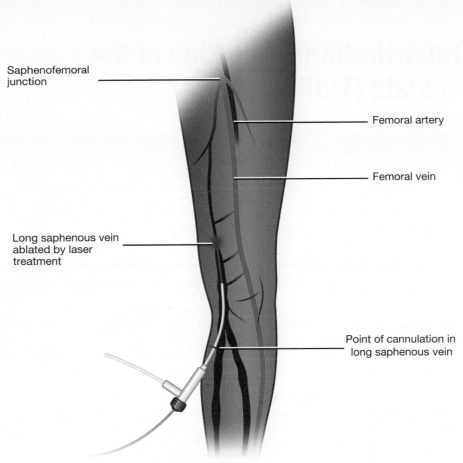

Endovenous ablation of the long saphenous vein.

Labels on figure:
- Saphenofemoral junction
- Femoral artery
- Femoral vein
- Long saphenous vein ablated by laser treatment
- Point of cannulation in long saphenous vein

Complications

EARLY
- Superficial thrombophlebitis.
- Bleeding.
- Haematoma.
- Thermal injury to the skin and surrounding tissues.

INTERMEDIATE AND LATE
- Infection of the wound or deeper soft tissues.
- Permanent skin discolouration secondary to thermal injury.
- Damage to the saphenous nerve resulting in numbness, chronic pain, or neuropathy.
- Deep vein thrombosis (DVT).
- Recurrence of varicosities.

Postoperative Care

INPATIENT
- EVRF/EVLT is usually performed as a day case, and patients are discharged once the local anaesthesia has worn off and pain is adequately controlled with simple analgesia whilst mobilising.

OUTPATIENT
- Compression stockings are worn for at least 7 days postoperatively.
- No routine follow-up is required unless the need for further intervention is considered likely.

Surgeon's Favourite Question

What does the term 'laser' stand for?

The term 'laser' is an acronym for 'light amplification by stimulated emission of radiation'.

59 Trans-Urethral Resection of the Prostate (TURP)

John Pascoe

Definition

Endoscopic removal of the inner portion of the prostate gland via the urethra.

Indications and Contraindications

INDICATIONS

- Benign prostatic enlargement causing bladder outflow obstruction and low urinary tract symptoms (LUTS) or urinary retention.
- Recurrent frank haematuria caused by prostatic pathology.
- Symptomatic relief in prostate cancer where radical prostatectomy is not possible (channel trans-urethral resection of the prostate (TURP)).

CONTRAINDICATIONS

- Active urinary infection.
- Coagulopathy.
- Where a TURP procedure would last longer than 60–90 minutes (e.g. grossly enlarged prostate).
- Presence of complex urethral disease preventing access.
- Patient not suitable for general or spinal anaesthesia.
- With prostates greater than 80 g, other surgical techniques such as holmium laser enucleation of prostate (HoLEP) should be considered.

Anatomy

GROSS ANATOMY

- The prostate is a walnut-sized exocrine gland surrounding the prostatic urethra in males.
- The prostate lies posterior to the pubic symphysis, inferior to the bladder, and anterior to the rectum.
- The ejaculatory ducts enter the postero-superior prostate, opening into the verumontanum (colliculus seminalis) of the urethra. Resection distal to the verumontanum during TURP increases the risk of damaging the urethral sphincter.

NEUROVASCULATURE

- The prostate's autonomic nerve supply arises from the inferior hypogastric plexus.
- The prostate receives its arterial supply from the inferior vesical artery (a branch of the internal iliac artery), which bifurcates into the:
  - Urethral artery—supplies the transitional zone of the prostate.
  - Capsular artery—supplies the glandular tissue of the prostate.
- The prostate drains via the prostatic plexus, which receives blood via the dorsal vein of the penis and then communicates with the pudendal and vesical plexuses. It drains into the internal iliac vein.

HISTOLOGY

- The prostate is composed of glandular and nonglandular (muscle or fibrous) tissue.
- It comprises four histological zones:
  1. Central—surrounds the ejaculatory ducts.
  2. Peripheral—most prostatic cancers arise here.
  3. Anterior fibromuscular stroma.
  4. Transitional—surrounds the urethra and is the site of benign prostatic hypertrophy (BPH); comprises two lateral and one median lobe.
- Hypertrophy of the transition zone causes obstruction of the prostatic urethra, compressing the peripheral fibromuscular tissue to create a surrounding 'surgical capsule'.

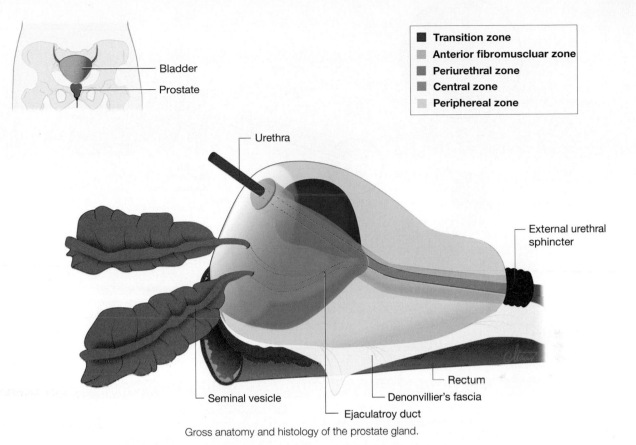

Transition zone
Anterior fibromuscluar zone
Periurethral zone
Central zone
Periphereal zone

Bladder

Prostate

Urethra

External urethral sphincter

Rectum

Denonvillier's fascia

Ejaculatroy duct

Seminal vesicle

Gross anatomy and histology of the prostate gland.

¹²₃ STEP-BY-STEP OPERATION

Anaesthesia: general or spinal.
Position: lithotomy.
Considerations: Preoperative antibiotics as per trust policy or previous urine cultures.
Steps:

1. The urethral meatus of the penis is lubricated with local anaesthetic gel (a narrow meatus may first require dilatation).
2. The resectoscope is passed into the lower urinary tract through the meatus, and continuous irrigation of the lower urinary tract is commenced.
3. As the resectoscope is passed throughout the lower urinary tract and into the bladder, all components of the tract are examined to exclude other pathology (e.g. tumours/urethral stricture/bladder calculi).
4. The verumontanum is identified and used as the distal landmark to avoid damage to the external sphincter.
5. Using a bipolar diathermy loop with a saline irrigation fluid, the prostate is resected (if using monopolar diathermy, glycine irrigation solution should be used to prevent the conduction of current through the fluid).
6. The Blandy method resects the median lobe first followed by resection of left lobe starting at 2 O'Clock and completing the resection of the left lobe to the median channel. Resection of the right lobe starts at 10 O'Clock and joins the resection of the median lobe. This method is thought to reduce bleeding.
7. The bladder is irrigated with an Ellik evacuator to retrieve the prostatic fragments for histological analysis.
8. Prior to the removal of instruments, the tract is carefully observed for bleeding, which is halted with coagulative diathermy.
9. A large-bore three-way catheter, e.g. 22F, is then inserted for postoperative bladder irrigation.

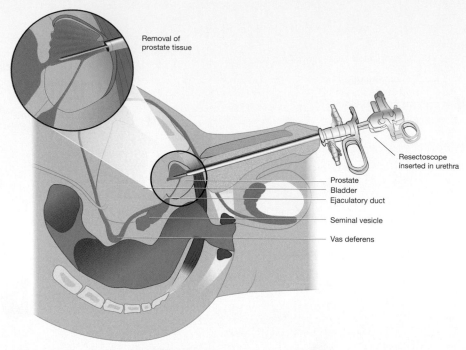

Removal of prostate tissue

Resectoscope inserted in urethra

Prostate
Bladder
Ejaculatory duct

Seminal vesicle

Vas deferens

Trans-urethral resection of the prostate gland.

 Complications

EARLY

- Haemorrhage and clot retention, commonly presenting as haematuria or loss of urine output.
- Urinary tract infection.
- Transurethral resection (TUR) syndrome—excessive absorption of irrigation fluid causing volume overload, electrolyte disturbance (hyponatraemia and hyperkalaemia), disseminated intravascular coagulopathy, and acute renal failure.
- Bladder perforation.

INTERMEDIATE AND LATE

- Urinary incontinence—injury to the external sphincter (can be temporary or permanent).
- Erectile dysfunction—injury to the prostatic plexus.
- Retrograde ejaculation—injury of the internal sphincter system.
- No improvement in symptoms.
- Urethral injury with resultant strictures.

Postoperative Care

INPATIENT

- The large-bore three-way catheter should remain in situ 6–24 hours postoperatively with continuous irrigation to remove blood clots and debris from the prostate and urethra. If bleeding persists, the catheter may remain in until the urine becomes clear.
- Patients are commonly discharged after 24–48 hours; however, TURP can be performed as a day-case procedure.
- A trial without catheter (TWOC) is attempted prior to discharge; if this fails, patients are recatheterised and discharged with the catheter in situ, and they return to clinical for a repeat TWOC in 1 week.

OUTPATIENT

- If the histology reveals prostate cancer, they are followed up accordingly.
- Patients should be advised they may still experience symptoms of increased urinary frequency and clots for up to 6 weeks.

? Surgeon's Favourite Question

What are the symptoms of BPH?

Mnemonic: LUTS are not FUN or WISE

Storage symptoms:
- Frequency
- Urgency
- Nocturia

Voiding symptoms:
- Weak stream
- Intermittency
- Straining
- Incomplete bladder emptying

Trans-Urethral Resection of Bladder Tumour (TURBT)

60

John Pascoe

Definition

Endoscopic access of the bladder via the urethra for diagnostic, staging, and therapeutic purposes.

 Indications and Contraindications

INDICATIONS
- To obtain histological confirmation of bladder malignancy and guide need for further treatment or surveillance.
- Removal of macroscopic noninvasive bladder tumours.
- Debulking of large tumours prior to further treatment (e.g. chemotherapy/radiotherapy).
- Palliation of symptoms in advanced disease.

CONTRAINDICATIONS
- Untreated urinary tract infection.
- Untreated coagulopathy.
- Patient not suitable for general or spinal anaesthesia.

Anatomy

GROSS ANATOMY
- The bladder is a highly distensible muscular structure lying posterior to the pubic symphysis.
- The bladder wall consists of four distinct layers:
  1. Mucosa—composed of transitional epithelium (urothelium).
  2. Lamina propria.
  3. Muscular layer—detrusor muscle/muscularis propria, the fibres of which are organised in three layers: inner longitudinal layer, middle circumferential layer, outer longitudinal layer.
  4. Perivesical soft tissue.
- The trigone is a triangular region of the bladder bordered by the internal urethral opening and the right and left ureteric openings. The superior border of the trigone (interureteric ridge) is folded and raised, lying between the ureteral orifices.
- The urethra runs from the neck of the bladder to the external urethral orifice. In females, it is approximately 4–5 cm long, running along the pelvic floor, and firmly attached to the anterior vaginal wall. In males, it is approximately 20 cm long, passing through the prostate, pelvic floor, perineal membrane, and penis. It is therefore divided into three sections: prostatic, membranous, and spongy.

NEUROVASCULATURE
- The parasympathetic fibres are motor to the detrusor muscle and inhibitory to the internal urethral sphincter.
- The sympathetic fibres innervate the neck and trigone of the bladder.
- The obturator nerve (L2–4) is responsible for sensation of the medial thigh and motor innervation of the hip adductors. Intraoperative stimulation of the obturator nerve during a TURBT can result in violent adductor muscle spasming, causing an increased risk of bladder wall perforation.
- The bladder receives its arterial supply via the superior and inferior vesical arteries (branches of the internal iliac arteries).
- Additional supply is from the obturator and inferior gluteal artery and the uterine and vaginal arteries in females.
- The venous drainage of the bladder is via a plexus terminating in the internal iliac veins.

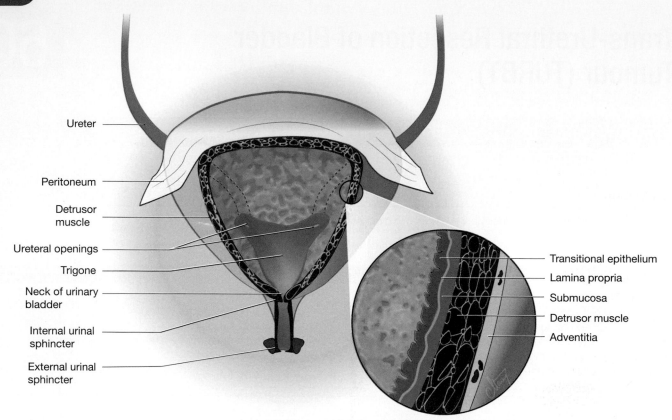

Gross anatomy and histology of the bladder.

Labels (left): Ureter, Peritoneum, Detrusor muscle, Ureteral openings, Trigone, Neck of urinary bladder, Internal urinal sphincter, External urinal sphincter

Labels (right): Transitional epithelium, Lamina propria, Submucosa, Detrusor muscle, Adventitia

1 2 3 STEP-BY-STEP OPERATION

Anaesthesia: general or spinal.
Position: lithotomy.
Considerations: Preoperative antibiotics as per trust policy or previous urine cultures.
Steps:

1. The urethra is lubricated with local anaesthetic gel; a narrow meatus may require dilatation.
2. A resectoscope is passed via the urethral meatus into the bladder, and continuous irrigation of the lower urinary tract is initiated (to allow for adequate distention for visualisation and access).
3. Once the resectoscope is within the bladder, the whole bladder is surveyed to identify the location, number, and size of tumours.
4. Using diathermy, the tumour is resected from the bladder with controlled and systematic swipes.
5. Further biopsies of the base of the resection site may be obtained to ensure muscle is in the specimen (for accurate staging and to identify muscle invasive bladder cancer).
6. Diathermy is used to coagulate any remaining bleeding points.
7. Following resection, the specimen is collected with a bladder syringe or Ellik evacuator.
8. A final survey of the lower urinary tract is performed to ensure haemostasis, and the resectoscope is removed.
9. A large-bore three-way catheter, e.g. 22F, is typically inserted for postoperative bladder irrigation.
10. At the end of the operation a single dose of a chemotherapeutic agent called mitomycin C is instilled in to the bladder.

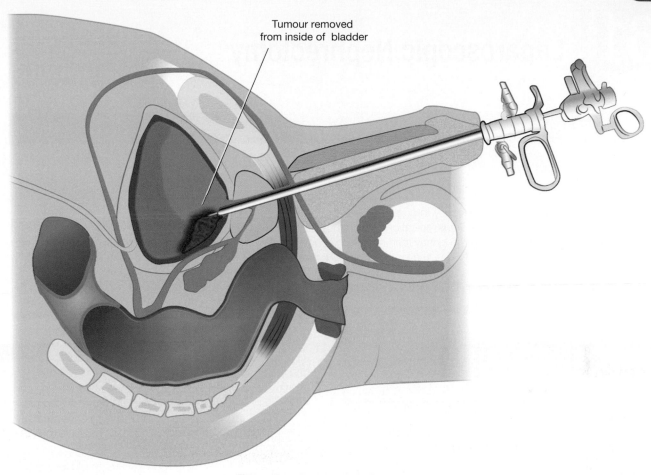

Tumour removed
from inside of bladder

Trans-urethral resection of the bladder.

 Complications

EARLY

- Bleeding.
- Urinary tract infection.
- Haemorrhage and clot retention, commonly presenting as haematuria or loss of urine output.
- Transurethral resection (TUR) syndrome—excessive absorption of irrigation fluid causing volume over-load, electrolyte disturbance (hyponatraemia and hyperkalaemia), disseminated intravascular coagulopathy, and acute renal failure.
- Bladder perforation.

INTERMEDIATE AND LATE

- Urinary incontinence (temporary or permanent) due to injury to the external urethral sphincter.
- Urethral injury with resultant strictures.
- Injury to the ureteric orifice causing ureteric obstruction.
- Recurrence of tumour.

Postoperative Care

INPATIENT

- The large-bore three-way catheter should remain in situ 6–24 hours after surgery with continuous irrigation to remove blood clots and debris from the prostate and urethra. If bleeding persists, the catheter may remain in until the urine becomes clear.
- Uncomplication procedures can be performed as a day case.

OUTPATIENT

- Further follow-up depends on histological findings and indications of surgery.

 Surgeon's Favourite Question

Where do squamous cell bladder cancers most commonly develop?

The urothelium of the trigone and lateral walls.

61

Laparoscopic Nephrectomy

John Pascoe

Definition

Surgical removal of all or part of the kidney through an open, laparoscopic, or robotic approach. Nephrectomy may be:
- Benign— performed for noncancerous indications (this removes the structures effected by the benign process).
- Radical—structures surrounding the kidney (peri-renal fascia, adrenal glands, peri-renal fat, and lymphatics) are also excised.
- Partial/nephron-sparing surgery (NSS)—the kidney is partially resected, preserving as much of the renal parenchyma as possible.
- Nephroureterectomy—removal of the kidney, the ureter and a cuff of bladder.

Indications and Contraindications

INDICATIONS
- Radical nephrectomy:
  - Primary renal malignancy, e.g. renal cell carcinoma (RCC)
  - Palliation for advanced/metastatic malignancy to relieve pain/haematuria/paraneoplastic syndrome.
- Benign nephrectomy:
  - Nonfunctioning kidney secondary to:
    - Stone disease.
    - Chronic and severe pyelonephritis that fails to respond adequately to medical management.
    - Hypertension secondary to renal artery disease (nephrosclerosis).
    - Congenital anomalies—polycystic kidney disease causing significant symptoms.
    - Living-donor transplantation (donor nephrectomy).
    - Trauma.
- Partial nephrectomy/NSS:
  - Small, solitary, localised tumours.
  - Same indications as for simple or radical nephrectomy where a simple or radical approach would result in renal failure—bilateral disease, single functioning kidney, existing/imminent renal impairment.
- Nephroureterectomy
  - Urothelial carcinoma affecting the renal pelvis or ureter.
  - Nonfunctioning kidney related to stone disease with ureteric stones in situ.

CONTRAINDICATIONS
- Patient not suitable for general anaesthesia.
- Patients with widespread metastatic disease where surgery is unlikely to offer significant survival benefit compared to oncological treatments or offer any palliative relief of symptoms.

Anatomy

GROSS ANATOMY
- The kidneys are paired retroperitoneal structures extending from the T12–L3 vertebral levels.
- The right kidney is positioned slightly lower than the left kidney due to the liver positioned superiorly on the right side.
- The kidneys, adrenals, and their surrounding peri-renal fat are enveloped by peri-renal (Gerota's) fascia, a dense connective tissue sheath.
- The renal parenchyma is divided into the outer cortex and the inner medulla, which feeds into the renal hilum, a recessed area containing the renal artery and vein, renal pelvis, hilar fat, and lymphatic tissue.

NEUROVASCULATURE

- The kidneys receive their innervation via the renal plexus with sympathetic fibres causing vasoconstriction.
- The kidneys receive their blood supply via the left and right renal arteries (branches of the abdominal aorta). Each renal artery branches into segmental vessels, which undergo multiple divisions, supplying the renal parenchyma and becoming the afferent glomerular arterioles.
- The right renal artery is lower than the left and has a longer course, passing posterior to the inferior vena cava (IVC) (the renal arteries run posterior to the veins).
- The kidneys drain into the left and right renal veins, which drain into the IVC.
- The left renal vein is longer and receives tributaries from the phrenic, adrenal, and gonadal veins.
- Lymphatic drainage is into the lateral aortic (lumbar) nodes.

HISTOLOGY

- The nephron is the functional unit of the kidney.
- Filtration commences at the renal corpuscle of the nephron (Bowman's capsule and glomerulus).
- The subsequent draining sequence is as follows: renal corpuscles → renal tubules → collecting ducts → papillae of renal pyramids → 10–12 minor calyxes → three to four major calyxes → renal pelvis.

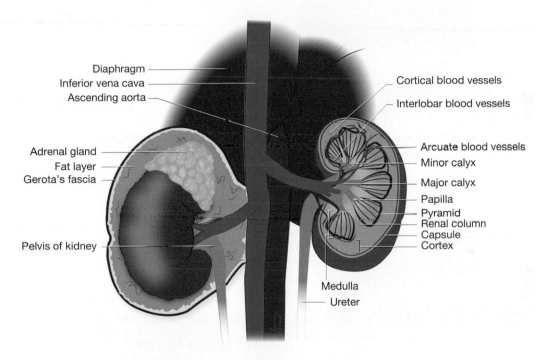

Diaphragm
Inferior vena cava
Ascending aorta
Cortical blood vessels
Interlobar blood vessels
Adrenal gland
Fat layer
Gerota's fascia
Arcuate blood vessels
Minor calyx
Major calyx
Papilla
Pyramid
Renal column
Capsule
Cortex
Pelvis of kidney
Medulla
Ureter

Gross anatomy and histology of the kidney.

①②③ STEP-BY-STEP OPERATION

Anaesthesia: general.
Position: lateral with the contralateral side leg flexed at knee and the ipsilateral leg straight.
Considerations: Antibiotics at induction.
Steps:

1. Pneumoperitoneum is achieved via an open cut down and a thorough laparoscopic examination is performed (identifying adhesions, excluding peritoneal metastases and demarcating relevant anatomy).
2. Further instrument ports are inserted under direct vision.
3. Adhesions to the abdominal wall are carefully dissected.
4. The colon is reflected medially by dissecting along the white line of Toldt.
5. The ureter is identified and lifted away from colon. The ureter is then dissected of surrounding tissue towards the level of the renal hilum.
6. The renal artery is ligated and divided, followed by the renal vein and then the ureter.
7. The kidney dissected from the abdominal wall.
8. The kidney is placed in an extraction bag and removed via an extension of a preexisting port site (the kidney and surrounding tissue is sent for histology).
9. The abdominal wall is then closed in layers—the fascia is closed with a continuous absorbable suture and the skin is closed with a continuous absorbable suture or staples.

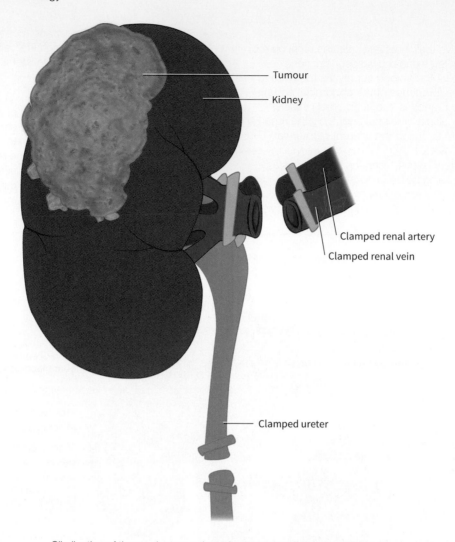

Tumour

Kidney

Clamped renal artery

Clamped renal vein

Clamped ureter

Clip ligation of the renal artery, vein and ureter prior to removal of the kidney.

Complications

EARLY
- Pneumothorax.
- Haemorrhage.
- Damage to adjacent organs/blood vessels.
- Renal impairment—usually transient due to intraoperative ischaemia/parenchymal loss.

INTERMEDIATE AND LATE
- Urinary fistula/leak.
- Incisional hernia.
- Infection.
- Tumour recurrence.

Postoperative Care

INPATIENT
- Bloods are checked the next morning and catheter is removed.
- Typically patients are discharged on day 2 post op.

OUTPATIENT
- Outpatient follow-up at 4–6 weeks to monitor recovery and renal function, and blood pressure. These parameters are then checked every 6–12 months.
- Strenuous activities should be avoided for 6 weeks postoperatively.
- Surveillance depends on the outcome of histology.

Surgeon's Favourite Question

What are the features of paraneoplastic syndrome in RCC?

Paraneoplastic syndrome comprises a cluster of widespread symptoms secondary to malignancy. RCC-induced paraneoplastic symptoms include hypercalcaemia, polycythaemia, Stauffer syndrome/hepatic dysfunction pyrexia, cachexia, and hypertension.

Scrotal Exploration and Orchidopexy

62

John Pascoe

Definition

Surgical exploration of the contents of the scrotum to assess and treat underlying pathology.

Indications and Contraindications

INDICATIONS
- Clinical or radiological suspicion of testicular torsion.
- Scrotal abscesses requiring drainage.
- Large symptomatic epididymal cysts.

CONTRAINDICATIONS
- Untreated coagulopathy.

Anatomy

GROSS ANATOMY
- The scrotum:
  - A dual-chambered pouch lying between the penis and anus responsible for housing the testes.
  - The scrotum consists of a thin layer of skin overlying the dartos muscle, which contracts and relaxes to bring the testes closer to and further away from the abdomen, controlling scrotal temperature for optimal sperm viability.
  - Deep to the dartos lie the external, middle, and internal spermatic fascia.
- The spermatic cord:
  - The spermatic cord starts at the deep inguinal ring, travels through the inguinal canal, and exits via the superficial inguinal ring to enter the testis.
  - It contains multiple key structures:
    - Three arteries—testicular, deferential, and cremasteric.
    - Three nerves—genital branch of the genitofemoral nerve, autonomic fibres, and the ilioinguinal nerve (note that the ilioinguinal nerve does not actually run within the cord, but alongside it).
    - Three supportive structures—vas deferens, pampiniform plexus, and lymphatic vessels.
    - Three coverings—external spermatic fascia, cremaster muscle/fascia, and internal spermatic fascia.

- The testes:
  - The testes are paired organs lying within the scrotum, separated by the scrotal septum.
  - The tunica vaginalis surrounds the testes in two layers (viscera and parietal). Deep to the tunica vaginalis lies the tunica albuginea, the tough, fibrous covering of the testes.
  - The testicular parenchyma is composed of 250–350 lobules, separated by septa of connective tissue that arise from the mediastinum testis (a vertical septum derived from the tunica albuginea).
  - The lobules contain seminiferous tubules, which join to form the rete testis, which in turn forms the efferent ducts that allow sperm to enter the epididymal head.
- Epididymis:
  - The epididymis is a highly convoluted tubule extending from the upper to the lower pole of the testis, where it becomes the vas (ductus) deferens.
  - The vas deferens joins the duct of the seminal vesicle to form the ejaculatory duct, which empties into the verumontanum of the urethra.

NEUROVASCULATURE
- The testes received their autonomic innervation via the testicular plexus.
- Arterial supply is from the testicular arteries, arising from the abdominal aorta.
- The testes drain through a network of 8–12 veins that form the pampiniform plexus. The plexus then converges to form the right (drains into the inferior vena cava) and left (drains into the renal vein) testicular veins.

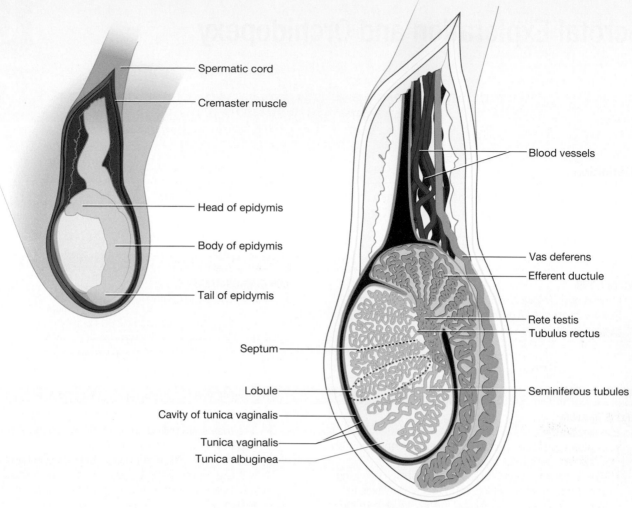

Spermatic cord

Cremaster muscle

Head of epidymis

Body of epidymis

Tail of epidymis

Blood vessels

Vas deferens

Efferent ductule

Rete testis

Tubulus rectus

Septum

Lobule

Cavity of tunica vaginalis

Tunica vaginalis

Tunica albuginea

Seminiferous tubules

Gross anatomy of the spermatic cord and testes.

₁₂₃ STEP-BY-STEP OPERATION

Anaesthesia: general.
Position: supine.
Steps:

1. The scrotal skin is stretched over the testis, and a midline raphe or bilateral transverse incision is made through the scrotal skin, the dartos muscle, and the spermatic fasciae.
2. After entering the ipsilateral scrotal compartment, the tunica vaginalis is incised.
3. The testis is then delivered out of the incision.
4. The spermatic cord and testis are examined for a twisted cord and a blue/black testicle.
5. If torsion is apparent, then the cord is untwisted and the affected testicle is wrapped in a warm swab (100% oxygen is then delivered to the patient by the anaesthetist).

6. Following a few minutes, perfusion to the testicle is reassessed by observing its colour, using Doppler to assess for adequate flow, and making a small incision in the tunica albuginea and observing for fresh bleeding.
7. If the testis is unsalvageable/nonviable, an orchidectomy is performed.
8. A 3 point fixation is undertaken for both salvaged and contralateral testes to prevent future torsion. The testis is secured to the medial, lateral and anterior walls of the scrotum with fine nonabsorbable sutures.
9. Haemostatic control is achieved, and the testis is repositioned into the hemiscrotum in the correct anatomical position (epididymis placed posteriorly, and sinus of testes placed laterally).
10. The dartos muscle and skin are closed in layers and a scrotal support is fitted postoperatively.

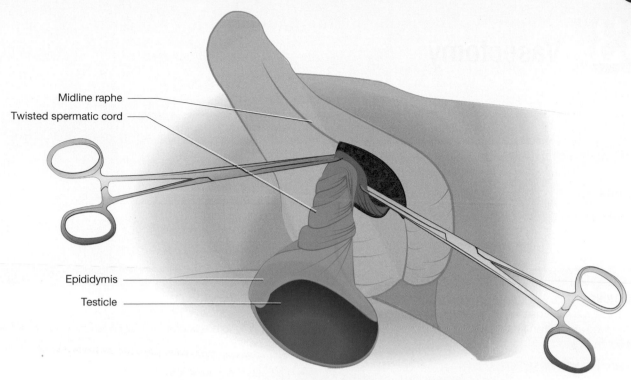

Midline raphe
Twisted spermatic cord

Epididymis

Testicle

Delivery of a testicle through a scrotal incision to assess viability.

Complications

EARLY
- Scrotal oedema or haematoma.
- Wound infection.
- Testicular infarction—this is a rare complication that has a similar clinical presentation to testicular torsion but occurs in the postoperative period.

INTERMEDIATE AND LATE
- Testicular atrophy—rare.
- Subfertility.

Postoperative Care

INPATIENT
- Patients are typically discharged on the day of surgery.

OUTPATIENT
- Follow-up appointment at 6–8 weeks.
- Testicular prosthesis may be requested at a later stage if orchidectomy performed.

Surgeon's Favourite Question

How does testicular torsion present?

Signs and symptoms of torsion include sudden-onset, severe testicular pain radiating to the lower abdomen, scrotal erythema/swelling, nausea/vomiting, high-riding testis with a transverse lie, and absent cremasteric reflex.

63 Vasectomy

John Pascoe

Definition

The surgical interruption of the vas deferens.

Indications and Contraindications

INDICATIONS

- Surgical male sterilisation as a means of contraception in men who are certain that they do not want to have further children.

CONTRAINDICATIONS

Absolute

- Patients who are uncertain they no longer want to father children.
- Scrotal infections.
- Untreated coagulopathy.

Relative

Most relative contraindications can be mitigated by vasectomy in the operating room either with or without general anaesthetic.

- Presence of hydrocoeles/varicocoeles that may interfere with the procedure.
- Previous orchidopexy—may have resulted in the blood supply being exclusively from the artery to vas, making vasectomy inappropriate.
- Anatomic variations that preclude the safe identification/isolation of the vas deferens.

Anatomy

GROSS ANATOMY

- The vas is a paired fibromuscular structure that travels within the spermatic cord.
- It transports spermatozoa from the epididymis to the ejaculatory ducts.
- When the vas reaches the seminal vesicles, it enlarges, terminating as the ampulla of the ductus, which then merges with the duct of the seminal vesicles, forming the ejaculatory ducts.
- The ejaculatory ducts enter at base of the prostate and terminate at the verumontanum.

NEUROVASCULATURE

- The vas receives sympathetic innervation from the pelvic plexus.

- The vas receives its arterial supply via the artery of the vas deferens (deferential artery), which is derived from the superior vesical artery (a branch of the internal iliac artery).
- The vas drains into the pelvic venous plexus.

HISTOLOGY

- The vas is comprised of three histological layers:
  1. Outer layer.
  2. Middle muscular layer—this layer of contractile smooth muscle wall of the vas propels semen during ejaculation through peristaltic motion.
  3. Internal mucosal layer—a layer of pseudostratified columnar epithelium containing apical stereocilia that enable forward propagation of sperm within the vas.

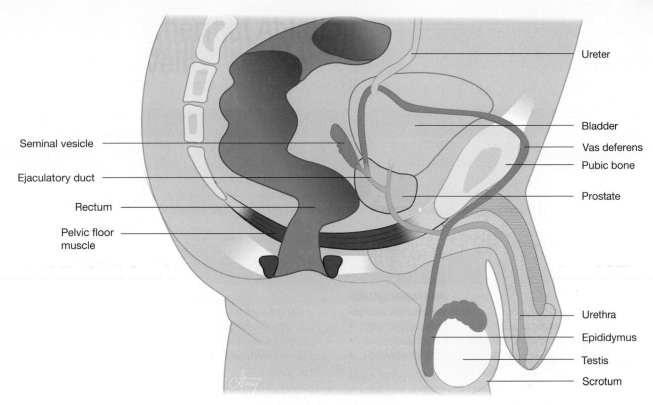

Course of the vas deferens.

Seminal vesicle

Ejaculatory duct

Rectum

Pelvic floor muscle

Ureter

Bladder

Vas deferens

Pubic bone

Prostate

Urethra

Epididymus

Testis

Scrotum

¹²₃ STEP-BY-STEP OPERATION

Anaesthesia: local.

Position: supine.

Considerations: The ambient temperature of the theatre should be checked to ensure it is adequately warm to prevent the cremasteric reflex.

Steps:

1. The external genitalia are examined, and the vas deferens is palpated. The penis is retracted superiorly to ensure an adequate view of the operative field.
2. Each vas deferens is identified and held by a three-point fixation technique using the thumb and the index and middle fingers.
3. A small bleb of local anaesthetic is used to numb the scrotal skin at the site of instrumentation/incision, and a deeper anaesthetic block is achieved by infiltrating along the spermatic cord to the level of the external ring bilaterally.
4. A small puncture incision is made through the median raphe of the scrotum, and vasectomy ringed forceps are used to retrieve the spermatic cord.

5. A portion of vas is carefully dissected from its surrounding fascia within the spermatic cord, with care being taken to ensure that the surrounding blood vessels are not stretched/ruptured.
6. The freed length of vas is cut.
7. The lumen of vas is occluded using electrocautery, and a 'barrier' of fascia is placed between the cut ends of the vas (fascial interposition). These steps reduce the risk of recanalisation.
8. In the 'open-ended' technique, the cut ends of the vas are left to retract to their natural positions (reduces epididymal congestion, vas granuloma formation, and development of postvasectomy pain syndrome).
9. The procedure is then repeated for the other vas using the same incision.
10. The wound edges rarely require closure with sutures, and antibacterial ointment and gauze are used as a dressing.

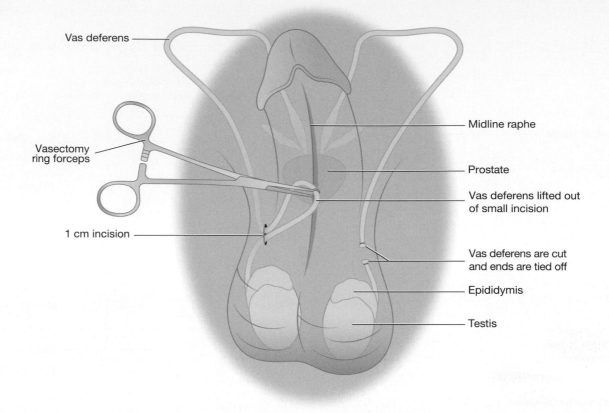

Vas deferens

Vasectomy ring forceps

1 cm incision

Midline raphe

Prostate

Vas deferens lifted out of small incision

Vas deferens are cut and ends are tied off

Epididymis

Testis

Cutting of a freed loop of vas deferens.

Complications

EARLY
- Bruising/haematoma.
- Iatrogenic damage to the spermatic vessels that compromises blood supply to the testicles.

INTERMEDIATE AND LATE
- Epididymal congestion causing pain and swelling.
- Infection.
- Sperm granuloma formation—usually occurs 2–3 weeks postoperatively and consists of a small nodule secondary to sperm leaking from the vas.
- Postvasectomy pain syndrome—occurs due to nerve damage and can occur immediately or later on.
- Persisting fertility—in the early period, this is usually due to unprotected sex before azoospermia is established; in the late period, failure can be due to spontaneous recanalisation of the vas.

Postoperative Care

INPATIENT
- Day-case procedure.
- Application of ice packs or support garments to the scrotum helps to reduce swelling and pain.

OUTPATIENT
- Patients are advised to lie supine as much as possible in the first 1–2 days postprocedure and limit themselves to light activities for the first week.
- Before patients can be certified as sterile, they need to have two negative sperm samples (azoospermia) obtained at least 3 months postvasectomy and at least 1 month apart. In the meantime, advise patients to use a second form of birth control.

? Surgeon's Favourite Question

Can a vasectomy be reversed?

Yes. This can be achieved through vasovasostomy (anastomosing the cut segments of the vas) or vasoepididymostomy (anastomosing the vas to the epididymis); however, it is best to describe a vasectomy as an irreversible procedure to patients.

Circumcision

John Pascoe

Definition

Surgical removal of the foreskin (prepuce) that covers the glans of the penis.

Indications and Contraindications

INDICATIONS

- Balanitis xerotica obliterans (BXO)—inflammatory condition causing scarring of the foreskin and adherence to the glans.
- Foreskin malignancy.
- Unsalvageable traumatic foreskin injury.
- Phimosis—severe narrowing of the foreskin orifice; can be congenital (rare) or a result of trauma, scarring, or infection.
- Paraphimosis—resulting from a tight foreskin and causing a tight constriction and resultant swelling of the glans.
- Recurrent balanitis and balanoposthitis—infection of the glans and foreskin (circumcision may be indicated in refractory cases where medical management has failed).

CONTRAINDICATIONS
Relative
- Chordee—deficient ventral skin causing angulation of the penile shaft (the foreskin may be required at a later stage for reconstruction in these instances).
- Untreated coagulopathy.

Anatomy

GROSS ANATOMY
- The penile shaft is composed of three columns of erectile tissue:
  - Corpus cavernosa × 2.
  - Corpus spongiosum × 1—within which the urethra runs. The distal extension of the corpus spongiosum covers the tips of the cavernosa and forms the glans of the penis.
- The three erectile structures are surrounded by deep penile (Buck) fascia, the dartos fascia, and the penile skin.
- The glans has a raised proximal rim called the corona. The sagittal slit, through which the urethra exits, sits at the tip of the glans.
- The foreskin, or penile prepuce, is a continuation of the penile skin, which at the corona becomes double-sided, and therefore retractable, and covers the glans of the penis.
- The frenulum is a Y-shaped band of connective tissue on the underside of the glans that tethers the foreskin to the glans.

NEUROVASCULATURE
- The dorsal nerve of the penis supplies the glans and foreskin (it is a terminal branch of the pudendal nerve S2–S4).
- Arterial supply is via the dorsal artery of the penis (a branch of the internal pudendal artery).
- The penis is drained via the superficial dorsal vein of the penis.

A. Unretracted foreskin

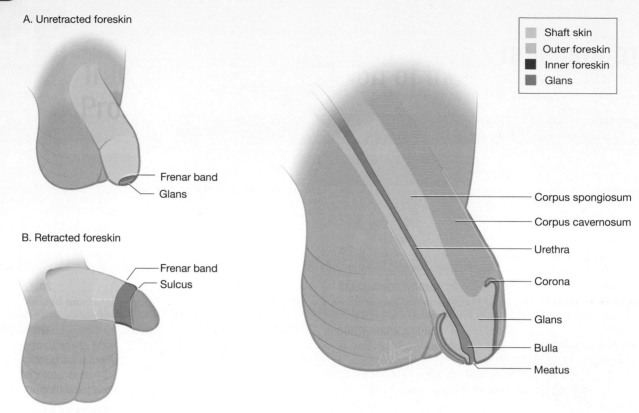

	Shaft skin
	Outer foreskin
	Inner foreskin
	Glans

Frenar band
Glans

B. Retracted foreskin

Frenar band
Sulcus

Corpus spongiosum
Corpus cavernosum
Urethra
Corona
Glans
Bulla
Meatus

Gross anatomy of the penis.

1 2 3 STEP-BY-STEP OPERATION

Anaesthesia: A dorsal penile nerve block is commonly used in conjunction with a general anaesthetic.

Position: supine.

Considerations: Various well-established surgical techniques are used: dorsal slit, sleeve, guillotine technique, or with aid of devices such as Plastibell, Mogen clamp, Gomco clamp, and The Shang Ring. The various devices are used in accordance with age and size of penis.

Steps:

1. The outer foreskin is marked circumferentially using a pen.
2. Sharp dissection is used to dissect through the outer layers of foreskin.
3. Mosquito clips are placed at the 2, 6, and 11 o'clock positions.
4. With bipolar diathermy scissors, a dorsal slit is performed to meet the circumferential incision.
5. The foreskin is inverted and an inner circumferential mucosal incision is made with a scalpel.
6. Using bipolar scissors, the skin is excised between the inner and outer incisions (the skin is sent for routine histology).
7. Haemostasis is achieved using bipolar forceps
8. The wound is closed using absorbable 3-0 sutures.
9. A box stitch is used over the frenular artery and haemostasis is observed.
10. A dressing of jelonet and soft gauze is fixed.

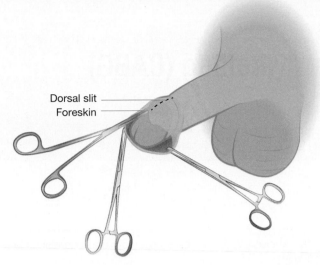
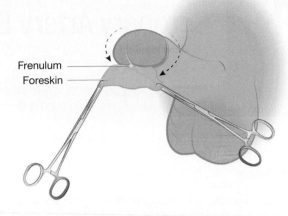

Dorsal slit
Foreskin

Frenulum
Foreskin

Surgical circumcision.

 Complications

EARLY
- Haemorrhage.
- Pain and discomfort.
- Bruising/swelling.

INTERMEDIATE AND LATE
- Meatal stenosis.
- Removal of too much or too little skin with resulting unsatisfactory cosmetic result.
- Change in sensation due to loss of hypersensitivity at the glans.
- Infection.

Postoperative Care

INPATIENT
- Circumcision is performed as a day-case procedure; patients are discharged once they have passed urine.

OUTPATIENT
- Petroleum-based ointments (e.g. Vaseline) can be applied regularly to the wound and glans to avoid irritation.
- Parents are advised that children should remain home from school for 1 week.
- Adults are advised to avoid sexual intercourse until fully healed (commonly 4–6 weeks).

? Surgeon's Favourite Question

When does the foreskin separate from the glans during normal development?

The foreskin is normally adherent to the glans in infancy and up to the first 3 years of life. It gradually spontaneously separates during this time, and by 3 years, 90% of boys will have a retractable foreskin.

65 Coronary Artery Bypass Grafting (CABG)

Charles Jenkinson

Definition

The use of a venous or arterial graft to bypass significant coronary artery stenosis to restore blood flow to the myocardium. Can be done open or with minimally invasive techniques such as robotic surgery.

Indications and Contraindications

INDICATIONS

- Multivessel disease is the main indication for coronary artery bypass grafting (CABG) over percutaneous coronary intervention (PCI) or medical management for improvement in long term outcomes, particularly in the context of left ventricular (LV) impairment, complex anatomy, or patients with diabetes and renal failure.
- Single/double vessel disease where:
  - There is significant left main (or proximal left anterior descending) disease.
  - There is a large amount of ischaemic myocardium.
  - Patients are unsuitable for long-term dual antiplatelet therapy.
- Unstable angina or angina that severely limits activity and cannot be controlled medically or with PCI.
- Ischaemia in a non-ST elevation myocardial infarction (NSTEMI) that is refractory to medication.
- An emergency CABG may be indicated in ST elevation myocardial infarction (STEMI) where PCI is not possible.

CONTRAINDICATIONS

- Patients with coronary artery disease that can be managed with PCI that do not otherwise have a survival advantage with surgery.
- Patients with significant comorbidities or frailty who are not operative candidates.
- Asymptomatic patients with stable coronary artery disease may not have survival benefit from surgery.

Anatomy

THE CORONARY ARTERIES

- The left main and right coronary arteries arise from the left and right aortic sinuses, distal to the aortic valve.
- Left main coronary artery (LMCA):
  - The LMCA branches to form the Left Circumflex Artery (LCx) which runs in the atrioventricular groove, and the Left Anterior Descending (LAD), which produces a series of diagonal arteries and gives off septal perforators to supply the left ventricle.
  - Obtuse Marginal (OM) atery branches arise from the LCx.
- Right coronary artery (RCA):
  - The RCA runs in the groove between the right atrium and ventricle.
  - Along its path, the RCA gives rise to the acute marginal arteries.

- 80% of individuals have a right dominant coronary circulation where the RCA continues as the Posterior Descending Artery (PDA). In a left dominant circulation, this artery usually arises from the LCx.
- Stenosis can occur at any site, but the most significant stenoses occur along the LAD and the LMCA, as these supply the majority of the left ventricular tissue.

GRAFT ANATOMY

- A section of blood vessel taken from one of three sites
- The internal mammary artery/internal thoracic artery (the most commonly used graft):
  - Branches from the subclavian artery proximal to the vertebral arteries.
  - The artery descends along the internal anterior chest wall parallel to edges of the sternum, where it branches

into the musculophrenic and superior epigastric arteries.
- The saphenous veins:
  - The long saphenous vein ascends the anteromedial thigh and drains into the femoral vein at the sapheno-femoral junction.

- The short saphenous vein ascends the posterior calf to drain into the popliteal vein.
- The radial artery:
  - Arises from the bifurcation of the brachial artery to then run distally along the anterior forearm.

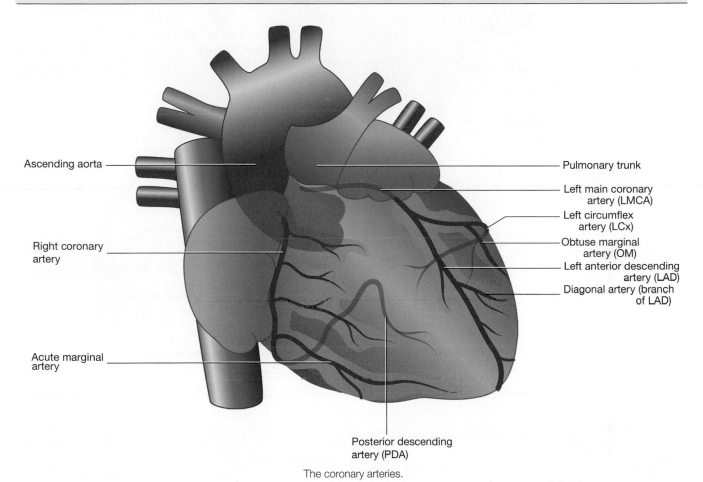

The coronary arteries.

STEP-BY-STEP OPERATION

Anaesthesia: general.
Position: supine.
Considerations: Two teams work simultaneously, with one exposing the heart and the second focusing on harvesting the graft. Minimally invasive techniques and 'off-pump' or 'beating heart' surgery can be used, often reserved for elderly patients with multiple comorbidities or patients with calcified aortas who may not tolerate the aortic manipulation required for cardiopulmonary bypass (CPB). Intraoperative transoesophageal echocardiogram (TOE) is often used.

Steps:
1. An incision is made in the midline of the chest, and the sternum is split using a sternal saw (median sternotomy).
2. Conduit to be used for bypass is harvested from the chest wall, the forearm, and/or the leg.
3. CPB is then established, directing the circulation through the bypass machine, which includes an oxygenation membrane and heat exchange pump.

Heparin is given to prevent clot formation within the CPB machine.
4. A cross-clamp is applied to the ascending aorta, and cardioplegia (usually a potassium-enriched solution) is administered, causing the heart to stop beating.
5. When the saphenous vein or radial artery grafts are used, the distal portion is anastomosed with the coronary artery at a point beyond the stenosed section of the vessel, and the proximal portion is most commonly anastomosed to the ascending aorta.
6. The left internal mammary artery is anastomosed beyond the point of stenosis.
7. The patient is rewarmed, and the cross-clamp is removed. This restores blood flow to the heart, washing out the cardioplegia. After a period of reperfusion, the patient is slowly weaned off cardiopulmonary bypass.
8. The sternum is commonly closed using sternal wires, and then the soft tissues of the chest are closed in layers.

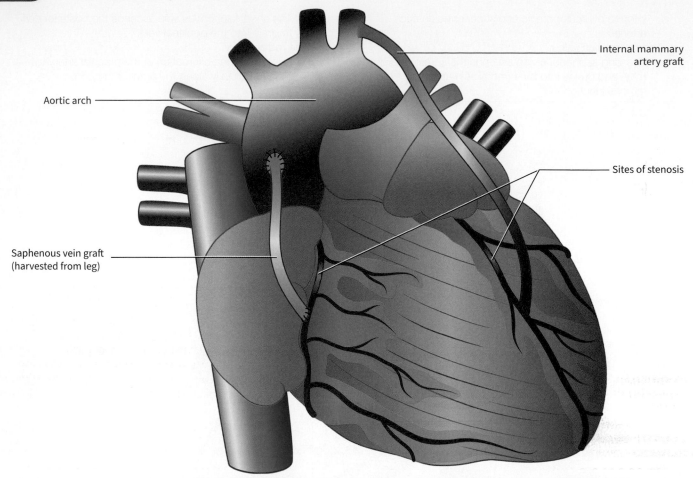

Aortic arch

Internal mammary artery graft

Sites of stenosis

Saphenous vein graft (harvested from leg)

Internal mammary artery bypass graft for stenosis of the left anterior descending and a saphenous vein bypass graft for stenosis of the right coronary artery.

Complications

EARLY

- Death.
- Neurological complications --stroke or transient ischaemic attack, delirium, cognitive decline, neuropsychiatric abnormalities, peripheral neuropathy (uncommon).
- MI (uncommon).
- Bleeding, which may warrant reoperation or transfusion.
- Acute kidney injury, sometimes requiring dialysis.
- Pleural effusion—may require drainage with an intercostal catheter.
- Arrhythmia, including atrial fibrillation (very common).
- Aortic dissection.
- Pericardial effusion and tamponade.

INTERMEDIATE AND LATE

- Deep sternal wound infection and mediastinitis.
- Leg wound complications—dermatitis, cellulitis, ulcers, greater saphenous neuropathy.
- Radial artery harvest can result in a self-limiting numbness and tingling in the distal forearm.
- Graft restenosis—more common in venous grafts.

Postoperative Care

INPATIENT

- The patient usually spends less than 24 hours on intensive care if no complications occur.
- The patient will be started on lifelong antiplatelets, statins, and blood pressure therapy to prevent the progression of ischaemic heart disease.

OUTPATIENT

- Cardiac rehabilitation—exercise, reducing risk factors, and dealing with emotional sequelae.
- Regular cardiology outpatient appointments with transthoracic echocardiograms.

Surgeon's Favourite Question

Why does aortic manipulation during the conduct of CPB result in complications?

Patients requiring CABG have atherosclerotic disease that also affects major vessels such as the aorta. Any underlying atheroma (calcified/noncalcified) along the ascending aorta has the potential when manipulated to lead to stroke or distal embolisation.

Aortic Valve Replacement/Repair

66

Charles Jenkinson

Definition

Surgical repair of a stenosed or regurgitating aortic valve or replacement with either a prosthetic or a biological valve.

Indications and Contraindications

INDICATIONS

- Symptomatic severe aortic stenosis (AS) or severe aortic regurgitation (AR).
- Asymptomatic patients with severe AS or AR and:
  - Require cardiac artery bypass graft surgery.
  - Having surgery on the aorta or other heart valves.
  - A left ventricular ejection fraction <50%.
  - An abnormal exercise test showing symptoms/signs attributed to AS.
  - Very severe aortic stenosis.
- Severe AR with left ventricular (LV) dilatation.
- Infective endocarditis resulting in a nonfunctioning valve—repair versus replacement depends on extent of valve disease.
- Indications for mechanical versus biological:
  - A bioprosthetic valve is made from either bovine (cow) pericardium, or porcine (pig) heart valves. These do not last as long as their mechanical counterparts, so they are often chosen in the elderly or in active individuals for whom lifelong anticoagulation is not an option for their lifestyle.
  - Modern mechanical valves are made of bileaflet discs of pyrolytic carbon that rotate to open or close with the flow of blood. There are no longer any valves made of metal in routine clinical use, so the term "metallic valve" should be avoided.

CONTRAINDICATIONS

- Asymptomatic patients with normal LV function.
- Patients who are unfit for surgery should be considered for:
  - Transcatheter aortic valve implantation (TAVI) – an endovascular technique used to replace aortic valves. This is becoming more common, and in lower risk patients as the technology continues to mature.
  - Aortic valve balloon angioplasty, where a balloon is blown up to open a stenosed aortic valve. This technique can also be used as a bridge to treatment in high risk patients when the LV has been impaired by longstanding aortic stenosis.

Anatomy

- The heart consists of four valves. The mitral (bicuspid) and tricuspid valves are atrioventricular valves. The aortic and pulmonary valves are classed as semilunar valves.

THE ATRIOVENTRICULAR VALVES

- Consist of two or three leaflets that open during diastole to allow blood flow into the ventricle and close to prevent the backflow of blood during systole.
- Papillary muscles are anchored to the ventricular walls. Chordae tendineae (fibrous cords) connect the papillary muscles to the valve leaflets. During systole, these structures prevent the atrioventricular valve leaflets from prolapsing into the atrium, thus ensuring valve closure and competence.

THE SEMILUNAR VALVES

- The semilunar valves sit at the base of the aorta and the pulmonary trunk. They open during systole to allow the flow of blood from the ventricles into their respective vessels; during diastole, the cusps meet to prevent the backflow of blood.
- The semilunar valves comprise three half-moon (hence 'semilunar') cusps.

THE AORTIC VALVE

- The left and right cusps contain the left and right aortic sinuses from which the coronary arteries derive, and a non-coronary sinus with no derivations.
- At the base of the aortic valve is a fibrous ring (a continuation of the cardiac skeleton). This structure may calcify with age, and calcification of the leaflets may impair their mobility, and/or cause restriction to blood flow.
- Around 2% of the population have a bicuspid (two-cusp) aortic valve, which has an increased risk of becoming stenosed at a much younger age, and is also associated with ascending aortic aneurysm.

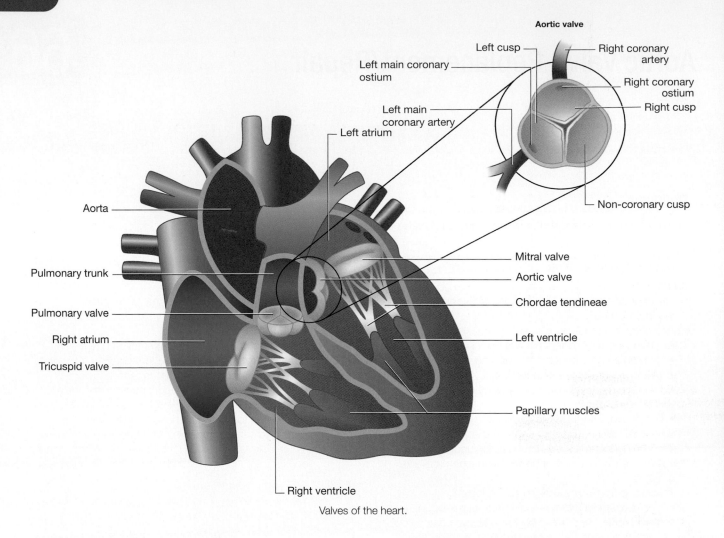

Aortic valve

Left cusp — Right coronary artery

Left main coronary ostium

Left main coronary artery — Right coronary ostium — Right cusp

Left atrium

Aorta

Pulmonary trunk

Pulmonary valve

Right atrium

Tricuspid valve

Mitral valve

Aortic valve

Chordae tendineae

Left ventricle

Papillary muscles

Non-coronary cusp

Right ventricle

Valves of the heart.

STEP-BY-STEP OPERATION

Anaesthesia: general.
Position: supine.
Considerations: The use of intraoperative transoesophageal echocardiography (TOE) is commonplace.
Steps:

1. An incision is made in the midline of the chest, and the sternum is split using a sternal saw (median sternotomy).
2. CPB is then established, directing the circulation through the bypass machine, which includes an oxygenation membrane and heat exchange pump. Heparin is given to prevent clot formation within the CPB machine.
3. A cross-clamp is applied to the ascending aorta, and cardioplegia (usually a potassium-enriched solution) is administered, causing the heart to stop beating.
4. Using a transverse incision from its root, the aorta is dissected, and the diseased valve is excised.
5. For replacement of the aortic valve due to calcification, the valve annulus is first decalcified and then the replacement valve is sewn in the annulus using a parachute technique.
6. Once the replacement or repair is complete, the aorta is closed using a nonabsorbable suture. TOE is commonly used to ensure no paravalvular leak.
7. The heart is restarted by removing the cross-clamp, allowing the cardioplegia to be washed out of the myocardium. The patient is slowly weaned off bypass following rewarming, and removal of air from the chambers of the heart.
8. The sternum is commonly closed using sternal wires, and then the soft tissues of the chest are closed in layers.

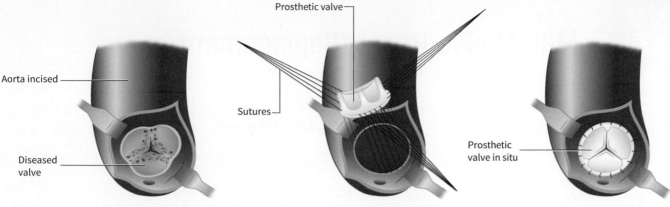

Replacement of a stenosed aortic valve.

 ## Complications

EARLY

- Death.
- Stroke or transient ischaemic attack.
- Bleeding, including requirement for transfusion.
- Infection, including deep sternal wound infection.
- Kidney failure (potentially requiring dialysis).
- Heart block due to the proximity of the conduction system, which may require a permanent pacemaker.
- Atrial fibrillation.

INTERMEDIATE AND LATE

- Endocarditis—occurrence of fever and a new murmur in a patient who has undergone valve replacement surgery is endocarditis until proven otherwise.
- Embolism or haemolysis—more common with mechanical valves.
- Structural valve deterioration—biological valves are prone to 'wearing out', especially in younger patients.

Postoperative Care

INPATIENT

- Intensive care for 24 hours if no other complications arise.
- Total hospital stay of 5–7 days.
- Transthoracic echocardiogram is often performed prior to discharge to ensure valve is functioning adequately.

OUTPATIENT

- Strenuous activities, including driving and full-time work, should be delayed until 4–6 weeks postoperatively to allow for the sternum to heal.
- Patients with mechanical valves will need lifelong anticoagulation with warfarin.
- Patients with biological heart valve replacements do not need lifelong anticoagulation and should be provided with warfarin for 3 months, then low dose aspirin once daily lifelong.
- Outpatient follow-up usually at 6 weeks to examine wounds and check medications.
- Yearly follow-up appointments if asymptomatic and have normal cardiac function.
- Antibiotic prophylaxis is required should the patient require dental or other invasive treatments.

Surgeon's Favourite Question

What is a commonly associated pathology with a bicuspid aortic valve?

Ascending aorta dilatation as part of bicuspid aortic valve aortopathy. This can occur due to either a biomechanical or connective tissue disorder mechanism. In patients with an aortic dimension >55 mm, or perhaps lower in the presence of high risk features (or during concomitant cardiac surgery), an aortic root replacement will be considered to prevent the risk of aortic dissection.

67

Mitral Valve Repair/Replacement

Charles Jenkinson

Definition

Surgical repair or replacement of the mitral valve due to severe stenosis (MS) or regurgitation (MR).

Indications and Contraindications

INDICATIONS

- Severe mitral stenosis (mitral valve area ≤1.5 cm^2) AND:
- Severe symptomatic mitral regurgitation
  - Surgery is indicated in asymptomatic patients with severe mitral regurgitation in the setting of:
    - Impaired LV function
    - LV dilatation
    - Pulmonary hypertension
    - New onset arrhythmia (i.e. atrial fibrillation)
  - Patient undergoing other cardiac surgery or cardio-pulmonary bypass for other indications
  - Asymptomatic, with high likelihood of achieving a durable repair
- Mitral valve repair is favoured over mitral valve replacement, where technically feasible. Complex pathology, especially severe rheumatic disease with calcified leaflets, may necessitate replacement over repair.
- Indications for mechanical versus biological replacement:
  - A bioprosthetic valve is made from either bovine (cow) pericardium, or porcine (pig) heart valves. These do not last as long as their mechanical counterparts, so they are often chosen in the elderly or in active individuals for whom lifelong anticoagulation is not an option for their lifestyle.
  - Modern mechanical valves are made of bileaflet discs of pyrolytic carbon that rotate to open or close with the flow of blood. There are no longer any valves made of metal in routine clinical use, so the term "metallic valve" should be avoided.
- In severe rheumatic disease or calcified valve leaflets, replacement is often preferred over repair.

CONTRAINDICATION

- In rheumatic mitral stenosis, percutaneous mitral balloon valvotomy is preferred when there is favourable valve morphology, at most mild regurgitation, and no left atrial thrombosis.
- Patients with significant comorbidities or frailty who are not operative candidates.

Anatomy

- The heart consists of four valves. The mitral (bicuspid) and tricuspid valves are atrioventricular valves. The aortic and pulmonary valves are classed as semilunar valves.

THE SEMILUNAR VALVES

- The semilunar valves sit at the base of the aorta and the pulmonary trunk. During systole, they allow the flow of blood from the ventricles into their respective vessels; during diastole, the cusps meet to prevent the backflow of blood.
- The semilunar valves comprise three half-moon (hence 'semilunar') cusps.

THE MITRAL VALVE

- The mitral valve serves as the conduit for blood flowing from the left atrium to the left ventricle.
- The valve has two leaflets that are anchored to a fibrous annulus, and there is a commissure on each side between the leaflets. During diastole, the valves allow the free flow of blood in one direction. During systole, the two leaflets come together to prevent the backflow of blood into the left atrium.
- Papillary muscles anchored to the ventricular walls are connected to chordae tendineae, prevent prolapse of the valve leaflets during systole. The high tensile strength of the chordae tendineae means that the valves remain shut against the flow of blood.

PATHOLOGY

- Mitral regurgitation is most commonly caused by a valve which prolapses into the left atrium during systole. This regurgitation occurs due to reasons including myxomatous degeneration of the valve, rupture of chordae tendineae, infection, or changes to the annulus geometry.
- Mitral stenosis is often secondary to rheumatic heart disease. This is becoming less common in high income countries, due to reduced rates of Streptococcus pyogenes (Group A) infections.

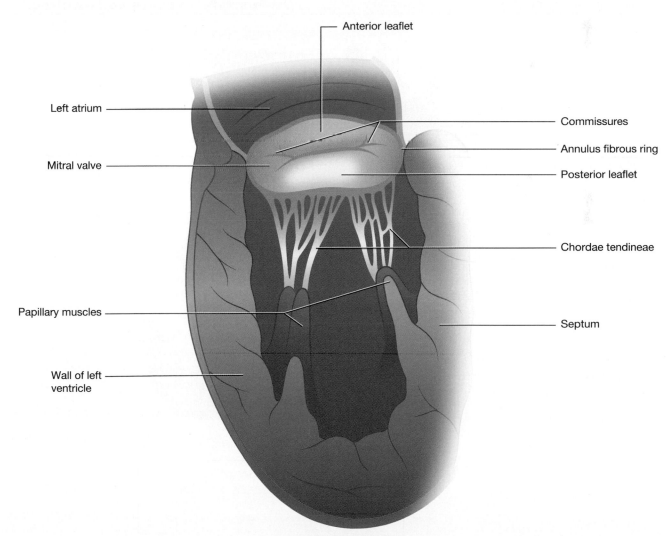

Anatomy of the mitral valve.

123 STEP-BY-STEP OPERATION

Anaesthesia: general.

Position: supine.

Considerations: The use of intraoperative transoesophageal ECHO (TOE) is commonplace.

Steps:

1. Using either a median sternotomy or a minimally invasive approach (right-sided anterior thoracotomy incision through the fourth intercostal space), the thoracic cavity is opened.
2. CPB is then established, directing the circulation through the bypass machine, which includes an oxygenation membrane and heat exchange pump. Heparin is given to prevent clot formation within the CPB machine.
3. A cross-clamp is applied to the ascending aorta, and cardioplegia (usually a potassium-enriched solution) is administered, causing the heart to stop beating.
4. There are various ways to approach the mitral valve, but a common one is to dissect the interatrial septum in the groove between the left and right atria, and then incise the left atrium.
5. Where feasible, the valve is repaired:
   a. Artificial chordae can be placed to improve valve coaptation.
   b. Excessive leaflet tissue resulting in prolapse can be resected.
   c. Loss of leaflet volume can be corrected using a patch of pericardium.
   d. Fusion of leaflets can be repaired by commissurotomy, where the junctions between leaflets are incised.
   e. An annuloplasty (a stiff prosthetic ring) is sutured into the circumference of the annulus to improve geometry and improve stability of the valve.
6. Where repair of the valve is not possible, it is replaced with a mechanical or bioprosthetic valve. TOE is commonly used to ensure no paravalvular leak.
7. The heart is restarted by removing the cross-clamp, allowing the cardioplegia to be washed out of the myocardium. The patient is slowly weaned off bypass following rewarming, and removal of air from the chambers of the heart.
8. The sternum is commonly closed using sternal wires, and then the soft tissues of the chest are closed in layers.

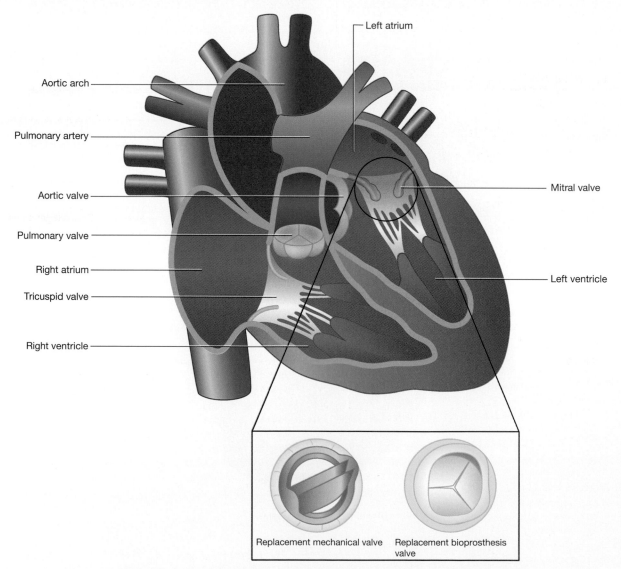

Replacement of a diseased mitral valve with either a mechanical or bioprosthesis valve.

Complications

EARLY

- Death.
- Stroke or transient ischaemic attack.
- Bleeding, including requirement for transfusion.
- Infection, including deep sternal wound infection.
- Kidney failure (potentially requiring dialysis).
- Heart block due to the proximity of the conduction system, which may require a permanent pacemaker.
- Atrial fibrillation
- Systolic anterior motion (SAM), the dynamic anterior movement of the mitral valve towards the interventricular septum that creates left ventricular outflow obstruction. This can lead to haemodynamic instability and intractable hypotension (requires medical therapy or prompt surgical revision).

INTERMEDIATE AND LATE

- Endocarditis—fever and a new murmur in a patient having undergone valve replacement surgery is endocarditis until proven otherwise.
- Embolism or haemolysis—more common with prosthetic valves.
- Deep sternal wound infections.
- Paravalvular leak.
- Graft failure—biological valves are prone to 'wearing out', especially in younger patients.
- Mortality.

Postoperative Care

INPATIENT

- Intensive care for 24 hours if no other complications arise.
- Total hospital stay of 5–7 days.

OUTPATIENT

- Strenuous activities, including driving and full-time work, should be delayed until 4–6 weeks postoperatively to allow for the sternum to heal.
- Patients with mechanical valves will need lifelong anticoagulation with warfarin and international normalised ratio (INR) monitoring.
- Patients with bioprosthetic heart valve replacements do not need lifelong anticoagulation and should be provided with warfarin for three months, then low dose aspirin lifelong.
- Outpatient follow-up usually at 6 weeks to examine wounds and check medications.
- Antibiotic prophylaxis is required should the patient require dental treatment.

? Surgeon's Favourite Questions

What is the functional classification of mitral valve regurgitation?

Carpentier's classification:

Type 1: Normal leaflet motion. [Note: A perforated valve, i.e.: infective endocarditis, may also be Type 1.]

Type 2: Excess leaflet motion (prolapse).

Type 3: Restricted leaflet motion (either restricted opening or closing motion).

This classification is important in identifying the exact pathology to help plan the surgery.

68

Thoracoscopic Pulmonary Lobectomy

Charles Jenkinson

Definition

The surgical removal of a lobe of a lung.

 Indications and Contraindications

INDICATIONS
- Lung cancer—primary (non–small cell lung cancer, large cell lung cancer, carcinoid) or metastatic, which is confined to one lobe.
- Bronchiectasis, chronic obstructive pulmonary disease (COPD), or a fungal infection, which is confined to a single lobe and is not responding to initial medical management.
- Rare indications:
  - Congenital cystic adenomatoid malformation (CCAM).
  - Uncontrollable bleeding (e.g. trauma).
  - Infarction.
  - Abscess.

CONTRAINDICATIONS
Relative
- Inadequate cardiopulmonary reserve—e.g. a predicted post-operative FEV1 of <60% or reduced diffusing capacity of the lung for carbon monoxide.

Absolute
- Tumours with distant metastases (Stage IV).
- High grade tumours, or tumours invading the chest wall or other structures (Stage IIIb+) - usually treated with chemotherapy and/or radiotherapy.

Anatomy

GROSS ANATOMY
- The right lung is composed of upper, middle, and lower lobes, while the left lung only consists of upper and lower lobes.
- The middle and lower lobes of the right lung are separated by the oblique fissure, which begins anteriorly in the sixth intercostal space at the costochondral junction and curves to end at the third thoracic vertebra.
- The upper and middle lobes of the right lung are separated by the horizontal fissure, which is at the level of the fourth intercostal space and meets the oblique fissure at the midaxillary line.
- The left lung is divided into the upper and lower lobes by the oblique fissure.

NEUROVASCULATURE
- The phrenic nerve descends through the thoracic cavity, immediately anterior to the hilum of the lung, to reach the diaphragm.
- Each lobe contains a hilum, the point of entry for the blood vessels and bronchus.
- Each lung has one pulmonary artery that branches to give lobar arteries. These lobar arteries then divide further into segmental arteries.
- Capillaries converge to form progressively larger veins. These eventually form the four pulmonary veins that drain back to the left atrium.
- The lung drains into the superficial and deep lymphatic plexuses. These plexuses converge to the bronchopulmonary nodes, located in the hilum, which then continue to the bronchomediastinal trunks and into the junction of the internal jugular and subclavian veins.

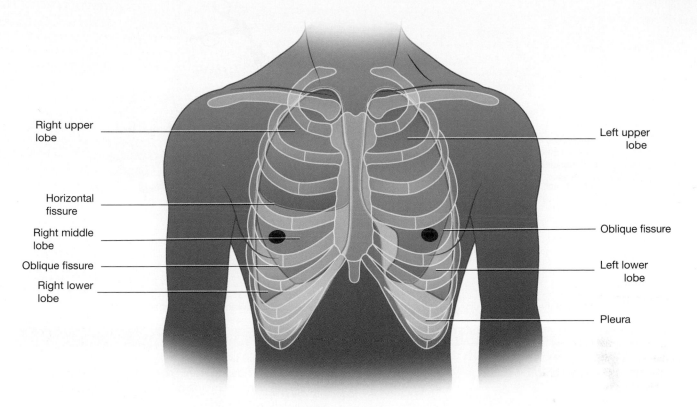

Lobes of the lungs.

123 STEP-BY-STEP OPERATION

Anaesthesia: general, with single-lung ventilation, using a double-lumen endotracheal tube, which allows for one lung to be deflated.

Position: either the left or right lateral decubitus position.

Considerations: Lobectomy can be performed as either an open approach or through video-assisted thoracoscopic approach (VATS), as described in the following.

Steps:

1. A large incision is made for the 'utility port'. When removing the lower lobes, the port is above the inferior pulmonary vein. For upper and middle lobes, the incision is above the superior pulmonary vein.

2. The thoracoscope is inserted through an incision into the seventh intercostal space in the anterior axillary line. Anterior and posterior ports are created for instruments.

3. The hilar lymph nodes are then either completely dissected with a complete mediastinal lymph node dissection (CMLND) or the sentinel lymph node is biopsied.

4. The lung is retracted to expose the hilum. Care is taken to identify the phrenic nerve.

5. The pulmonary vein is identified, dissected and stapled. The pleura within the fissure is then dissected so that the pulmonary arteries are exposed. The pulmonary arteries are dissected until the appropriate branches are identified. These branches are freed and stapled, which also allows for greater visualisation of the bronchus.

6. The bronchus is stapled and divided, after test-inflating the remaining lobes to ensure that they are not compromised by the planned point of resection.

7. Staples are placed along the line of the fissure until the lobe is completely freed.

8. The lobe is then placed in a drawstring bag and removed through the utility port.

9. An 'air' test is performed by the anaesthetist, wherein the remaining lung is inflated to check for air leaks.

10. To complete the procedure, chest drains are inserted, the muscle layers are approximated, and the incision is closed in layers.

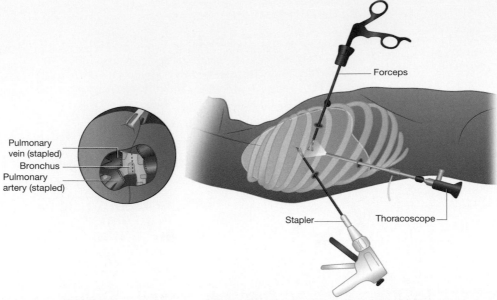

Stapling of the pulmonary vein, artery, and bronchus during a video-assisted thoracoscopic approach lobectomy.

Complications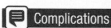

EARLY

- Arrhythmias—atrial fibrillation/flutter.
- Chyle leak.
- Atelectasis.
- Respiratory failure.
- Intercostal nerve damage which may lead to chronic pain (post-thoracotomy syndrome)
- Conversion to pneumonectomy may occur if the lung cancer spread is too great and the cancer resection margins involve the major vessels of the heart.
- Lobar torsion is a rare complication and occurs because of the increased space within the thorax. The remaining lobe(s) twists, causing decreased venous drainage, requiring an emergency thoracotomy to untwist the lobe.
- Prolonged, >7 days, postoperative air leak.
- Pneumonia.
- Empyema.
- Surgical site infection.
- Bronchopleural fistula. This presents the same symptoms as a pneumothorax and results in prolonged chest drain insertion.

INTERMEDIATE AND LATE

- Recurrence of cancer – this risk is reduced by administering adjuvant chemotherapy in tumours pathologically staged at T2a or greater.

Postoperative Care

INPATIENT

- Pain control can be administered by a regional catheter or patient-controlled analgesia.
- Postoperative chest X-ray is used to confirm that there is no pneumothorax.
- The chest drain should be removed 24–48 hours postoperatively.
- The patient is usually discharged 3–5 days postoperatively.

OUTPATIENT

- Follow-up depends upon the indication for resection, but for cancers, surveillance follow-up with history, examination, chest X-ray (CXR), and/or CT every 6 months for first two years, and then annually for the next 5 years for most types of tumour.

Surgeon's Favourite Questions

Is a rising fluid level within the pleural space of the resected lobe, as seen on a postoperative CXR, acceptable?

This is not acceptable within the context of a lobectomy, as it may suggest the development of a chyle leak (especially if it occurs in the very early post-operative period), or an empyema (infection within the pleural space). These two conditions may require further surgical management. A rising fluid level is an expected finding after a pneumonectomy.

Percutaneous Patent Foramen Ovale Repair

69

Charles Jenkinson

Definition

The closure of a patent foramen ovale (PFO) by a percutaneous approach.

 Indications and Contraindications

INDICATIONS
- Cyanosis in a newborn caused by a PFO.
- Stroke risk reduction secondary to a PFO.
- Migraines caused by a PFO.

CONTRAINDICATIONS
- Eisenmenger's syndrome—a PFO enlarges over time, leading to pulmonary hypertension that causes the reversal of flow of blood through the shunt and subsequent cyanosis. Closure of the PFO is not curative.
- In patients >60 years old with stroke due to PFO (antiplatelet therapy is preferred).
- Presence of IVC filter.
- Coagulopathy.
- Use of long-term anticoagulants for other reasons.
- Vascular, cardiac, or PFO anatomy unsuitable for device placement.

Anatomy

- An atrial septal defect (ASD) is a congenital malformation where the tissue that forms the interatrial septum fails to properly form and thus allows for blood to pass between the left and right atria.
- A PFO is the failure of closure of the foramen ovale after birth.
- In utero, the foramen ovale is an important shunt that is formed during the fourth week of gestation. Its function is to divert semioxygenated blood away from the pulmonary circulation (right atrium) into the systemic circulation (left atrium).
- Following birth, due to the increasing pressure in the left atrium overcoming the pressure in right atrium, the foramen ovale closes.
- Progressively, the septum fuses. In the first years of life, a rounded depression (fossa ovalis) is the only remaining remnant of the foramen ovale.
- In up to 20% of the population, the foramen ovale remains patent throughout life and remains asymptomatic during normal physiological activities.

215

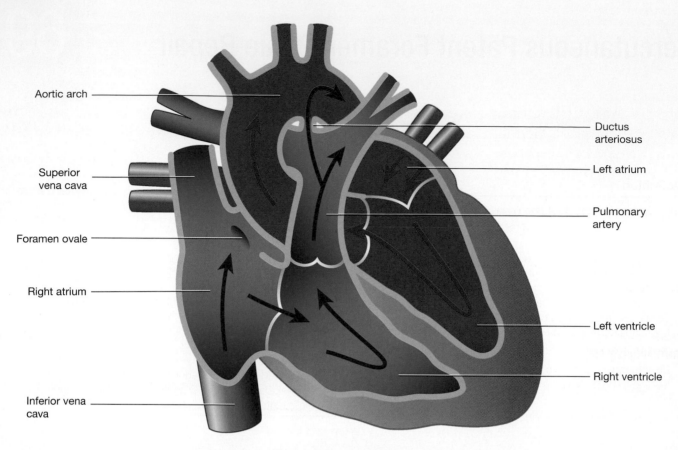

Physiological cardiac shunts.

Aortic arch

Superior
vena cava

Foramen ovale

Right atrium

Inferior vena
cava

Ductus
arteriosus

Left atrium

Pulmonary
artery

Left ventricle

Right ventricle

1 2 3 STEP-BY-STEP OPERATION

Anaesthesia: sedation or general anaesthetic.
Position: supine.
Considerations: Transoesophageal ECHO (TOE) is used to guide the catheter into position.
Steps:

1. A vascular sheath is placed into the femoral vein, and IV heparin is administered.
2. A catheter is inserted into the femoral vein and passed upwards to the IVC.
3. The catheter is then passed into the right atrium and through the PFO into the left atrium.
4. Under ultrasound guidance, a balloon is inflated to grade the size of the PFO.
5. A correctly sized closure device is selected.
6. A guide wire with a large sheath is used to position the occlusion device and is passed up and positioned in the left upper pulmonary vein.

7. The occlusion device contains two self-expandable discs (made from Nitinol wire mesh), which will sit against either side of the septal wall. The guide wire is pulled back, and the left atrial disc opens like an umbrella and sits against the septum. The right atrial disc is expanded in the same way, which fully occludes the septal defect.
8. Throughout the procedure, air must be continuously removed from the catheter to prevent air embolisation.
9. An echocardiogram confirms that the device is positioned correctly. The occlusion device can then be released from the guide wire.
10. The guide wire is removed, and the wound is dressed.

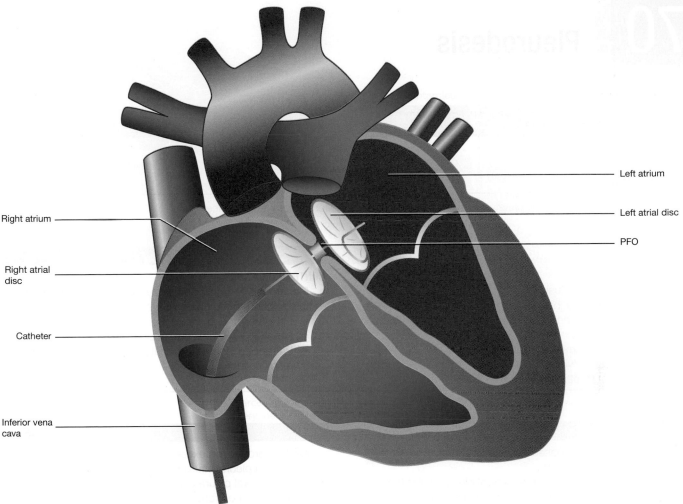

Right atrium

Right atrial disc

Catheter

Inferior vena cava

Left atrium

Left atrial disc

PFO

Deployment and expansion of a patent foramen ovale occlusion device across a patent foramen ovale.

 ## Complications

EARLY
- Air embolism (<5%) can be caused by introduction of air from the catheter and can be identified by ST elevation on ECG.
- Arrhythmias—new-onset atrial fibrillation is most common (4%).
- Cardiac perforation—rare but potentially fatal complication (through tamponade).

INTERMEDIATE AND LATE
- Thrombus formation.
- Device migration, erosion, embolisation, or thrombosis causing recurrent ischaemic stroke.
- Residual shunt on echo (20% of cases), which require further monitoring and follow-up.

Postoperative Care

INPATIENT
- PFO closure can be day-case surgery, but patients usually stay overnight for cardiac monitoring and to have a postoperative echocardiogram.

OUTPATIENT
- Patients usually take dual antiplatelets, aspirin lifelong, and clopidogrel for 3–6 months.
- An echocardiogram is performed after 4 weeks and again after a further 6 months.

? Surgeon's Favourite Questions

What is the difference between an ASD and a PFO?

An ASD is a congenital defect, while a PFO is failure of the foramen ovale to close (i.e. it is not a congenital defect of the heart and is confined to the fossa ovalis). ASDs can be larger and may affect the atrioventricular fibrous skeleton.

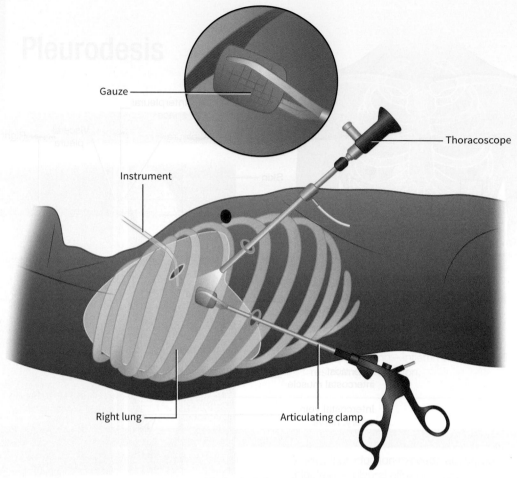

Mechanical pleurodesis.

Complications

EARLY
- Chest pain.
- Fever through mild systemic inflammatory response.
- Tachycardia.
- Hypoxaemia rarely progressing to respiratory failure/acute respiratory distress syndrome.

INTERMEDIATE AND LATE
- Infection (e.g. empyema).
- Cardiac: hypotension, arrhythmias, myocardial infarction.
- Pneumothorax.
- Empyema.
- The pleura can take from a few weeks to a few months to become fully adherent.
- Failure requiring repeat pleurodesis.

Postoperative Care

INPATIENT
- The chest drain is kept in place, often for a minimum of two to three days, and then until there is no air leak, and drainage is less than 200 mL in 24 hours in order to maintain apposition of pleural surfaces.
- Patients are encouraged to mobilise early, as this will lead to lower incidence of chest infections.
- Early discharge is important for patients with malignant pleural effusion, as this group of patients usually have a limited life expectancy, and this therapeutic procedure's main aim is to improve quality of life.

OUTPATIENT
- A follow-up appointment will often be undertaken 4-6 weeks after surgery with a CXR to confirm success of the procedure, and to check wounds.

Surgeon's Favourite Question

What other procedure could be done concurrently with a VATS pleurodesis for a patient with recurrent pneumothoraces?

A bullectomy, which involves stapling off any areas of the lung surface with 'blebs', which are a source of recurrent pneumothoraces, as these are areas of lung wall weakness.

Thoracotomy

Charles Jenkinson

Definition

A surgical procedure to gain access to the pleural space, or structures within the chest: heart, lungs, oesophagus, thoracic aorta, or anterior thoracic spine.

Indications and Contraindications

INDICATION

- Any pulmonary resections, mediastinal operations, or oesophageal operations that are unsuitable to a minimally invasive approach.
- Surgical approach to the posterior mediastinum and vertebral column (e.g. scoliosis surgery or descending thoracic aorta surgery).
- Emergency trauma surgery to manage correctable causes of shock: decompressing cardiac tamponade, managing exsanguinating cardiac or vascular injuries, and evacuating air embolism.
- As a conversion from failure of video-assisted thoracoscopic surgery (VATS).

CONTRAINDICATIONS

- In the context of trauma, thoracotomy is likely to be futile if >10 minutes prehospital CPR, there are no signs of life or massive nonsurvivable injuries.

Anatomy

GROSS ANATOMY

- Thoracotomy can be divided into three different approaches; the choice of approach is based on the aim of surgery being performed:
  - Posterolateral thoracotomy is used to access the posterior mediastinum, lung, and oesophagus.
  - Anterolateral thoracotomy is used for unilateral lung transplant, some heart procedures, or for open chest massage, especially in the setting of trauma.
- Layers of the thoracic wall: subcutaneous tissue, external intercostal muscle, internal intercostal muscle, innermost intercostal muscle, parietal pleura, interpleural space, visceral pleura, and the lung.

NEUROVASCULATURE

- The intercostal neurovascular bundle runs in the costal groove on the inferior border of the rib and contains, from top to bottom, vein, artery, nerve ('VAN'). These structures run deep to the intercostal muscles and are covered by the parietal pleura.
- Muscles of the chest wall
  - Lateral: latissimus dorsi and serratus anterior.
  - Anterior: pectoralis major and minor.
  - Posterior: trapezius, rhomboid major and minor.

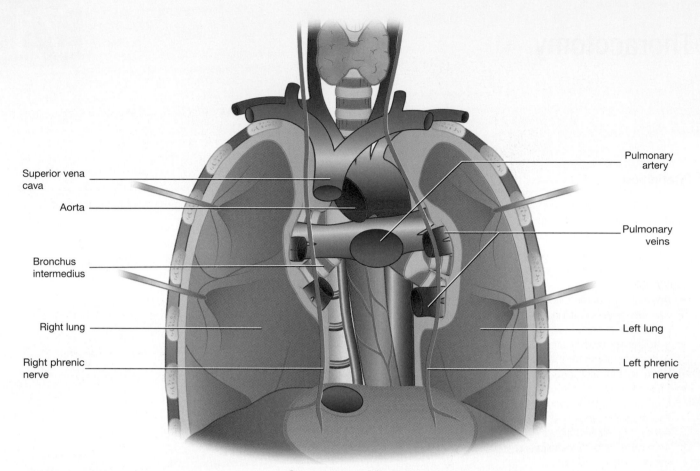

Superior vena cava

Aorta

Bronchus intermedius

Right lung

Right phrenic nerve

Pulmonary artery

Pulmonary veins

Left lung

Left phrenic nerve

Gross anatomy of the thorax.

¹²₃ STEP-BY-STEP OPERATION

Anaesthesia: general, with a double lumen endotracheal tube that allows for one lung to be deflated.

Position: The most common approach is the postero-lateral approach, which requires the lateral decubitus position.

Steps:

1. A skin incision is made from the fifth intercostal space (just below level of nipple) and runs from the anterior axillary line and extends posteriorly to below the tip of the scapula.
2. The incision is continued cranially between the medial border of the scapula and the vertebral spinous processes and continues to the level of the spine of scapula.
3. The latissimus dorsi is divided, and serratus anterior is identified and retracted.
4. To avoid damage to the underlying intercostal neuro-vascular bundle, the intercostal muscles just above the sixth rib are divided.
5. Prior to entering the pleural cavity, the lung is deflated.
6. The intrathoracic procedure of choice is then undertaken.
7. Chest drains are inserted.
8. Muscle layers are approximated, and the wound is closed in layers.

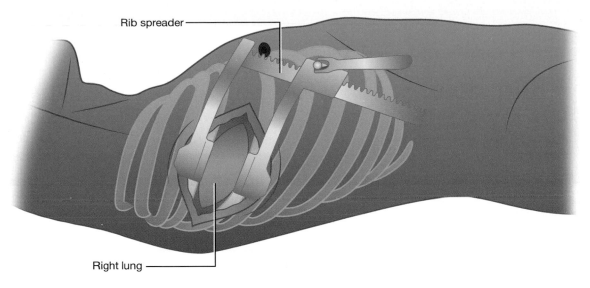

Posterolateral thoracotomy to expose the right lung.

Complications

EARLY
- Atelectasis.
- Respiratory failure.
- Bleeding.

INTERMEDIATE AND LATE
- Pneumothorax (made less common with the placement of a chest drain).
- Infection.
- Arrhythmias.
- Pulmonary oedema.
- Thoracotomy pain syndrome (chronic pain).
- Cardiac herniation (if pericardium disrupted).
- Right heart failure (with extensive lung resection).

Postoperative Care

INPATIENT
- Inpatient course is largely dependent upon indication for thoracotomy and postoperative complications, but generally chest tube management and removal as guided by clinical assessment and/or chest X-rays.
- Regular physiotherapy and early mobility are recommended.

OUTPATIENT
- Specific follow-up and typical duration of hospital stay will be guided based on the indication and type of surgery performed.

Surgeon's Favourite Question

In the lateral decubitus position, poor positioning may lead to shoulder displacement. What are the structures that may be at risk if this occurs?

The brachial plexus (lower four cervical nerves and first thoracic nerve, C5, C6, C7, C8, T1). Injury can cause pain, numbness, weakness, and/or loss of movement in the shoulder, arm, or hand.

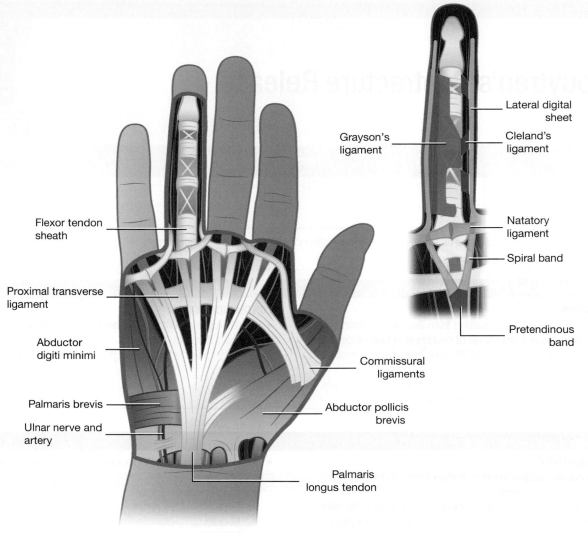

Lateral digital sheet

Grayson's ligament

Cleland's ligament

Natatory ligament

Spiral band

Pretendinous band

Flexor tendon sheath

Proximal transverse ligament

Abductor digiti minimi

Palmaris brevis

Ulnar nerve and artery

Commissural ligaments

Abductor pollicis brevis

Palmaris longus tendon

Components of the palmar aponeurosis.

STEP-BY-STEP OPERATION

Anaesthesia: general or regional.
Position: supine with arm on board with tourniquet.
Steps:

1. Make either a Z-plasty or Brunner incision running down the affected digit and, if affected, into the webspace.
2. Elevate the skin flaps above the central cords; these should be slightly thicker than subdermal.
3. Excise any longitudinal cord tissue.
4. Blunt-dissect the neurovascular bundle away from the central cords all the way to the extent of the distal interphalangeal joint.
5. Now that the cords have been freely dissected, reassess for any further flexion deformity:
   a. Boutonniere deformity of the proximal interphalangeal joint—splint in full extension for 6 weeks.
   b. Volar plate contracture—release the tough ligament tissue with sharp dissection.
6. Assess the perfusion of fingers by releasing the tourniquet. If the finger fails to perfuse:
   a. Blunt-dissect away tissue to directly observe the arteries supplying the affected digits.
   b. Flex the finger to the original position and reassess blood flow.
   c. Bathe the vessel in verapamil or glyceryl trinitrate (GTN) solution and reassess blood flow.
7. Close the Z-plasty or Brunner incision with either absorbable interrupted or continuous sutures.
8. If the wound is unable to be closed, a skin graft is considered or the wound is left open to heal by secondary intention.

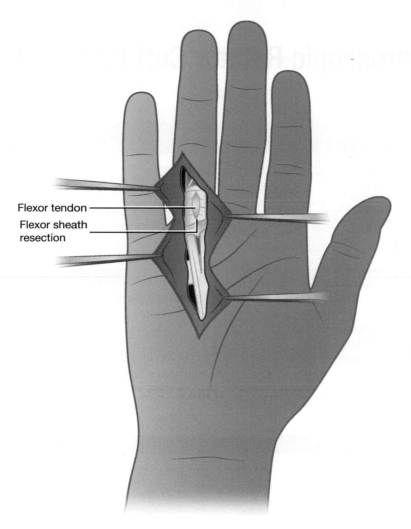

Flexor tendon
Flexor sheath
resection

Excision of longitudinal cord tissue.

Complications

EARLY
- Vascular injury (including those related to the use of a tourniquet).
- Digital nerve injury—paraesthesia of the affected digit.
- Skin loss or failure of flap resulting in requiring a skin graft.
- Local pain (due to digital nerve injury and neuromas).
- Wound infection.

INTERMEDIATE AND LATE
- Recurrence (25%, repeat surgery is often less successful).
- Complex regional pain syndrome (nociceptive sensitisation causing allodynia and vasomotor dysfunction).
- Stiffness and incomplete correction.

Postoperative Care

OUTPATIENT
- Hand should be splinted in full extension for 1 week. Dressings are then removed and hand therapy commenced.
- The affected digit should be splinted in full extension, at night, for 3 months.
- Outpatient follow-up appointment in 6–8 weeks or via hand physiotherapists.

Surgeon's Favourite Question

What patient demographic is commonly affected by idiopathic Dupuytren's?

Dupuytren's disease typically affects elderly men of northern European descent.

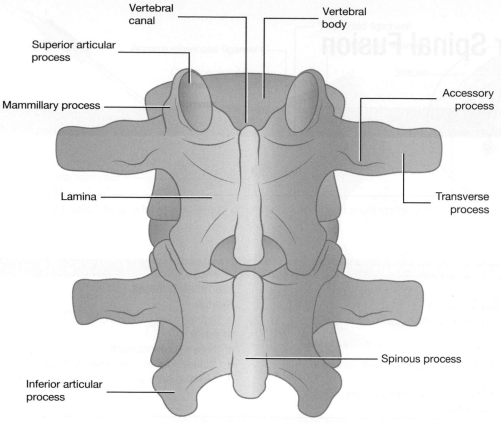

Gross structure of the thoracic vertebra.

Labels (clockwise from top):
- Vertebral canal
- Vertebral body
- Superior articular process
- Accessory process
- Mammillary process
- Transverse process
- Lamina
- Spinous process
- Inferior articular process

1·2·3 STEP-BY-STEP OPERATION

Anaesthesia: general.
Position: prone.
Steps:

1. A 3–4-cm midline incision is made directly over the spinous process running between the paraspinal muscles.
2. The large muscles of the back are retracted, and the lumbar dorsal fascia overlying the spinous processes is cauterised.
3. To create more space to visualise nerve roots, a high-speed burr is used to perform a laminectomy.
4. If needed, a discectomy can be performed to allow for nerve root decompression.
5. For an instrumented fusion, metal plates, screws, or rods can be used to hold two vertebrae until they fuse. Bone grafts may still be inserted into the intervertebral space to further promote fusion.
6. For a noninstrumented fusion, a bone graft is prepared, either allografted (donor bone) or autografted from the patient's iliac crest. This requires a second incision over the site of bone grafting.
7. The prepared bone graft fragments are then packed into the anterior and lateral aspects of the disc space. An inter-body spacer is inserted, and the posterior aspect of the space is sealed with bone graft fragments.
8. Using Floseal (a liquid coagulant), complete haemostasis of the operative site is confirmed. It is vital that this is achieved in order to prevent epidural haematoma formation.
9. The operative site is closed with absorbable sutures—first the lumbar dorsal fascia, then the subcutaneous tissues, followed by the skin.

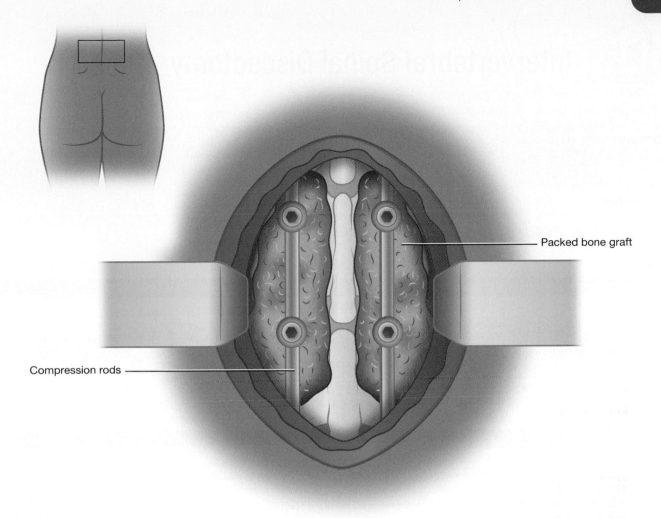

Compression rods and bone graft for lumbar spinal fusion.

Complications

EARLY
- Bleeding and epidural haematoma formation.
- Nerve injury, which may cause leg pain and weakness, saddle anaesthesia, and bladder or bowel dysfunction.
- Paralysis.
- Dural tear and cerebrospinal fluid (CSF) leakage causing orthostatic headache.

INTERMEDIATE AND LATE
- Infection.
- Chronic pain at graft site (10%).
- Osteoarthritis at vertebral joints on either side of fusion due to altered movement and stress.
- Failure to relieve symptoms.

Postoperative Care

INPATIENT
- The patient remains in hospital for 2–3 days.
- Full weight-bearing is encouraged with physiotherapy, which continues for many months.
- Patients need to be counselled about preventing the risks of deep vein thrombosis (DVT), as pharmaceutical thromboprophylaxis is avoided due to the risk of epidural haematoma formation.

OUTPATIENT
- Follow-up appointment 6–8 weeks postoperatively.

Surgeon's Favourite Question

How many vertebrae are there?

The vertebral column consists of 33 vertebrae: 7 cervical, 12 thoracic, 5 lumbar, 5 sacral (fused together), and 4 coccygeal (fused together).

80 Intervertebral Spinal Discectomy

Gareth Rogers

Definition

Debridement and excision of a symptomatic extruded intervertebral disc.

 ## Indications and Contraindications

INDICATIONS
- Cauda equina syndrome (CES) (a surgical emergency).
- Symptomatic intervertebral disc prolapse potentially stenosing the spinal canal/compressing the spinal nerve root.

CONTRAINDICATIONS
Relative
- Clinical signs and radiological findings discrepancy.
- Mechanical (rather than sciatic) back pain.
- Inadequate conservative treatment.

Anatomy

VERTEBRAL COLUMN
- The vertebral column consists of 33 vertebrae: 7 cervical, 12 thoracic, 5 lumbar, 5 sacral (fused together), and 4 coccygeal (fused together). Vertebrae are separated by intervertebral discs.
- The spinal cord runs within the vertebral canal, from the foramen magnum to vertebral level L1/2 (in adults). Below this is the cauda equina, comprising the remaining nerve roots and descending the vertebral canal before exiting at the appropriate level.
- The vertebral column is supported by several ligaments: the anterior and posterior longitudinal ligaments, the ligamenta flava, the interspinous ligaments, and the supraspinous ligament. Running along the vertebral column are the erector spinae muscles.

VERTEBRAE
- Each vertebra can be divided into two sections. The anterior vertebral body functions to bear most of the load. The posterior vertebral arch protects and allows the spinal cord and nerve roots, along with the central vessels, to pass through it.
- The posterior vertebral arch consists of laminae, pedicles, and a spinous process, as well as transverse processes in thoracic vertebrae.
- At each vertebral level, there is an intervertebral foramen located between the inferior vertebral notch of the vertebra above and the superior vertebral notch of the vertebra below. Spinal nerves travel out of these foramina to innervate peripheral structures.
- Between the vertebrae lie the intervertebral discs, consisting of an outer annulus fibrosus and an inner nucleus pulposus. The intervertebral discs are avascular in adults.

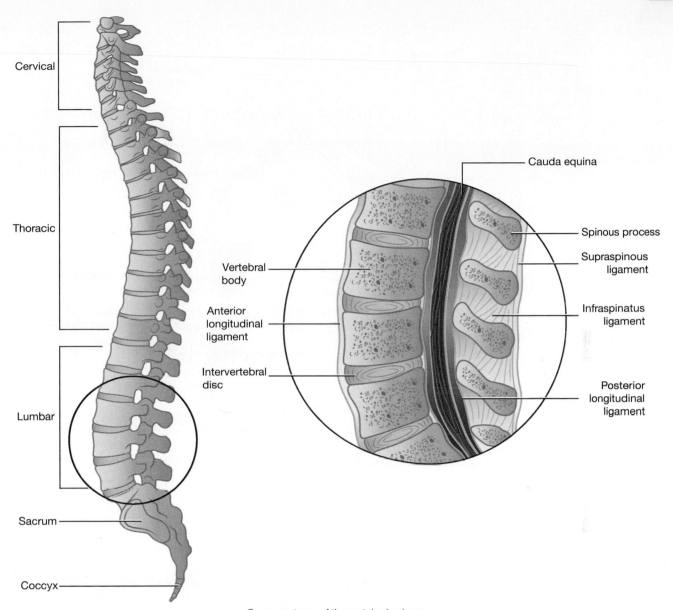

Gross anatomy of the vertebral column.

STEP-BY-STEP OPERATION

Anaesthesia: general. Hypotensive anaesthetic techniques create less venous ooze during the procedure.

Position: knee-to-chest position.

Steps:

1. Intraoperative imaging is used to localise the affected vertebral level.
2. A 6–9-cm incision is made along the line of the spinous processes, through skin, followed by fascia.
3. The spinal muscles running beside the spinous processes are retracted.
4. A high-speed burr is used to perform a laminotomy. This is where the inferior part of the lamina of the vertebra above and the superior part of the lamina of the vertebra below are removed.
5. The ligamentum flavum is removed.
6. The cauda equina/spinal cord needs to be carefully retracted out of the field of view.
7. Through the widened intervertebral foramen, the protruding disc is identified, dissected, and removed using a micrograsper or forceps. It is important that the prolapsed part of the disc is removed completely to avoid recurrence.
8. Absolute haemostasis must be achieved.
9. The wound is washed and closed in layers.

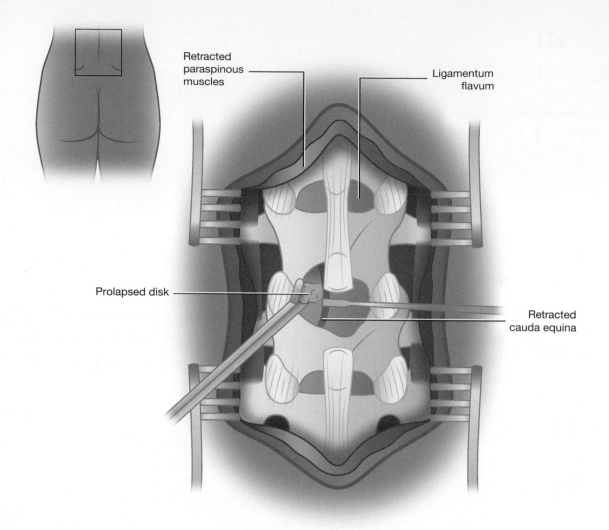

Excision of a prolapsed intervertebral disk.

Complications

EARLY

- Bleeding, which may lead to an epidural haematoma.
- Fracture.
- Nerve root damage, which may result in leg pain and weakness, saddle anaesthesia, and bladder or bowel dysfunction.
- Paralysis.
- Posterior longitudinal ligament injury.
- Wrong level surgery.
- Dural tear and cerebrospinal fluid (CSF) leakage causing orthostatic headache.

INTERMEDIATE AND LATE

- Residual disc prolapse.
- Infection.
- Fibrotic scar tissue formation.
- Recurrent prolapse.

Postoperative Care

INPATIENT

- Pain control via patient-controlled analgesia (PCA).

OUTPATIENT

- Early mobilisation with a specific exercise programme via physiotherapy.
- Dressing change and/or suture removal after 7 days by general practice nurse.
- Follow-up appointment in 4–6 weeks.

Surgeon's Favourite Question

What are the symptoms of CES?

Classically presents with worsening low back and leg pain, leg weakness, saddle anaesthesia (decreased sensation on the inner thighs and buttocks), altered function of the bladder and bowel, and sexual dysfunction.

Total Hip Replacement (THR) via the Posterior Approach

81

Gareth Rogers

Definition

Replacement of the femoral head and acetabulum with a surgical prosthesis.

Indications and Contraindications

INDICATIONS
- End-stage arthritis (inflammatory or degenerative) following failure of conservative and medical interventions.
- Avascular necrosis of the femoral head.
- Patients with an intracapsular neck of femur fracture who are:
  - Mobilising with a single stick or less.
  - Are not cognitively impaired and would be able to follow postoperative total hip replacement (THR) precautions.
- Are medically fit for both the anaesthesia and the procedure.

CONTRAINDICATIONS
Absolute
- Severe dementia or psychiatric disease—unable to comply with hip precautions.
- Systemic infection.

Relative
- Age.
- Obesity.

Anatomy

GROSS ANATOMY
- The hip joint comprises two articulating surfaces: the head of the femur and the acetabulum of the pelvis, which form a stable ball-and-socket synovial joint.
- The articular surfaces are lined by hyaline cartilage.
- The acetabulum:
  - The acetabulum comprises the acetabular fossa, the location for attachment of the ligamentum teres, and the lunate surface, which surrounds the fossa and articulates with the femur.
  - The lunate surface is horseshoe shaped and is open at the inferior aspect, forming the acetabular notch, which houses the transverse acetabular ligament (TAL).
  - The ligamentum teres connects the acetabular fossa to the head of femur at the fovea.
  - The acetabular labrum deepens the acetabulum, enhancing the stability of the joint.

- The joint capsule attaches to the pelvis via the margins of the acetabulum, the transverse ligament, and the margin of the obturator foramen, and to the femur via the intertrochanteric line anteriorly and the intertrochanteric crest posteriorly.

NEUROVASCULATURE
- The hip joint is innervated by branches from the femoral, obturator, and superior gluteal nerves, as well as the nerve to the quadratus femoris.
- Vascular supply to the hip joint arises from the profunda femoris artery via the medial and lateral femoral circumflex arteries (the main supply travelling beneath the capsule).
- The femoral head receives minimal blood supply from the artery of the ligamentum teres, which is not clinically significant.
- Additional arteries supplying the hip joint include the superior and inferior gluteal arteries and the first perforating branch of the deep artery of the thigh.

251

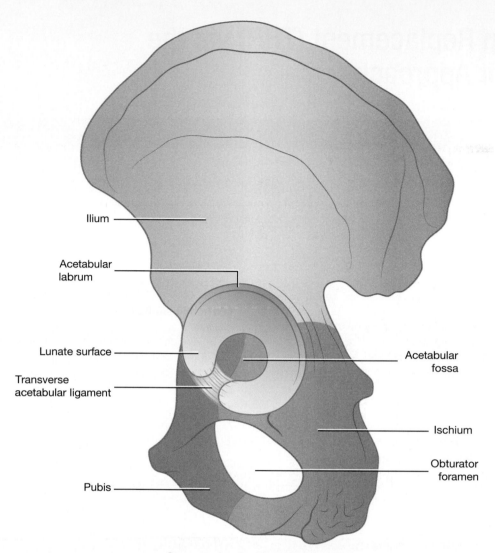

Ilium

Acetabular labrum

Lunate surface

Transverse acetabular ligament

Pubis

Acetabular fossa

Ischium

Obturator foramen

Structures forming the acetabulum.

[123] STEP-BY-STEP OPERATION

Anaesthesia: general or spinal.

Position: lateral position with the affected leg flexed to 90 degrees.

Consideration: Antibiotics and tranexamic acid are administered at induction.

Steps:

1. A 15-cm curved longitudinal incision is made centred over the posterior tip of the greater trochanter extending distally in line with the femur and proximally by 7 cm. The subcutaneous tissue is then incised.

2. A small incision is made into the tensor fascia lata, revealing vastus lateralis and gluteus maximus.

3. The fibres of gluteus maximus are split and haemostasis is observed.

4. The leg is then internally rotated, and stay sutures are placed in the short external rotators (piriformis and obturator internus).

5. The short external rotators are detached from their insertion into the greater trochanter; these are then reflected protecting the sciatic nerve.

6. The joint capsule is palpated, a 'T'-shaped incision is made into the joint capsule, and the hip is then dislocated.

7. An osteotomy is performed to separate the femoral head from the neck of the femur.

8. The acetabulum is prepared with clearance of soft tissue and sequential reaming of the bone. Once prepared, either a cemented or uncemented acetabular cup is sited.

9. The femur is prepared by creating an entry point in the postero-lateral aspect of the femoral canal. The femur is then sequentially reamed and the canal rasped to fit the shape of the implant.

10. A trial is performed with a 'dummy' stem prosthesis to assess stability, range of movement, and leg length. The appropriate size implant (cemented or uncemented) is then implanted.

11. The wound is washed. The deep layer of the external rotators and joint capsule is closed with nonabsorbable sutures, and the superficial subcutaneous tissue is closed with absorbable sutures.

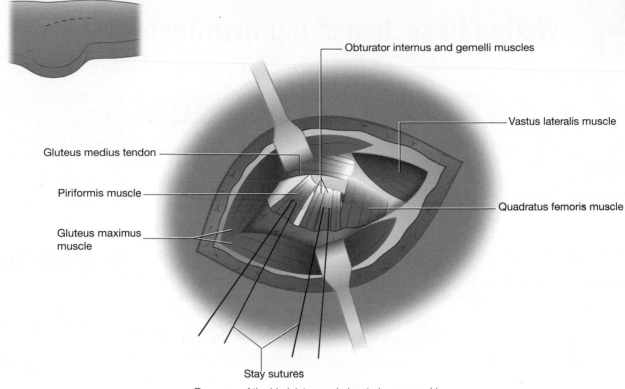

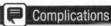

Obturator internus and gemelli muscles

Vastus lateralis muscle

Gluteus medius tendon

Piriformis muscle

Quadratus femoris muscle

Gluteus maximus muscle

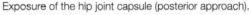

Stay sutures

Exposure of the hip joint capsule (posterior approach).

Complications

EARLY
- Bleeding and haematoma.
- Damage to the sciatic nerve and, less commonly, the femoral nerve.
- Fracturing of the femoral shaft during insertion of the femoral component.

IMMEDIATE AND LATE
- Dislocation (usually within the first 6 weeks).
- Infection of the prosthetic joint or superficial tissues—can be either acute or chronic.
- Loosening (may be due to infection or wear particles).
- Periprosthetic fracture—often due to trauma in elderly patients with osteoporosis.
- Leg length discrepancy.

Postoperative Care

INPATIENT
- Check AP pelvis and lateral of hip X-rays.
- Early mobilisation with weight-bearing status determined by the prosthesis used.
- Hip precautions—avoid crossing legs or excessive flexion of the hips.

OUTPATIENT
- Venous thromboembolic (VTE) prophylaxis for 1 month.
- Follow-up appointment in 6 weeks.

? Surgeon's Favourite Question

What are the classifications of hip replacement?

- Hemiarthroplasties:
  - Cemented
  - Uncemented
- THRs:
  - Cemented
  - Uncemented
  - Hybrid
  - Reverse hybrid

82 Wedge Resection of Ingrown Toenail

Gareth Rogers

Definition

Marginal excision of the nail plate and nail fold to treat an ingrown toenail (onychocryptosis).

Indications and Contraindications

INDICATIONS
- Failure of conservative management.

CONTRAINDICATIONS
- Ingrown toenail on both the lateral and medial sides. Excision on both sides will leave the toenail too thin, and therefore it may be more appropriate to completely remove the toenail (total nail avulsion).
- Active local infection or abscess.

Anatomy

GROSS ANATOMY
- The nail plate is composed of hard, keratinised squamous cells attached to the nail bed inferiorly.
- The nail fold is where the nail plate proximally attaches to the underlying tissues and consists of the dorsal roof superiorly and the ventral floor inferiorly. The ventral floor is the site of the germinal matrix. The germinal matrix is responsible for the majority of nail production.
- The eponychium (cuticle) is the distal portion of the nail fold.
- The paronychium is the soft tissue along the lateral borders of the nail plate.
- The sterile matrix is the distal portion of the nail bed and is tightly adherent to both the overlying nail plate and the underlying periosteum. Along with the dorsal roof, it is a secondary site of nail production.
- The nail plate is loosely attached to the germinal matrix but is densely attached to the sterile matrix.
- Nails grow at roughly 3–4 mm per month (0.1 mm/day).

PATHOLOGY
- Onychocryptosis involves an abnormally wide or incurved nail plate, classically affecting the lateral aspect of the big toe.
- Onychocryptosis causes trauma to the surrounding soft tissue, resulting in pain, inflammation, and/or chronic infection.

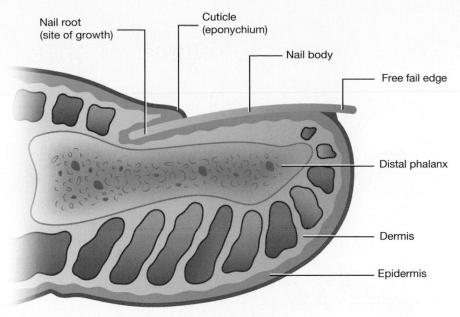

Anatomy of the nail bed.

1 2 3 STEP-BY-STEP OPERATION

Anaesthesia: regional is achieved using a ring block at the base of the toe with 1% lidocaine. Local anaesthetic should not contain adrenaline due to the risk of avascular necrosis.

Position: supine/sitting.

Steps:

1. A tourniquet is wrapped around the base of toe to ensure a bloodless field for optimal visualisation of structures.
2. Blunt dissection is used to separate the nail plate from the surrounding soft tissues.
3. Scissors cut vertically along the depth of the nail plate roughly 3–5 mm parallel to the affected lateral border.
4. The nail plate and the underlying germinal centre are avulsed.
5. An oblique 0.5-cm incision at the base of the nail is made to expose and excise the germinal matrix.
6. Two 1-minute applications of 90% liquid phenol are applied to the exposed nail bed (sterile matrix) and nail fold (germinal matrix). This causes cellular destruction, which prevents nail regrowth (matrixectomy).
7. The operative site is washed with normal saline.
8. The site is dressed with a nonadherent dressing, then gauze, and is secured with tape.

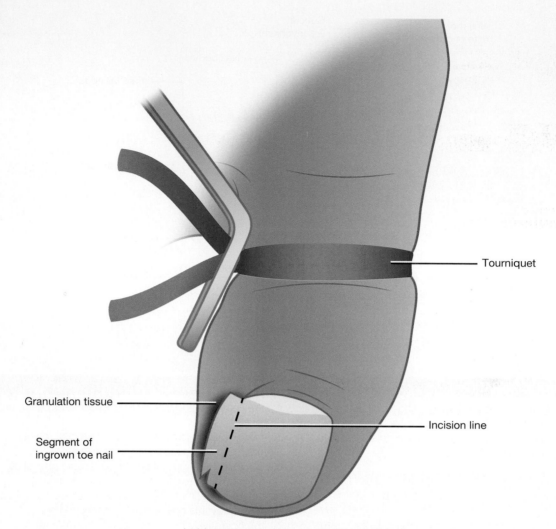

Tourniquet

Granulation tissue

Incision line

Segment of
ingrown toe nail

Incision to expose and excise the germinal matrix.

Complications

EARLY
- Bleeding.
- Pain and discomfort.
- Local skin burns from phenol.

INTERMEDIATE AND LATE
- Recurrence of ingrown toenail.
- Narrower nail.
- Infection.

Postoperative Care

OUTPATIENT
- Dressing removed after 48 hours in clinic. Redressed with simple dressing.
- Review of wound in 2 weeks by a GP nurse.

? Surgeon's Favourite Question

What are the surgical techniques for treatment of ingrown toenails?

Wedge nail resection or total nail avulsion. These can be performed in combination with matrixectomy (removal/destruction of sterile and germinal matrix to prevent nail regrowth).

Carpal Tunnel Decompression

83

Gareth Rogers

Definition

Decompression of the median nerve as it passes through the carpal tunnel of the wrist, by transection of the flexor retinaculum.

Indications and Contraindications

INDICATIONS

- Symptoms of carpal tunnel syndrome (CTS) for >6 months, with failure of conservative management.
- Functional weakness or atrophy of the muscles supplied by the median nerve in the hand.

CONTRAINDICATIONS

- Pregnancy—CTS often resolves spontaneously following delivery.

Anatomy

GROSS ANATOMY

- The flexor retinaculum (a thick layer of connective tissue) is anchored to the scaphoid tuberosity and trapezium on the radial side and then transverses the carpal tunnel to attach to the pisiform bone and hook of hamate on the ulnar side.
- Contents of the carpal tunnel:
  - Four tendons of flexor digitorum superficialis and the four tendons of flexor digitorum profundus (surrounded by a single synovial sheath).
  - Tendon of flexor pollicis longus (surrounded by its own synovial sheath).
  - The median nerve.
- Structures surrounding the carpal tunnel:
  - The tendon of flexor carpi radialis runs within the flexor retinaculum.
  - Superficial to the flexor retinaculum and on the ulnar side of the ventral wrist runs the ulnar artery and nerve.
  - Superficial to the flexor retinaculum and running down the midline of the ventral wrist is the tendon of palmaris longus (absent in 14% of the population).

NEUROVASCULATURE

- Within the forearm the median nerve courses between the muscle bellies of flexor digitorum profundus and flexor digitorum superficialis where two branches are emitted— the anterior interosseus nerve (supplies the deep muscles of the forearm) and the palmer cutaneous nerve (innervation of the skin of the lateral palm).
- After passing into the carpal tunnel, the median nerve branches into the recurrent branch of the median nerve (RBMN) and the palmar digital nerves.
- The RBMN supplies motor innervation to the thenar eminence (opponens pollicis, abductor pollicis brevis, and flexor pollicis brevis).
- The RBMN runs a variable course at risk of damage during surgery and therefore should always be identified prior to the transection of the flexor retinaculum.
- The palmar digital branch of the median nerve is responsible for the innervation of the palmar surface and fingertips of the lateral three and a half digits.

CARDINAL LINES

- Kaplan's cardinal line runs from the apex of the first web space to the ulnar side of the ventral surface of the hand.
- An innominate line runs from the radial border of the ring finger to the wrist crease.

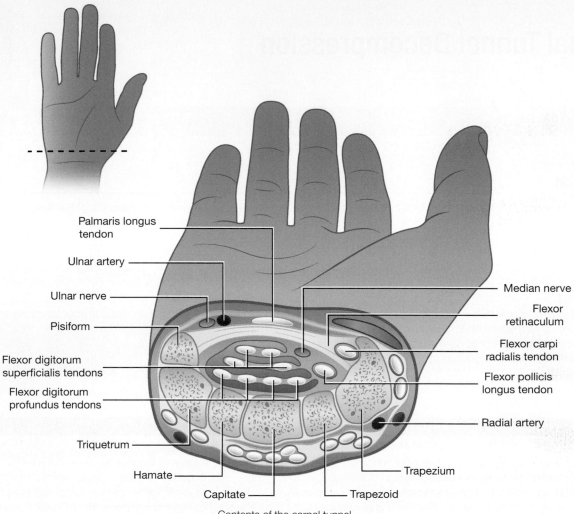

Contents of the carpal tunnel.

Labels (clockwise from upper left):
Palmaris longus tendon
Ulnar artery
Ulnar nerve
Pisiform
Flexor digitorum superficialis tendons
Flexor digitorum profundus tendons
Triquetrum
Hamate
Capitate
Trapezoid
Trapezium
Radial artery
Flexor pollicis longus tendon
Flexor carpi radialis tendon
Flexor retinaculum
Median nerve

①②③ STEP-BY-STEP OPERATION

Anaesthesia: regional block or local anaesthetic infiltration.
Position: supine with the arm rested on an arm board.
Steps:

1. An incision is marked from intersection of Kaplan's cardinal line and the innominate line running from the radial border of the ring finger, to the level of the wrist crease. This site of incision minimises the risk of damage or scarring of the underlying median nerve.
2. The skin is incised and subcutaneous tissue retracted to expose the underlying longitudinal fibres of the palmar fascia.
3. A self-retaining retractor is inserted for exposure, and a scalpel is used to incise the palmar fascia along the full length of the skin incision site.
4. The flexor retinaculum is exposed and inspected for any anatomical variations in the RBMN.
5. Fibres of palmaris brevis are dissected off the flexor retinaculum.
6. A small incision is made through the flexor retinaculum, through which a McDonald retractor is inserted and is used to elevate the flexor retinaculum, separating it from the underlying structures.
7. With the retractor in place, under direct vision, a scalpel is used to dissect the distal segment of the ulnar aspect of the flexor retinaculum (close to the hook of hamate).
8. Tissue scissors are then used to dissect the more proximal segment of the ulnar aspect of the flexor retinaculum.
9. The contents of the carpal tunnel are inspected, and the release of the median nerve is confirmed.
10. Using nonabsorbable sutures, only the skin is closed. A pressure dressing is applied to control haemostasis.

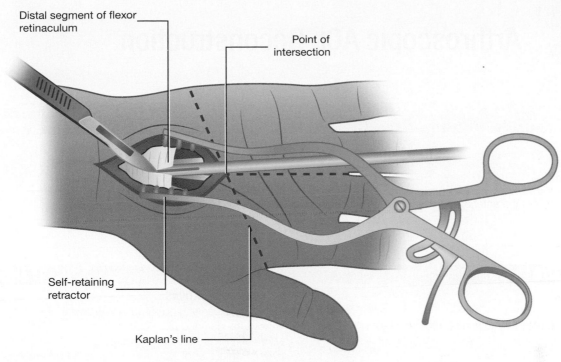

Distal segment of flexor retinaculum

Point of intersection

Self-retaining retractor

Kaplan's line

Dissection of the flexor retinaculum.

Complications

EARLY
- Bleeding.
- Palmar discomfort.

INTERMEDIATE AND LATE
- Infection.
- Excessive fibrosis leading to movement restriction.
- Nerve damage: most commonly affecting the RBMN (which results in thenar wasting), the median nerve itself (loss of flexor grip strength), or, in very rare cases, the ulnar nerve.
- Recurrence of CTS symptoms, either from failure to sufficiently expand the volume of the carpal tunnel or recurrence of pathology.
- Complex regional pain syndrome due to nociceptive sensitisation, resulting in allodynia and vasomotor dysfunction.

Postoperative Care

OUTPATIENT
- Simple analgesia for pain relief.
- Gentle hand therapy exercises to reduce stiffness.
- Remove pressure dressing at 2 days.
- Wound review at 2 weeks in the community by GP nurse.
- No routine outpatient appointment required.

[?] Surgeon's Favourite Questions

Which structure is compressed in CTS, and how does this relate to the typical clinical presentation?

Median nerve—sensory changes in median nerve distribution (thumb, index, and half of the middle finger) and weakness of the LOAF muscles (lateral lumbricals, opponens pollicis, abductor pollicis brevis, and flexor pollicis brevis).

84

Arthroscopic ACL Reconstruction

Gareth Rogers

Definition

Surgical repair of the anterior cruciate ligament (ACL) of the knee, usually following traumatic rupture.

Indications and Contraindications

INDICATIONS

- Unstable knee with ACL tear.
- Multiligament injury to knee ± meniscal tear.

CONTRAINDICATIONS

- ACL tear with no symptomatic instability.
- Low demand or elderly patient.
- Significant arthritis of knee.
- Partial tear of ACL.
- Lack of motivation to complete the long rehabilitation programme.

Anatomy

GROSS ANATOMY

- The knee joint is a hinge-type synovial joint composed of three compartments: the patellofemoral compartment and the medial and lateral femorotibial compartments.
- Ligaments:
  - The knee has four main stabilising ligaments: the anterior and posterior cruciates (ACL and PCL) and the medial and lateral collateral ligaments.
  - The ACL runs from the posterolateral intercondylar eminence of the femur to just anterior to the inter-condyloid eminence of the tibia, blending in with the anterior horn of the medial meniscus.
  - The ACL consists of three bundles: an anteromedial, an intermediate, and a posterolateral. It functions to limit anterior translation and medial rotation of the tibia and posterior translation and lateral rotation of the femur. The overall ligament is fully taut in knee extension. However, some bundles are taut in interme-diate and flexed positions.

NEUROVASCULATURE

- The knee receives sensory and motor innervation from the femoral, sciatic, and obturator nerves.
- The femoral nerve provides musculocutaneous branches to the quadriceps muscles and, distal to the knee, gives off the saphenous nerve.
- The sciatic nerve descends in the posterior compartment of the upper leg, innervating the hamstring muscles. It enters the popliteal fossa and divides into the tibial nerve and the common peroneal nerve.
- The vascular supply to the knee joint is from genicular arteries and branches of the femoral and popliteal arteries.

TENDON GRAFT TYPES

- Autografts: harvested from the patient.
  - Bone-patellar tendon-bone (B-PT-B) graft.
  - Hamstring tendon graft—the tendons of gracilis and semitendinosis.
- Allografts: harvested from a deceased donor:
  - Quadriceps tendon.
  - Achilles tendon.
  - Synthetic grafts.

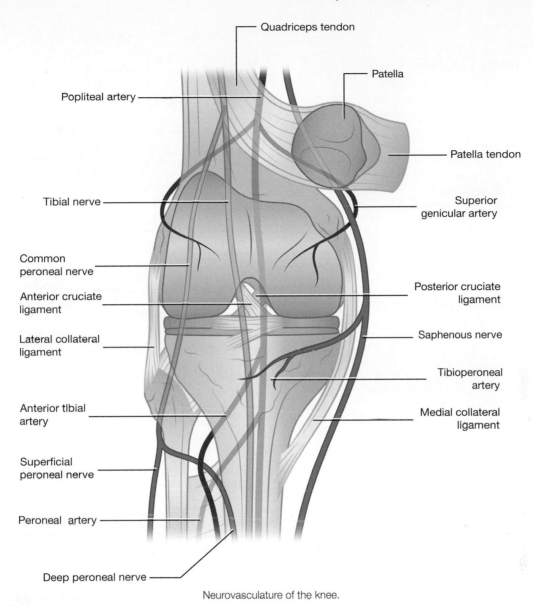

Neurovasculature of the knee.

Labels:
- Quadriceps tendon
- Popliteal artery
- Patella
- Patella tendon
- Tibial nerve
- Superior genicular artery
- Common peroneal nerve
- Posterior cruciate ligament
- Anterior cruciate ligament
- Saphenous nerve
- Lateral collateral ligament
- Tibioperoneal artery
- Anterior tibial artery
- Medial collateral ligament
- Superficial peroneal nerve
- Peroneal artery
- Deep peroneal nerve

1 2 3 STEP-BY-STEP OPERATION

Anaesthesia: general.
Position: supine with a thigh tourniquet and leg held in the flexed position.
Considerations: Intravenous antibiotics.
Steps:

1. Standard arthroscopic portals established anteromedially and anterolaterally.
2. After an evaluation of surrounding structures, a motorised shaver is used to completely remove the remaining ACL alongside the footprint of the ACL insertion into the tibia and femur.
3. For graft harvesting, a 4-cm incision is made either into the posteromedial aspect of the knee (hamstring graft) or anteriorly below the patella (patellar tendon graft). Once harvested, the graft is trimmed to size.
4. Using appropriate instrumentation, tunnels are made in the tibia and femur in the line of the ACL. The tunnel begins in the upper part of the external tibia and exits in the intercondylar eminence at the site of the ACL attachment.
5. To widen the tunnel, a guide pin is inserted and drilled over with a cannulated drill. A guide pin is then drilled into the femoral ACL attachment site. A cannulated drill is used to widen the tunnel.
6. Sutures are passed through the tunnels and are used to pull the prepared graft through the tibial tunnel and the femoral tunnel.
7. The graft is anchored to the femur first and then the tibia under physiological tension with interference screws.
8. The wounds are closed with absorbable sutures with the knee in flexion.
9. A pressure cuff is applied proximal to the operation site for 3 days.
10. A Bledsoe brace is applied for 14 days to control the range of movements.

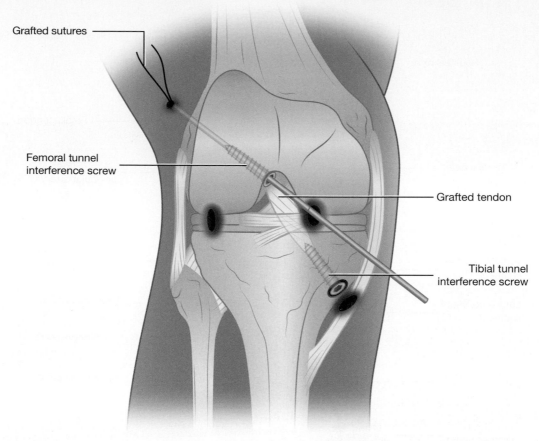

Grafted sutures

Femoral tunnel
interference screw

Grafted tendon

Tibial tunnel
interference screw

Anchoring of an anterior cruciate ligament graft.

Complications

EARLY
- Swelling and stiffness.
- Common fibular and saphenous nerve injury resulting in hypoaesthesia and foot drop. These occur especially if a hamstring from the medial side of the thigh is harvested.
- Numbness.

INTERMEDIATE AND LATE
- Deep vein thrombosis (DVT) or pulmonary embolism (PE).
- Infection.
- The graft tendon may stretch or loosen, which can progressively result in an unstable knee.
- The graft may fail, resulting in an unstable knee (less than 10%) requiring surgical revision.
- Limited range of movement.
- Pain (18% suffer from pain, especially when crouching or kneeling).

Postoperative Care

INPATIENT
- Pain control, elevation, and mobilise full weight-bearing in a brace.

OUTPATIENT
- Dressing change at 2 weeks in general practice.
- Follow-up appointment in 6 weeks.
- A week after surgery, the initial rehabilitation begins (6 weeks). The patient is encouraged to weight bear as much as tolerated. It can take 4–6 months for normal activity to resume.

? Surgeon's Favourite Question

Which tendons are commonly used as grafts for this surgery?

Gracilis, semitendinosus, and patellar tendons.

Total Knee Replacement (TKR)

85

Gareth Rogers

DEFINITION

Replacement of the knee joint with a surgical prosthesis.

Indications and Contraindications

INDICATIONS

- End-stage arthritis (inflammatory or degenerative) following failure of conservative and medical interventions.
- Knee pain and stiffness interfering with quality of life.
- Can be performed as a primary procedure in patients with a nonsalvageable distal femur fracture.
- Post-traumatic non/malunion of a distal femur fracture.

CONTRAINDICATIONS

Absolute
- Systemic infection.
- Septic arthritis.
- Overlying soft tissue infection.

Relative
- Age.
- Obesity.
- Comorbidities.

Anatomy

GROSS ANATOMY

- The knee joint is a hinge-type synovial joint composed of three compartments: the patellofemoral compartment and the medial and lateral femorotibial compartments.
- The knee has four main stabilising ligaments:
  - Anterior cruciate ligament (ACL)—runs from the posterolateral intercondylar eminence of the femur to just anterior to the intercondyloid eminence of the tibia, blending with the anterior horn of the medial meniscus. The ACL consists of three bundles: an anteromedial, an intermediate, and a posterolateral. It functions to limit anterior translation and medial rotation of the tibia and posterior translation and lateral rotation of the femur. The overall ligament is fully taut in knee extension. When taught, it prevents posterior dislocation of the tibia.
  - Posterior cruciate ligament (PCL)—runs from the posterior intercondylar eminence of the tibia and inserts into the anteromedial femoral condyle.
  - Medial collateral ligament—runs from the femoral medial epicondyle inserting into the medial tibial condyle blending with the medial meniscus.
  - Lateral collateral ligament—originates at the lateral femoral epicondyle and inserts into the lateral surface of the head of the fibula.

BIOMECHANICS

- Axis of the native knee:
  - The mechanical axis of the leg runs from the centre of the hip to the centre of the ankle and bisects the centre of the knee.
  - The anatomical of the leg runs through the centre of the long bones of the leg.
  - The anatomical axis of the femur is 6 degrees from the mechanical axis; however, the anatomical axis of the tibia matches its mechanical axis.
  - The joint line is highly variable; however, the tibial articular surface is 3 degrees varus from the mechanical axis and the femoral articular surface is 3 degrees valgus from the mechanical axis.
  - In combination the femoral joint line is in 9 degrees of valgus relative to the anatomic axis (6 degrees from the mechanical axis to anatomical axis and 3 degrees from the mechanical axis to the femoral joint line). For the tibial component, the joint line is 3 degrees of varus relative to the anatomic axis (0 degrees from the tibial anatomical axis to the mechanical axis, and 3 degrees from the mechanical axis to the tibial joint line).
- Mechanical total knee replacement (TKR) alignment:
  - The aim of a mechanically aligned TKR is to restore the normal mechanical axis of the leg and not to restore the anatomical axis of the leg.

PATHOLOGY

- It is the wear of articular surfaces and subsequent loss of joint space, osteophyte formation, subchondral cysts, and sclerosis that demonstrate osteoarthritis on weight-bearing radiographs of the knee.

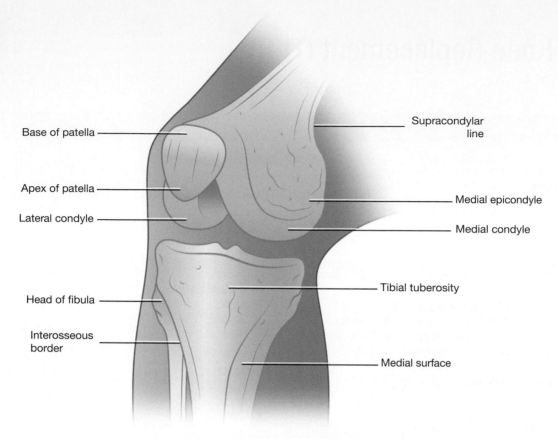

Base of patella

Apex of patella

Lateral condyle

Head of fibula

Interosseous border

Supracondylar line

Medial epicondyle

Medial condyle

Tibial tuberosity

Medial surface

Articulating components of the knee joint.

123 STEP-BY-STEP OPERATION

Anaesthesia: general or spinal.

Position: supine position with the knee flexed in a foot bolster with a side support.

Considerations: Antibiotics and tranexamic acid are administered at induction. A tourniquet may be used.

Steps:

1. For a medial parapatellar approach, a midline incision starting from 2 cm superior to the patella to 1 cm below the tibial tuberosity is made through the skin and down to muscle.

2. The vastus medialis oblique (VMO) is detached from its insertion into the quadriceps tendon and patella. The knee is extended, and the patella is either dislocated laterally or retracted. The knee is then flexed, and the fat pad and the menisci are excised.

3. With the knee flexed and using an extramedullary referencing system, the anatomical/mechanical axis the tibia is identified and the resection guide attached to the proximal tibia and then set to the appropriate amount of tibia to be resected (2–9 mm). Using an oscillating saw, the proximal tibia is resected.

4. With the knee in flexion, to prepare the femur, an intramedullary alignment rod is inserted through a drill hole at the apex of the intercondylar notch and the femoral alignment guide attached and set to 6 degrees.

5. Once aligned, the femoral cutting jig is applied to the alignment guide and the distal femoral resection made.

6. The femoral sizer is applied and set to the appropriate amount of external rotation; once measurements are completed and marked, the jig is removed and the femoral cutting block applied.

7. Using an oscillating saw, the anterior cortex, posterior condyles, the posterior chamfer, and anterior chamfer cuts are made.

8. Trial femur and tibia components are positioned with various sizes inserted, and stability in flexion and extension is assessed.

9. The patella may be resurfaced, trialled with a patella button, and tracking assessed.

10. Once satisfied, the appropriate component sizes are cemented into the prepared surfaces.

11. The wound is washed and closed in layers—first the capsule, followed by the fat and skin. The wound is dressed with a simple dressing and a crepe bandage.

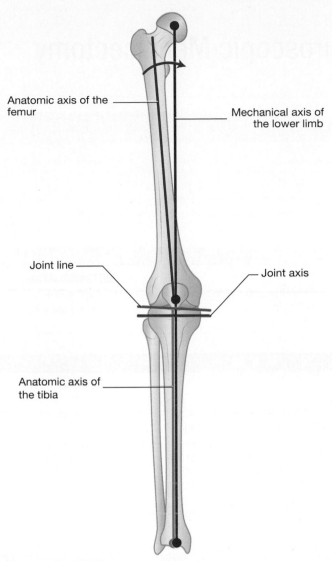

Alignment of the native knee.

Anatomic axis of the femur

Mechanical axis of the lower limb

Joint line

Joint axis

Anatomic axis of the tibia

Complications

EARLY
- Bleeding and haematoma.
- Popliteal artery injury.
- Fracture of the tibia or femur.
- Rupture of patellar tendon.

INTERMEDIATE AND LATE
- Deep vein thrombosis and pulmonary embolus.
- Infection—superficial or deep.
- Loosening, which may be due to infection or wear particles.
- Periprosthetic fracture—often due to trauma in elderly patients with osteoporosis.
- Failure of prosthesis.

Postoperative Care

INPATIENT
- Check antero-posterior and lateral knee radiographs day 1 postoperatively.
- VTE prophylaxis (normally extended for 1 month).
- Early mobilisation.

OUTPATIENT
- Follow-up appointment in 6 weeks.

Surgeon's Favourite Question
What artery can be damaged during the tibial cut?

Popliteal artery.

86

Arthroscopic Meniscectomy

Gareth Rogers

Definition

Arthroscopic-guided trimming of the medial or lateral meniscus of the knee.

Indications and Contraindications

INDICATIONS
- Large or moderate tear in the outer zone of the meniscus.
- Symptomatic meniscal tears causing pain, locking, limited function, or reduced range of movement.

CONTRAINDICATIONS
- Asymptomatic tears.
- Knee joint infection.

Anatomy

GROSS ANATOMY
- Articulations:
  - The tibio-femoral articulation is between the medial and lateral femoral condyles and the corresponding tibial plateaus.
  - The patellofemoral joint is between the patella (a sesamoid bone) and the anterior surface of the femur.
  - The articulation between the tibia and femur forms a synovial filled hinged knee joint.
  - Movements at the knee are flexion, extension, and external rotation.
- Femur:
  - The femoral condyles are separated by an intercondylar fossa—the area of attachment for the anterior and posterior cruciate ligaments.
  - The medial femoral condyle is larger and more circular than the lateral femoral condyle. This difference in size and curvature, which means that during flexion of the knee, the medial femoral condyle stays stationary whilst the lateral femoral condyle rolls back on the tibia (posterior rollback), results in external rotation of the femur on the tibia.
- Tibia:
  - The tibial plateau consists of medial and lateral condyles separated by an intercondylar fossa.
  - The intercondylar region is the site of the menisci and distal attachment of the anterior and posterior cruciate ligaments.
- Patella:
  - A triangular-shaped sesamoid bone located on the anterior aspect of the knee joint and articulating with the femur.
  - At the base of the patella (the most superior aspect) is insertion of the quadriceps tendon which envelopes the patella, and at the apex of the patella is the origin of the patella tendon which inserts onto the tibial tuberosity forming the extensor mechanism of the knee.
- Menisci:
  - The menisci are crescent-shaped fibrocartilaginous structures attached to the intercondylar area of the tibia. The role of the menisci is to improve the congruency of the articulating surfaces whilst functioning as shock absorbers.
  - The menisci are connected anteriorly by the transverse ligament.
  - The medial meniscus is also attached to the medial collateral ligament and to the capsule of the knee joint, decreasing its mobility and increasing its vulnerability to injury.
  - The lateral meniscus is smaller than its medial counterpart and due to its lack of ligamentous attachments is relatively mobile.

NEUROVASCULATURE
- The joint is innervated by the obturator, femoral, tibial, and common fibular nerves.
- The blood supply to the knee joint arises from an anastomosis created by branches of the descending genicular artery (from the femoral artery), popliteal artery, and anterior and posterior tibial arteries.

Pathology
- Commonly present either secondary to sporting injuries in younger athletic patients or to degeneration in older patients.
- Meniscal tears can be classified depending on the location of the tear:
  - Red zone—the outer one-third of the meniscus which is vascularised.
  - Red-white zone—the middle one-third of the meniscus.
  - White zone—the inner one-third of the meniscus which is relatively avascular.
- Meniscal tears can alternatively be classified based on the pattern of tear:
  - Vertical/longitudinal.
  - Bucket handle—a vertical meniscal tear which displaces centrally towards the notch—a common cause of a 'locked' knee.
  - Radial.
  - Horizontal.
  - Root.

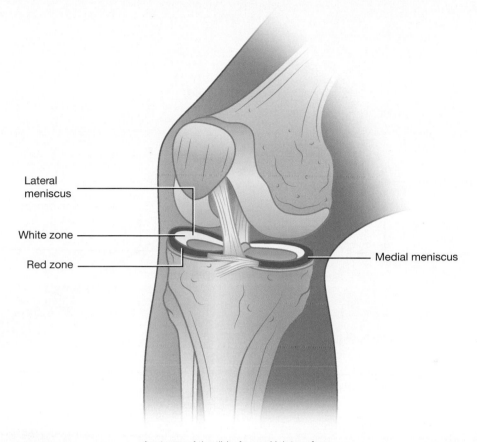

Anatomy of the tibio-femoral joint surface.

Lateral meniscus

White zone

Red zone

Medial meniscus

1/2/3   STEP-BY-STEP OPERATION

Anaesthesia: general or spinal anaesthesia
Position: supine with the thigh and knee flexed.
Considerations: A tourniquet may be used to restrict blood flow and improve the view through the arthroscope.
Steps:

1. For the anterolateral port site, an incision is made lateral to the patella tendon, and inferior to the distal pole of the patella, a port with a trocar is passed through the incision and inserted into the joint space.
2. The arthroscope is then inserted through the anterolateral port and into the medial compartment of the knee; then under direct vision, a hypodermic needle is inserted medial to the patella tendon and inferior to the patella. The needle should be visible in the medial compartment just superior to the level of the medial meniscus.
3. A diagnostic arthroscopy is performed in which the suprapatellar pouch, the under-surface of the patella, trochlear groove, the lateral and medial gutters, the medial compartment, the ACL/PCL, and the lateral compartment are examined.
4. To examine, grade, and prepare the damaged menisci, a probe is inserted through the anteromedial port and is used to probe and pull at the menisci assessing stability.
5. If the zone of the meniscal tear lends itself to repair, then an arthroscopic repair will be performed instead of a meniscectomy.
6. Arthroscopic punches, graspers, and synovators/burrs are used inserted to trim and remove the damaged portion of the meniscus.
7. The meniscal rim is smoothed with a shaver.
8. The knee is flushed with saline at the end of the procedure, and the surrounding structures, including the collateral medial collateral ligament and the ACL/PCL, are inspected for intraoperative damage.
9. The port sites are infused with local anaesthetic.
10. The port sites can be left open or closed with sutures (with the knee in flexion), and a bulky wool and crepe dressing is then applied to the knee.

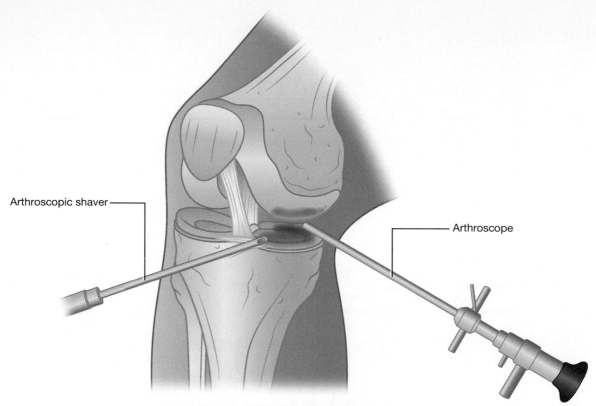

Arthroscopic shaver

Arthroscope

Arthroscopic debridement of the medial meniscus.

 Complications

EARLY

- Common peroneal nerve injury, which may result in numbness below the knee or foot drop.
- Haemarthrosis.
- Cartilage, meniscal, or ligamentous damage.
- Retained meniscal remnants—which may cause the knee to lock.

INTERMEDIATE AND LATE

- Infection.

Postoperative Care

INPATIENT

- Typically performed as a day-case procedure.
- Analgesia.
- Early mobilisation with the use of crutches.
- Elevation when immobile to reduce swelling and risk of deep vein thrombosis (DVT).

OUTPATIENT

- Progressive weight-bearing exercises, with a return to everyday activities at 2 weeks.
- Return to active sports at 4–6 weeks.
- Outpatient follow-up appointment at 6 weeks.

 Surgeon's Favourite Question

What is 'O'Donoghue's unhappy triad'?

O'Donoghue's unhappy triad comprises anterior cruciate ligament (ACL) tear and medial collateral ligament (MCL) injury (tear or sprain) with a medial meniscal tear. It often results from valgus stress with rotation of the knee in contact sports trauma.

Cephalomedullary Femoral Nail (CMN)

87

Gareth Rogers

Definition

Fixation of a femoral fracture with an intramedullary nail and a head screw.

Indications and Contraindications

INDICATIONS

- Subtrochanteric fractures.
  - Diaphyseal femoral fractures.
  - Painful pathological lesions prone to fractures where most of the femur needs to be stabilised.
  - Reverse oblique intertrochanteric fractures.

CONTRAINDICATIONS

- Imminent death, although a cephalomedullary femoral nail (CMN) is offered as a palliative treatment for pain control.
- Sclerotic bone conditions resulting in dense bone where entry into and reaming the canal are difficult.
- Proximal prothesis e.g. THR.

Anatomy

GROSS ANATOMY

- The proximal femur is composed of the head, neck, and proximal shaft.
- The intertrochanteric ridge runs from superior-lateral to inferior-medial between the greater and lesser trochanters.
- The neck-shaft angle is 130 ± 7 degrees in adults, with approximately 10 degrees of anteversion.
- Muscular attachments of the femur:
  - The vastus lateralis originates from the greater trochanter (GT) and inserts into the patella as part of the quadriceps tendon, a common tendon formed by the rectus femoris, vastus medialis, intermedius, and lateralis.
  - The obturator internus, the superior and inferior gemelli, the piriformis, and the gluteus medius and minimus muscles all insert into the GT.
  - The iliopsoas originates from the iliac fossa and the lumbar spine and inserts into the lesser trochanter.

NEUROVASCULATURE

- The sciatic nerve originates from L4–S3 and descends in the leg, innervating the hamstring muscles. Within the popliteal fossa, it divides into the common peroneal nerve and the tibial nerve.
- The femoral nerve derives from the rootlets of L2–L4 and divides within the thigh into anterior and posterior branches. The anterior branch supplies the anterior cutaneous surface and the sartorius. The posterior branch is responsible for the innervation of the quadriceps muscles.
- The arterial supply to the femoral head is retrograde via the medial (predominantly) and lateral circumflex arteries.
- The vascular supply to the femoral head from the artery of the ligamentum teres is insignificant.
- Lying in close proximity with the proximal femur are the sciatic, femoral, and pudendal nerves.

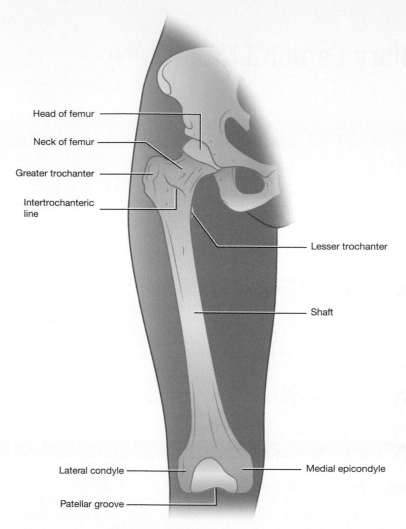

Head of femur

Neck of femur

Greater trochanter

Intertrochanteric line

Lesser trochanter

Shaft

Lateral condyle

Medial epicondyle

Patellar groove

Gross anatomy of the femur.

STEP-BY-STEP OPERATION

Anaesthesia: general or spinal.

Position: supine on a traction table with the fractured leg in traction and the contralateral hip in stirrup.

Considerations: Cephalomedullary nails are inserted with the aid of a portable image intensifier (II). Antibiotics and tranexamic acid are administered at induction.

Steps:

1. Using the traction table, the fracture is first reduced by closed technique using the II. If unable to achieve closed reduction, an incision is made over the fracture site and an open reduction is performed before proceeding with the remainder of the procedure.

2. The entry point of the nail is identified using fluoroscopy, and a 2–3 cm longitudinal incision is made proximal to the tip of the GT. Sharp dissection is then used through the fascia lata and blunt dissection down on to the GT.

3. An awl (curved canulated guide) is then inserted 2–3 mm medial to the tip of the GT on anteroposterior (AP) view and at the centre of the GT on lateral view. Once position is confirmed on II, the ball-tipped guidewire is inserted through the awl and down to the centre of the femoral canal bypassing the fracture site.

4. The awl is removed and an entry reamer is passed over the ball tip guide wire.

5. Dependent on the level of the fracture, a standard length nail may be preselected (a short or intermediate nail) or in the case of a diaphyseal/subtrochanteric fracture, a measure may be used in order to select a nail with a longer length.

6. Sequential reamers are passed across the guidewire and down the cortex to allow for the passage of the nail (the canal is reamed 1–1.5 mm greater than the desired nail diameter).

7. The nail and a locking jig are built and inserted under II. The guide wire is then removed.

8. The head screw guide wire is inserted through the proximal locking jig into the centre of the femoral head (on AP/lateral images) under II to ensure adequate tip-apex distance. The guidewire is then measured and overdrilled, and the head screw is then inserted. Using a flexible driver, the proximal rotational locking screw is fully tightened then loosened by half a turn.

9. Depending on the length of the nail, the nail can either be locked through the jig (short and intermediate nails) or free hand using II (long nails).

10. Final images and then obtained, the wound is irrigated and closed in layers—absorbable sutures are used for tensor fascia lata (TFL) and deep dermis, absorbable sutures or clips for subcutaneous tissue/skin.

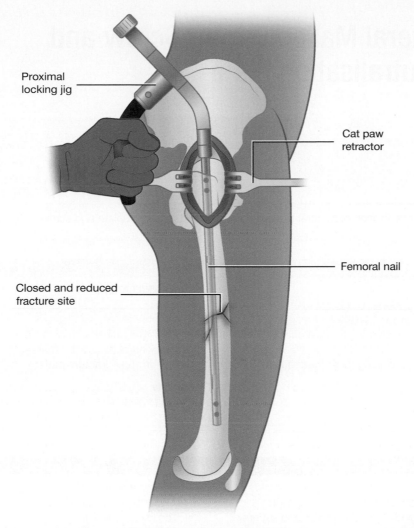

Proximal locking jig

Cat paw retractor

Femoral nail

Closed and reduced fracture site

Proximal jig to insert a femoral nail.

 Complications

EARLY
- Peripheral neuropathy (direct or tractional) affecting the pudendal, sciatic, or femoral nerves, which can result in paralysis of the supplied muscles and neuralgia or paraesthesia of the innervated cutaneous surfaces.
- Myocardial infarction and stroke at time of surgery due to fat embolism or thrombosis.

INTERMEDIATE AND LATE
- Infection.
- Implant failure.
- Deep vein thrombosis (DVT) and pulmonary embolism (PE).
- Nonunion—multifragmentary subtrochanteric fractures.
- Mortality—average 1-year mortality rates are highly dependent on comorbidities.

Postoperative Care

INPATIENT
- Full blood count and renal function tests the next day.
- Physiotherapy/occupational therapy—patients should be mobilising and fully weight-bearing from day 1 postoperatively unless there are concerns regarding the strength of the construct.
- Review within 72 hours by an orthogeriatrician.
- Nutritional and falls review.

OUTPATIENT
- Thromboprophylaxis continued for up to 1 month postoperatively.
- For subtrochanteric fractures and in cases of prophylactic nailing follow-up appointments until union has been confirmed with X-rays.

? Surgeon's Favourite Question

What are the two key factors that ensure nailing works properly?

True reduction of the fracture prior to nailing and entry point of initial guide wire to ensure good position of the nail.

88 Lateral Malleolus Lag Screw and Neutralisation Plate

Gareth Rogers

Definition

Open reduction and internal fixation of a lateral malleolar (fibular) fracture using a plate and screw.

Indications and Contraindications

INDICATIONS
- Unstable fractures (e.g. weber B & C fractures of the distal fibular, bimalleolar and trimalleolar fractures).
- Displacement of fracture following nonoperative management.
- Open ankle fractures—providing there is adequate soft tissue coverage.

CONTRAINDICATIONS
Relative
- Peripheral vascular disease.
- High-risk patient with poor bone quality—in these patients a locking plate may be more appropriate
- Comminuted fracture pattern.

Absolute
- Patients suitable for nonoperative management (e.g. undisplaced stable ankle fracture).

Anatomy

GROSS ANATOMY
- The ankle, or the talocrural joint, is the articulation between fibula, tibia, and talus. The inferior and superior tibiofibular syndesmoses hold the tibia and fibula together and form part of the soft tissue stabiliser of the joint.
- The medial and posterior malleoli (of the tibia) and the lateral malleolus (the base of the fibula) are all palpable on clinical examination.
- Ligaments of the ankle joint:
  - Four different groups of ligaments stabilise the ankle joint: lateral ligaments, medial ligaments, syndesmosis, and subtalar ligaments.
  - The lateral group of ligaments comprise the anterior talofibular ligament, calcaneofibular ligament, lateral talocalcaneal ligament, and posterior talofibular ligament.
  - The medial group of ligaments consists of the two parts of the deltoid ligament (superficial and deep).
  - The syndesmosis is the membranous band distally between the fibula and tibia. It is made up of three ligaments: anteroinferior tibiofibular ligament, posteroinferior tibiofibular ligament, and interosseous tibiofibular ligament.
- The lateral malleolus:
  - The lateral malleolus is formed by the distal fibula and provides attachment for the posterior and anterior talofibular ligaments and the lateral ligament complex.
  - Passing anterior to the lateral malleolus are the tendons of extensor digitorum longus and peroneus tertius.
  - Passing posterior to the lateral malleolus are the tendons of peroneus brevis and longus and, more posteriorly, the sural nerve, which descends along the posterolateral aspect of the leg to innervate the overlying cutaneous surface.

NEUROVASCULATURE
- The superficial peroneal nerve is at risk during the surgical approach to the fibula, as it leaves the lateral muscle compartment 10–12 cm above the tip of the distal fibula to run superficial to the anterior compartment, where it provides motor innervation to the peroneus longus and brevis.

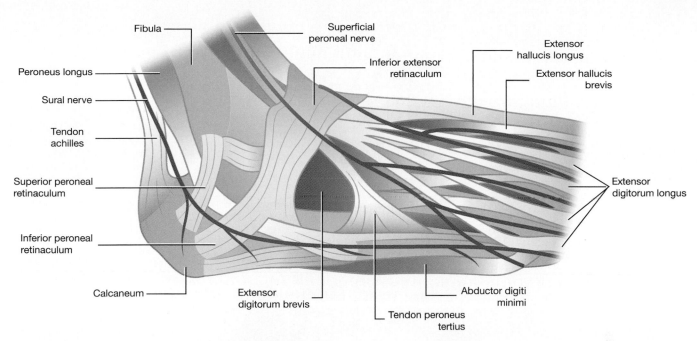

Anatomy of the lateral malleolus and surrounding nerves.

1·2·3 STEP-BY-STEP OPERATION

Anaesthesia: general or regional.

Position: supine position, with a tourniquet; a sandbag is under the ipsilateral buttock.

Considerations: The procedure is guided by a portable image intensifier (II). Antibiotics are administered at induction.

Steps:

1. For the direct lateral approach, a 5–10-cm incision is made along the lateral surface of the fibula, from the distal tip and extending proximally.

2. The subcutaneous fat is divided and the deep fascia incised. Special attention is paid to avoid the superficial peroneal nerve, which is at risk if the incision reaches within 10 cm of the proximal tip of the fibula.

3. The fracture site is exposed, evacuated of haematoma and periosteum around the fracture site is elevated.

4. Using pointed reduction clamps, the fracture is then reduced under direct vision.

5. Using a drill guide, a 3.5-mm hole is drilled perpendicular to the fracture site into the near cortex only, then the 2.5-mm drill guide is inserted through the near cortex hole and a 2.5-mm hole is drilled into the far cortex.

6. The drill hole is measured, and a 3.5 mm lag screw is inserted, compressing the fracture (a lag screw).

7. A one-third tubular plate is positioned over the fracture site and using plate clamps, is held in position.

8. The most distal hole is drilled first, using a 2.5-mm drill piece into the near cortex only. The depth is measured, and a cancellous screw is inserted.

9. The most proximal hole is then drilled with a 2.5-mm drill piece, this time passing through both cortices. The depth is measured and a cortical screw is inserted. This process is then repeated for the adjacent holes.

10. Final images are obtained. The wound is then washed, the deep fascia and subcutaneous tissue are closed with absorbable sutures, and the skin is closed with absorbable sutures or clips.

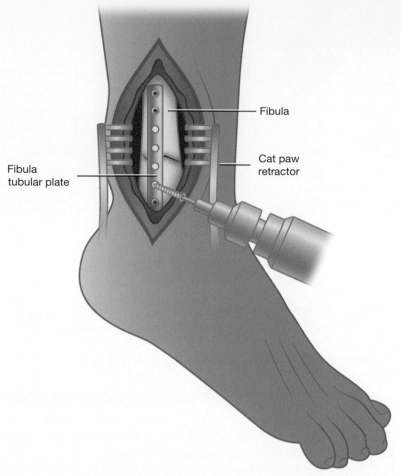

Fixation of a neutralisation plate to the fibula.

Complications

EARLY

- Damage to the superficial peroneal nerve or sural nerve, causing sensory loss over dorsal and lateral surfaces of the foot.
- Compartment syndrome (when the pressure within a muscle compartment rises above arterial pressure, resulting in reduced tissue perfusion, ischaemia, and necrosis).

INTERMEDIATE AND LATE

- Wound dehiscence and infection.
- Deep vein thrombosis (DVT) and pulmonary embolism (PE).
- Malunion or nonunion of the fracture.
- Metal work prominence/irritation.
- Ankle stiffness.
- Early ankle arthritis.

Postoperative Care

OUTPATIENT

- Weight-bearing status is dependent on bone quality and quality of fixation.
- 2-week fracture clinic review: X-ray and wound check.
- 6-week fracture clinic review: X-ray and full weight-bearing with outpatient physiotherapy.

Surgeon's Favourite Question

How would you assess for a syndesmotic injury?

Stress syndesmosis under II intraoperatively by forced external rotation of the ankle. If syndesmosis opens up, then add syndesmotic screws to stabilise and allow healing of syndesmosis.

Lower Limb Fasciotomy

Gareth Rogers

Definition

Decompression of the fascial compartments of the lower limb to relieve vascular tamponade and restore perfusion.

Indications and Contraindications

INDICATIONS

- Acute lower limb compartment syndrome—when the pressure within a compartment of the lower limb exceeds the tissue perfusion pressure. Untreated, it has the potential to result in irreversible muscle damage, nerve damage, and death.
- Fasciotomies of the lower limb may be performed prophylactically by vascular surgeons following re-perfusion procedures of the lower limb.

CONTRAINDICATIONS

- Delayed diagnosis of compartment syndrome—there is little benefit obtained in fasciotomies performed more than 12–24 hours after the onset of symptoms, as irreversible tissue damage has usually occurred by this point.

Anatomy

- The leg has four compartments: anterior, lateral, superficial posterior, and deep posterior.
- The compartments are separated by four fascial layers: the interosseous membrane, the transverse intermuscular septum, the anterior intermuscular septum, and the posterior intermuscular septum.
- Superficial posterior compartment:
  - The superficial posterior compartment is separated from the lateral compartment by the posterior intermuscular septum and from the deep posterior compartment by a transverse intermuscular septum.
  - The superficial posterior compartment contains the soleus, gastrocnemius, and plantaris muscles.
  - There are no major neurovascular structures in this compartment.
- Deep posterior compartment:
  - The deep posterior compartment is separated from the superficial posterior compartment by the transverse intermuscular septum and from the anterior compartment by the interosseous membrane.
  - The deep posterior compartment contains the tibialis posterior, popliteus, flexor hallucis longus, and flexor digitorum longus.
  - Importantly, the tibial nerve and the posterior tibial artery descend in the posterior compartment.
- The lateral compartment:
  - The lateral compartment is bounded by the anterior intermuscular septum (anteriorly), the posterior intermuscular septum (posteriorly), and the fibula (medially).
  - It is supplied by the superficial peroneal nerve, which arises from the bifurcation of the common peroneal nerve as it winds around the head of the fibula.
- The anterior compartment:
  - The anterior compartment is bounded medially by the lateral surface of the tibia and laterally by the extensor surface of the fibular and anterior intermuscular septum. It is separated from the deep posterior compartment by the interosseus membrane.
  - It contains the deep peroneal nerve and the anterior tibial artery as it descends the lower legs before transitioning into the dorsalis pedis artery on the dorsal surface of the foot.

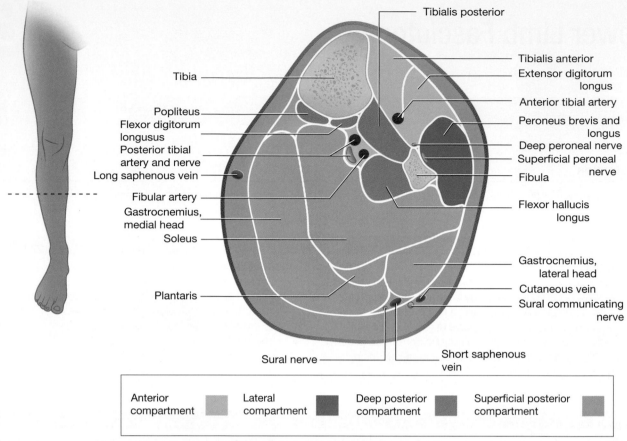

Tibialis posterior

Tibialis anterior

Extensor digitorum longus

Anterior tibial artery

Peroneus brevis and longus

Deep peroneal nerve

Superficial peroneal nerve

Fibula

Flexor hallucis longus

Gastrocnemius, lateral head

Cutaneous vein

Sural communicating nerve

Tibia

Popliteus

Flexor digitorum longusus

Posterior tibial artery and nerve

Long saphenous vein

Fibular artery

Gastrocnemius, medial head

Soleus

Plantaris

Sural nerve

Short saphenous vein

Anterior compartment	Lateral compartment	Deep posterior compartment	Superficial posterior compartment

Compartments of the lower limb.

🔢 STEP-BY-STEP OPERATION

Anaesthesia: general.

Position: supine, with a sandbag to rotate the leg for approach to the posterolateral aspect of the leg.

Steps:

1. Two 15–18-cm longitudinal incisions are made; the two incisions are separated by an 8-cm bridge of skin.
2. The first incision is over the anterolateral aspect of the leg 2 cm anterior to the fibula and runs from the level of the tibial tubercle to 6 cm above the ankle.
3. The superficial peroneal nerve is then identified as it distally penetrates the deep fascia.
4. The fascia overlying the anterior compartment is then incised for the length of the incision, decompressing it. The intermuscular septum is incised along its full length, decompressing the lateral compartment.
5. The second incision runs over the anteromedial aspect of the leg 2 cm posterior to the medial border of the tibia and runs from the level of the tibial crest to 6 cm above the ankle.

6. The saphenous nerve and vein are identified and protected. Caution is applied with the most distal aspect of the incision as intermuscular perforators are found at 5, 10, and 15 cm from the intermalleolar line, preservation of these structures is vital as they may later be required for perforator flaps for soft tissue coverage.
7. The fascia deep to the saphenous vein and overlying the superficial compartment is then incised, decompressing the superficial posterior compartment and exposing the gastrocnemius and soleus muscles.
8. The head of soleus is then freed from its origin, decompressing the deep posterior compartment.
9. Ensure vascularisation of muscles. Warm saline swabs can be used to encourage vasodilation. Necrotic tissues are debrided.
10. Wounds should be left open and covered with nonadhesive dressings.

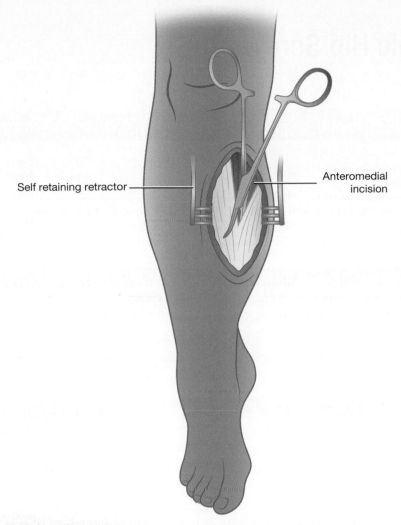

Self retaining retractor

Anteromedial
incision

Incising the fascia of the posterior compartment, allowing for decompression.

Complications

EARLY

- Saphenous (loss of sensation in the medial leg) and superficial peroneal nerve injury (inability to evert the foot and loss of sensation over the dorsum of the foot).
- Exposure of tibia or fibula if incisions are too anterior or lateral.
- Rhabdomyolysis—the excessive release of myoglobin and electrolytes caused by the rapid breakdown of skeletal muscle. These obstruct renal tubules, resulting in renal failure.
- Damage to intermuscular perforators which may later be required as a blood supply for soft tissue coverage.

INTERMEDIATE AND LATE

- Wound infection and delayed healing.
- Chronic venous insufficiency.
- Amputation may be required if fasciotomy is unsuccessful.

Postoperative Care

INPATIENT

- Commonly admitted to a HDU/ITU environment for post-monitoring.
- Second look in theatre at 48–72 hours ± debridement of nonviable tissue.
- Wound closure if possible, otherwise will need soft tissue coverage with skin graft or flap.
- Monitor and treat any renal failure from rhabdomyolysis—patients may require haemofiltration.

? Surgeon's Favourite Question

Why are young men especially prone to compartment syndrome?

Greater muscle mass.

90 Dynamic Hip Screw (DHS)

Gareth Rogers

Definition

Fixation of an extracapsular neck of femur fracture with a plate and a sliding screw to allow dynamisation and predictable fracture healing.

Indications and Contraindications

INDICATIONS
- Extracapsular intertrochanteric neck of femur fractures.
- Nondisplaced intracapsular neck of femur fractures.

CONTRAINDICATIONS
- Unstable fracture configurations (e.g. reverse oblique, multifragmentary, or subtrochanteric).
- Imminent death, although a dynamic hip screw (DHS) is offered as a palliative treatment for pain control.

Anatomy

GROSS ANATOMY
- The proximal femur is composed of the head, neck, and proximal shaft.
- The intertrochanteric ridge runs supero-lateral to infero-medial between the greater and lesser trochanters (LTs).
- The neck-shaft angle is 130 ± 7 degrees in adults, with approximately 10 degrees of anteversion.
- Muscular attachments of the femur
  - The extensor mechanism of the knee is composed of the vastus lateralis, vastus intermedius, vastus medialis, and rectus femoris (the quadriceps) inserting into the tibial tuberosity through the sesamoid patella.
  - Obturator internus, the superior and inferior gemelli, the piriformis, and the gluteus medius and minimus muscles all insert into the greater trochanter.
  - Iliopsoas originates from the iliac fossa and lumbar spine and inserts into the LT.
  - The tensor fascia lata (TFL) muscle inserts into the tibia through a tough aponeurosis—the ilioibial tract—which runs on the lateral aspect of the thigh inserting into the lateral condyle of the tibia.

NEUROVASCULATURE
- Lying in close proximity with the proximal femur are the sciatic, femoral, and pudendal nerves.
- The sciatic nerve originates from L4–S3 and descends the leg, innervating the hamstring muscles. Within the popliteal fossa, it divides into the common peroneal nerve and the tibial nerve.
- The femoral nerve derives from the rootlets of L2–L4 and within the thigh divides into anterior and posterior branches. The anterior branch supplies the anterior cutaneous surface and sartorius. The posterior branch is responsible for the innervation of the quadriceps muscles.
- The arterial supply to the femoral head is retrograde via the medial (predominantly) and lateral circumflex arteries branches of the profunda femoris.
- The supply to the femoral head from the artery of the ligamentum teres is insignificant.

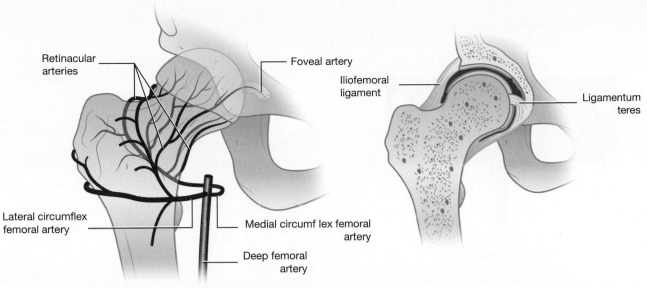

Retinacular arteries

Foveal artery

Iliofemoral ligament

Ligamentum teres

Lateral circumflex femoral artery

Medial circumf lex femoral artery

Deep femoral artery

Vasculature and ligaments of the hip.

123 STEP-BY-STEP OPERATION

Anaesthesia: general or spinal.

Position: supine on a traction table with the fractured leg in traction and the contralateral hip up in a stirrup.

Considerations: A DHS is inserted with the aid of a portable image intensifier (II). Antibiotics and tranexamic acid are administered at induction.

Steps:

1. Using the traction table, closed reduction is performed under II control.
2. Using the II, the level of the LT is identified and marked.
3. A longitudinal lateral incision is made just proximal to the LT through skin and subcutaneous tissue down to the level of TFL.
4. The fibres of TFL are then split in-line with the incision.
5. The vastus lateralis is then either split or elevated to expose the lateral femur.
6. Using a fixed 135-degree guide, a guide wire is inserted under image guidance through the neck of the femur and into the centre of the femoral head (on both anteroposterior [AP] and lateral views), the distance between the tip of the guidewire and apex of the femoral head should be <25 mm.
7. The length of the guide wire is measured, and a hip screw 5 mm shorter than the guide wire length is selected.
8. A triple-barrelled reamer is placed over the guide wire to make way for both the lag screw and the barrel of the plate. The lag screw is inserted under II guidance.
9. A 135-degree four-hole plate is slid over the lag screw. The most distal hole is drilled, the depth measured, and a bicortical screw inserted; this process is then repeated for the remaining three holes.
10. Final images are obtained, and the wound is washed and then closed in layers—an absorbable suture is used for to repair TFL and to close the deep dermal layer and either an absorbable suture or clips are used to close skin/subcutaneous tissue.

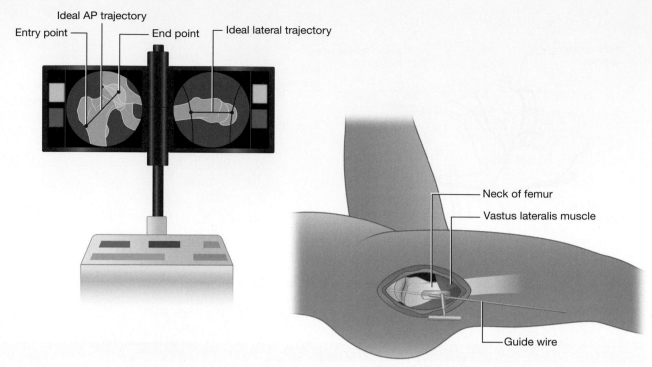

Insertion of guide wire through the femoral neck and into the head for a dynamic hip screw.

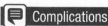 Complications

EARLY

- Peripheral neuropathy (direct versus tractional)—pudendal, sciatic, or femoral nerve damage that can result in paralysis of the supplied muscles and neuralgia or paraesthesia of the supplied cutaneous surfaces.
- Myocardial infarction and stroke at time of surgery due to fat embolism, thrombosis, or blood loss

INTERMEDIATE AND LATE

- Infection.
- Implant failure due to varus collapse.
- Avascular necrosis if fixation is used for undisplaced intracapsular neck of femur fractures (9–18%).
- Deep vein thrombosis (DVT) and pulmonary embolism (PE).
- Malunion in case of collapse.
- Mortality—average 1-year mortality rates are 10–20%.

Postoperative Care

INPATIENT

- Full blood count and renal function tests the next day.
- Physiotherapy/occupational therapy—patients should be mobilising and fully weight-bearing from day 1 postoperatively unless there are concerns regarding the strength of the construct.
- Review within 72 hours by an orthogeriatrician.
- Nutritional and falls review.

OUTPATIENT

- Thromboprophylaxis continued for up to 1 month postoperatively.
- No follow-up routinely required for extracapsular fractures; however, if a DHS is used in the fixation of a non-displaced intracapsular fracture, the patient is routinely followed up to ensure the fracture has united and has not gone on to develop AVN.

? Surgeon's Favourite Question

What makes a DHS dynamic?

The lag screw used to fix the femoral head slides into the barrel of the plate, allowing compression and healing at the fracture site and enabling healing as the patient weight-bears and mobilises after fixation. If this did not happen, the fracture fragments would remain separated and a high rate of nonunion would occur.

Cemented Hip Hemiarthroplasty

Gareth Rogers

Definition

Replacement of femoral head and neck with a stemmed implant in the treatment of displaced intracapsular fractured neck of femur (NOF).

Indications and Contraindications

INDICATIONS

- Displaced intracapsular NOF fractures where the viability of head is unlikely (Garden III and IV fractures) in patients who are:
  - Unable to walk outdoors without using more than a single stick.
  - Cognitively impaired and would be unable to follow postoperative THR precautions.
  - Not medically fit for either the anaesthesia or the procedure.

CONTRAINDICATIONS
Relative

- Imminent death, although hip hemiarthroplasty is offered as a palliative treatment for pain control.
- Extracapsular fractures where fixation is the treatment of choice.
- A THR should be considered in patients with a NOF fracture who are:
  - Able to walk independently not using more than one stick.
  - Are not cognitively impaired
  - Are medically fit for both the anaesthetic and the procedure.

Anatomy

GROSS ANATOMY

- The hip joint comprises two articulating surfaces: the head of the femur and the acetabulum of the pelvis, which form a stable ball-and-socket synovial joint.
- The articular surfaces are lined by hyaline cartilage.
- The acetabulum:
  - The acetabulum comprises the acetabular fossa, the location for attachment of the ligamentum teres, and the lunate surface, which surrounds the fossa and articulates with the femur.
  - The lunate surface is horseshoe shaped and is open at the inferior aspect, forming the acetabular notch, which houses the transverse acetabular ligament (TAL).
  - The ligamentum teres connects the acetabular fossa to the head of femur at the fovea.
  - The acetabular labrum deepens the acetabulum, enhancing the stability of the joint.
  - The joint capsule attaches to the pelvis via the margins of the acetabulum, the transverse ligament, and the margin of the obturator foramen, and to the femur via the intertrochanteric line anteriorly and the intertrochanteric crest posteriorly

NEUROVASCULATURE

- The hip joint is innervated by branches from the femoral, obturator, and superior gluteal nerves, as well as the nerve to the quadratus femoris.
- Vascular supply to the hip joint arises from the profunda femoris artery via the medial and lateral femoral circumflex arteries (the main supply travelling beneath the capsule).
- The femoral head receives minimal blood supply from the artery of the ligamentum teres, which is not clinically significant.
- Additional arteries supplying the hip joint include the superior and inferior gluteal arteries and the first perforating branch of the deep artery of the thigh.

PATHOLOGY

- Anteriorly the intertrochanteric line and posteriorly the intertrochanteric crest demarcate the margins of the joint capsule.
- A displaced intracapsular NOF fracture will result in disruption to the retrograde blood supply to the head of the femur. Disruption to this blood supply means that attempts to fix an intracapsular NOF fracture carry a significant risk of avascular necrosis of the femoral head; therefore, patients with these fracture patterns undergo arthroplasty of the hip joint.

Musculature of the hip in relation to the sciatic nerve.

¹²₃ STEP-BY-STEP OPERATION

Anaesthesia: general or spinal.

Position: lateral position with the affected leg facing up.

Consideration: Antibiotics and tranexamic acid are administered at induction.

Steps:

1. For the modified Hardinge approach, a 10-cm longitudinal incision is centred posterior to the tip of the greater trochanter (GT) extending in line with the femur distally and proximally curving slightly posterior—care is taken to not extend the incision too proximally due to risk of damage to the superior gluteal artery and nerve. The subcutaneous tissue is incised and swept away to expose tensor fascia lata (TFL).

2. A small incision is made into TFL and the leg is abducted, and using scissors, the fibres of TFL are split in-line with the incision. Using blunt dissection, the trochanteric bursa are cleared to view gluteus medius, the GT and vastus lateralis.

3. Using diathermy, an omega incision is made starting from the proximal edge of vastus lateralis running around the GT to the insertion of the gluteus medius tendon; from here, a radial cut is made down through gluteus medius, minimus, and the joint capsule down to the level of the neck of the femur. During this stage, the leg is rotated externally ensuring all tissues are raised in a single flap from the level of the GT and NOF to the level of the lesser trochanter (LT).

4. Following soft tissue release and with external rotation, the hip is dislocated.

5. Using a bone saw, the neck is osteotomised at the level required from the implant, and the femoral head is removed from the acetabulum with a corkscrew and measured for size.

6. A box-chisel is used to prepare the femur by making an entry point in the postero-lateral aspect of the femoral canal.

7. The femoral canal is then reamed with differing sizes of taper pin reamers. Broaches are then inserted into the femoral canal to shape it to the prosthesis. A trial reduction may be performed to assess stability, positioning, leg length equality, and movement of the hip.

8. A cement restrictor is sized and inserted, and the canal is washed and dried with a swab.

9. Cement is then inserted into the femoral canal, and the femoral implant is inserted in the predetermined position. Once the cement has set, the hip is then reduced and stability assessed.

10. The wound is washed. The deep layer of external rotators, the joint capsule deep dermal tissue, is closed with nonabsorbable sutures, and the subcutaneous tissue/skin is closed with absorbable sutures or clips.

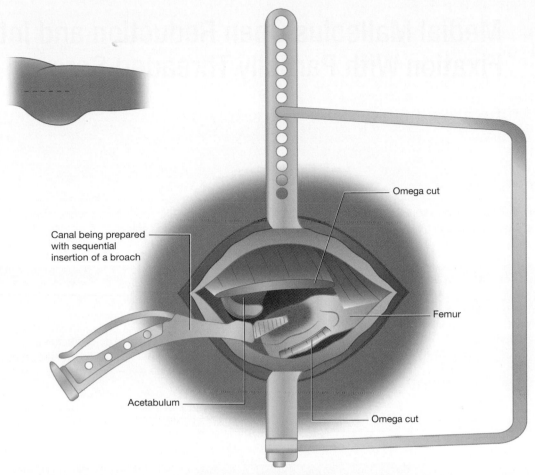

Omega cut

Canal being prepared with sequential insertion of a broach

Femur

Acetabulum

Omega cut

Rasping of the femoral canal.

Complications

EARLY

- Peripheral neuropathy (direct or tractional) affecting the pudendal, sciatic, or femoral nerves, which can result in paralysis of the supplied muscles and neuralgia or paraesthesia of the innervated cutaneous surfaces.
- Myocardial infarction and stroke at time of surgery due to fat or cement embolus or blood loss.
- Intraoperative fracture of the femur.
- Dislocation.
- Leg length discrepancy.

INTERMEDIATE AND LATE

- Infection of either the skin or soft tissues.
- Prosthetic joint infection (PJI).
- Deep vein thrombosis (DVT) and pulmonary embolism (PE).
- Mortality—average 1-year mortality rate is 14–36%, highly dependent on comorbidities.

Postoperative Care

INPATIENT

- Check X-ray of the hip joint.
- Full blood count and renal function blood tests the next day.
- Physiotherapy/occupational therapy—patients should be mobilising and fully weight-bearing from day 1 postoperatively.
- Review within 72 hours by an orthogeriatrician.
- Nutritional and falls review.

OUTPATIENT

- Thromboprophylaxis for 1 month postoperatively.
- Routine follow-up is not usually required.

Surgeon's Favourite Question

What sign may result if the innervation to the abductor muscles is damaged during the modified Harding approach?

A positive Trendelenburg sign indicates abductor dysfunction which may occur due to damage to the superior gluteal nerve and artery—responsible for innervation and supply of gluteus medius and minimus.

92 | Medial Malleolus Open Reduction and Internal Fixation With Partially Threaded Screws

Gareth Rogers

Definition

Fixation of an isolated displaced fracture of the medial malleolus using two partially threaded cancellous screws; in cases of bimalleolar ankle fractures can be used in conjunction with the lateral approach to the ankle.

Indications and Contraindications

INDICATIONS
- Unstable fractures involving the medial malleolus.
- Displacement following nonoperative management.
- Open ankle fractures.

CONTRAINDICATIONS
Absolute
- Fractures suitable for nonoperative management, including undisplaced stable ankle fractures.
- Comminuted fracture—these fractures may require ORIF with an antiglide plate or a tension suture.

Relative
- Patients with peripheral vascular disease.
- Osteoporotic bone.

Anatomy

GROSS ANATOMY
- The ankle or the talocrural joint is the articulation between fibula, tibia, and talus. The inferior and superior tibiofibular syndesmoses hold the tibia and fibula together and form part of the soft tissue stabiliser of the joint.
- The medial and posterior malleoli (parts of the tibia) and the lateral malleolus (the base of the fibula) are all palpable on clinical examination.
- Four different groups of ligaments stabilise the ankle joint: lateral ligaments, medial ligaments, syndesmosis, and subtalar ligaments.
  - Lateral ligaments comprise the anterior talofibular ligament, calcaneofibular ligament, lateral talocalcaneal ligament, and posterior talofibular ligament.

- The medial ligaments consist of the two parts of the deltoid ligament (superficial and deep).
- The syndesmosis is the membranous band distally between the fibula and tibia. It is made up of three ligaments: anteroinferior tibiofibular ligament, posteroinferior tibiofibular ligament, and interosseous tibiofibular ligament.

NEUROVASCULATURE
- The tibial nerve and posterior tibial artery lie posterior to the medial malleolus.
- The anterior tibial artery (which continues in the foot as the dorsalis pedis artery) and the deep peroneal nerve pass anterior to the ankle joint.

Distal Radius Volar Locking Plate

93

Gareth Rogers

Definition

Open reduction and internal fixation of unstable or displaced distal radius fracture using a volar locking plate with screws.

Indications and Contraindications

INDICATIONS
- Unstable displaced fracture of the radius.
- Intraarticular fracture.
- Fracture with associated nerve or vessel damage.
- Delayed presentation.
- Failed conservative management.
- Mal- or nonunion of fracture.

CONTRAINDICATIONS
Absolute
- Very distal fractures where purchase into distal fragments for plate attachment is not achievable.

Relative
- Severe soft tissue injury is a relative contraindication, as these patients may first require wound debridement and external fixation.

Anatomy

GROSS ANATOMY
- The wrist joint:
  - The wrist joint is a synovial joint composed of the articulation between the radius and an articular disc formed by the adjacent surfaces of the distal ulnar, scaphoid, lunate, and triquetrum bones.
  - The complex arrangement of articulations allows for a range of movements: abduction, adduction, flexion, and extension.
  - The wrist joint capsule is supported by the palmar radiocarpal, palmar ulnocarpal, and dorsal radiocarpal ligaments. There is additional ligament support from the radial and ulnar collateral ligaments.
- Muscles at the wrist joint:
  - Flexor carpi radialis (FCR) originates from the medial epicondyle of the humerus and inserts into the base of the second and third metacarpals. It is innervated by the median nerve, and it flexes and abducts the wrist.
  - Flexor pollicis longus (FPL) originates from the anterior surface of the radius and the adjacent portion of the interosseous membrane and inserts into the base of the distal phalanx of the thumb. It is innervated by the median nerve and is responsible for flexion of the thumb.

- Pronator quadratus originates from the anterior surface of the ulna and inserts on to the anterior surface of the radius. Innervated by the median nerve, it enables pronation of the forearm.

NEUROVASCULATURE
- The median nerve (CT–T1) enters the anterior compartment of the forearm through the cubital fossa; it then descends the forearm between the muscle bellies of flexor digitorum superficialis and profundus. Within the forearm, the median nerve divides into the anterior interosseus nerve (AIN) and the palmar cutaneous nerve (PCN), after which the median nerve enters the hand by passing through the carpal tunnel. In the hand, the median nerve then divides into the recurrent branch and palmar digital branch.
- The radial artery leaves the forearm by passing around the lateral surface of the wrist and onto the posterolateral aspect of the hand.
- The ulnar nerve and ulnar artery leave the forearm and enter the palmar surface of the hand by passing over the flexor retinaculum of the wrist.
- The radial and ulnar artery anastamopse in the hand to form the superficial and deep palmar arches.

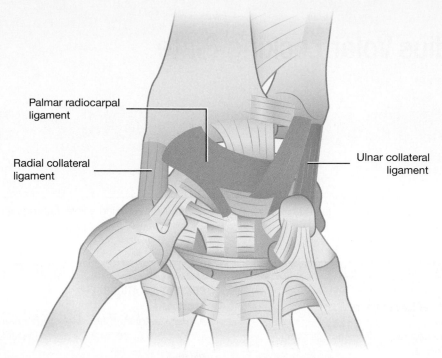

Palmar radiocarpal ligament

Radial collateral ligament

Ulnar collateral ligament

Ligament components of the wrist joint capsule.

STEP-BY-STEP OPERATION

Anaesthesia: general and/or local nerve blocks to the ulnar, radial, and median nerves.

Position: supine with the affected limb on an arm board.

Considerations: Prophylactic antibiotics are administered at induction. The procedure is guided by a portable image intensifier (II). A tourniquet may be used to produce a bloodless surgical field.

Steps:

1. For the FCR approach, a longitudinal volar incision is made in the plane between FCR and the radial artery centred over the fracture site.
2. Subcutaneous tissue is incised and the tendon of FCR exposed. The tendon of FCR is retracted ulnarly (protecting the median nerve) exposing the floor of FCR.
3. The floor of FCR is incised to reveal FPL. The tendon of FPL is retracted ulnarly and the radial artery is retracted radially.
4. Pronator quadratus is dissected along its radial insertion to expose the fracture.
5. The fracture is then reduced under direct vision and confirmed with II.
6. A percutaneous wire through the radial styloid process may be used to temporarily fixate the fracture.
7. An appropriately sized volar locking plate is placed across the fracture and is temporarily held in place by drilling a K-wire through a distal screw hole and then through a screw hole overlying the diaphyseal portion of the fracture. The position is then checked with the II.
8. The plate is first fixed proximally and then distally with a compression screw, positional K-wires are removed.
9. Subsequent screw holes both distally and proximally are then filled with a combination locking and nonlocking screws. The final position is then assessed.
10. The wound is irrigated and closed in two layers with absorbable sutures. Depending on the quality of bone and fixation, the patient may then either be placed in a below elbow back slab cast or alternatively in 'bulky' bandages for wound protection.

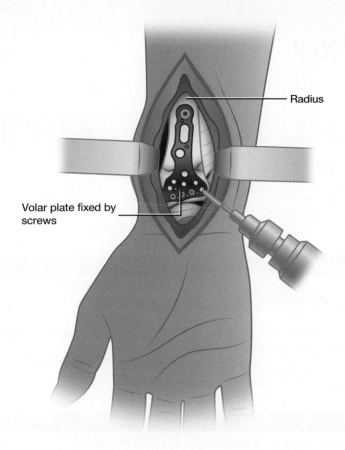

Radius

Volar plate fixed by screws

Fixation of distal radius fracture with a volar locking plate.

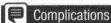 Complications

EARLY

- Radial artery injury, which in the absence of an ulnar artery has the potential to result in vascular insufficiency of the hand. The presence of an ulnar artery can be confirmed with the Allen's test.

IMMEDIATE AND LATE

- Infection.
- Median nerve injury resulting in carpal tunnel syndrome type symptoms.
- Tendon injury most commonly affecting the tendon of either FPL or extensor pollicis longus; damage to either structure results in weakness and requires repair.
- Mal- or nonunion of the fracture.
- Stiffness/post-traumatic arthritis.
- Complex regional pain syndrome (nociceptive sensitisation causing allodynia and vasomotor dysfunction).

Postoperative Care

OUTPATIENT

- Fracture clinic at 2 weeks for review of wound and simple exercises.
- Repeat X-rays at 6 weeks at which point the patient may be discharged to the care of physiotherapy.

 Surgeon's Favourite Question

Why is the volar approach preferred to dorsal?

Due to plate irritation of extensor tendons.

94

Tibial Nail

Gareth Rogers

Definition

Internal fixation of a tibial fracture with an intramedullary nail.

Indications and Contraindications

INDICATIONS

- Management of acute closed and open tibial shaft fractures (>5 cm from the articular surface).
- Minimally displaced tibial fractures with an intact fibula.
- Salvage procedure for mal- or nonunion of a tibial fracture following failed management.

CONTRAINDICATIONS

- Intraarticular fractures extending into the ankle or knee joint.
- Existing tibial deformity precluding the use of a straight nail.
- An undisplaced fracture that may be managed nonoperatively.

Anatomy

- The tibia is a major weight-bearing long bone and forms the articular surfaces of both the ankle and knee joints. It is connected to the fibula via the superior and inferior tibiofibular syndesmoses.
- The tibia is surrounded by the four muscle compartments of the leg: anterior, lateral, superficial posterior, and deep posterior.
  - The superficial posterior compartment is separated from the lateral compartment by the posterior intermuscular septum and from the deep posterior compartment by a fascial layer. The superficial posterior compartment contains the soleus, gastrocnemius, and plantaris muscles. There are no major neurovascular structures in this compartment.
  - The deep posterior compartment is separated from the anterior compartment by the interosseous
  membrane. It contains the tibialis posterior, popliteus, flexor hallucis longus, and flexor digitorum longus, along with the tibial nerve and the posterior tibial artery.
- The lateral (peroneal) compartment is bounded anteriorly by the intermuscular septum, posteriorly by the posterior intermuscular septum, and medially by the fibula. It contains peroneus longus, peroneus brevis and the superficial peroneal nerve.
- The anterior compartment is bounded medially by the lateral surface of the tibia, laterally by the extensor surface of the fibula, and posteriorly by the anterior intermuscular septum. It contains tibialis anterior, extensor digitorum longus, extensor hallucis longus, peroneus tertius and the anterior tibial artery together with the deep peroneal nerve.

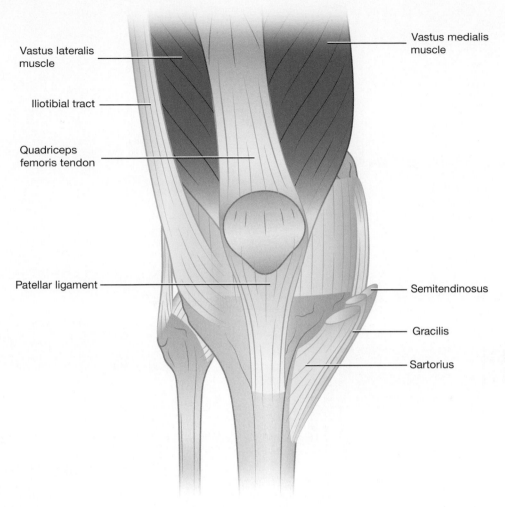

Muscular insertions of the tibia.

Labels:
- Vastus lateralis muscle
- Iliotibial tract
- Quadriceps femoris tendon
- Patellar ligament
- Vastus medialis muscle
- Semitendinosus
- Gracilis
- Sartorius

1 2 3 STEP-BY-STEP OPERATION

Anaesthesia: general or spinal (regional blocks should be avoided to monitor patients post-operatively for signs of compartment syndrome).

Position: supine; the fracture is reduced either with the aid of an assistant flexing the knee over a triangular block (free hand) or by using a traction table.

Considerations: Intramedullary nails are inserted with the aid of a portable image intensifier (II). Antibiotics are administered at induction.

Steps:

1. A longitudinal incision is made from the tibial tuberosity to the patellar. The patellar tendon is identified using blunt dissection and retracted to expose the ventral edge of the tibial plateau. In the transpatellar approach, the patellar tendon is split.

2. The fracture is then reduced using a variety of methods. It is important that the fracture reduction is maintained until both distal and proximal and distal locking screws have been placed.

3. Using an II, the tibial entry point is made in line with the axis of the intramedullary canal with the lateral tubercle of the intercondylar eminence, on a lateral film the entry point should be on the ventral edge of the tibial plateau (precise entry point varies between manufacturers).

4. The guide wire is inserted, and the cannulated entry reamer is then used to open the proximal tibia.

5. The entry guide wire is exchanged for a reaming rod, over which sequential reamers are passed and used to ream the cortex to allow passage of the nail (usually up to 2 mm greater than nail diameter).

6. Using a measure, the guide wire is measured and the appropriate length and diameter nail are selected and assembled.

7. The nail is inserted over the guide wire and positioned using an II.

8. Using the II, the distal nail is locked freehand with two locking screws.

9. The proximal locking jig is used to lock the proximal nail with two to three locking screws.

10. Soft tissue is closed in layers, and a pressure dressing is applied.

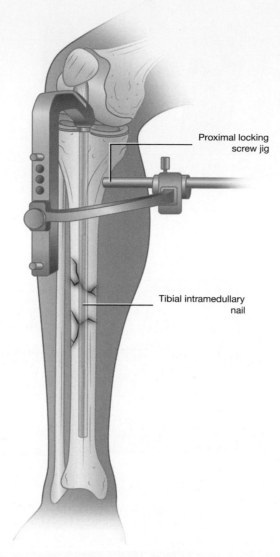

Proximal locking
screw jig

Tibial intramedullary
nail

Tibial nail locking jig.

 Complications

EARLY
- Bleeding.
- Compartment syndrome (when the pressure within a muscle compartment rises above arterial pressure, resulting in reduced tissue perfusion, ischaemia, and necrosis).

INTERMEDIATE AND LATE
- Infection, affecting 1% of patient with closed fractures, increasing to 6% in open fractures.
- Mal- or nonunion.
- Anterior knee pain.
- Deep vein thrombosis (DVT) and pulmonary embolism (PE).
- Stiffness of knee and ankle.
- Metal work prominence or irritation.

Postoperative Care

INPATIENT
- Thromboprophylaxis.
- Weight-bearing as tolerated.
- Physiotherapy consisting of a range of motion exercises to the knee and ankle.

OUTPATIENT
- Dressing change and suture/staple removal after 14 days by a GP nurse.
- Outpatient appointment in 4–6 weeks with tibial radiographs.

? Surgeon's Favourite Question

What would you do if fracture healing is not progressing as expected?

Review patient factors affecting healing—nutrition, smoking, poor circulation, noncompliance, etc. Remove static locking screws and dynamise the nail to aid fracture healing as early as possible. Consider ultrasonic stimulation. Consider bone grafting.

Split-Thickness Skin Graft (STSG)

95

Georgios Pafitanis

Definition

The harvesting of the epidermis and variable thickness of dermis from an area of the body and transplanted onto another area of the body. STSGs can be thick (0.45–0.75 mm) or thin (0.2–0.45 mm).

Indications and Contraindications

INDICATIONS
- Burns.
- Wounds that cannot be closed primarily.

CONTRAINDICATIONS
- Infected wounds.
- Bones and tendons stripped of periosteum and paratenon (devascularised tissues).

Anatomy

- The skin is formed of two layers:
  1. Epidermis—superficial and avascular.
  2. Dermis.
- The epidermis:
  - Composed of stratified squamous epithelium and provides a physical barrier to the external environment.
  - Keratinocytes are the predominant epidermal cell type.
  - Since the epidermis is devoid of blood vessels, nutrients reach this layer via diffusion from the underlying dermis.
- The dermis:
  - The dermis is a complex layer containing structural components such as collagen, blood vessels, hair follicles, sweat glands, and cells, including fibroblasts and other immune cells.
  - The dermis is responsible for nourishing the epidermis, as harbouring epithelial cells are able to replenish the epidermis should the need arise (e.g. in the lining of hair follicles).
- Larger blood vessels and nerves, fat, and connective tissue compose the subcutaneous tissue layer.

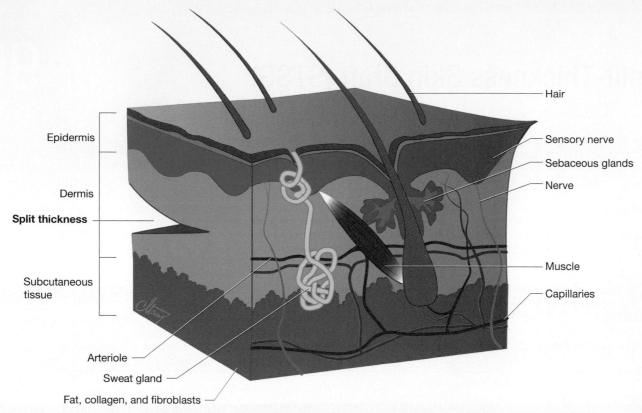

Epidermis

Dermis

Split thickness

Subcutaneous
tissue

Arteriole

Sweat gland

Fat, collagen, and fibroblasts

Hair

Sensory nerve

Sebaceous glands

Nerve

Muscle

Capillaries

Layers and components of the skin and underlying subcutaneous tissue.

1 2 3 STEP-BY-STEP OPERATION

Anaesthesia: general, regional, or local, dependant on whether skin grafting is being performed as a sole procedure or as part of a more complex operation.

Position: dependant on the harvest and recipient sites.

Steps:

1. Both the donor site and the harvest instrument are lubricated using Aquagel, paraffin, or normal saline.

2. The graft can be harvested using an electric or air-powered dermatome or a Watson or Humby knife (nonelectric) with an assistant flattening the donor site by providing proximal and distal traction.

   A. Using an electric or air-powered dermatome:
   - The device is set to the required thickness.
   - Power is switched on before the dermatome contacts the skin.
   - The dermatome is pressed firmly on the skin at 45 degrees and advanced slowly in one smooth passage.
   - Power is only switched off when the dermatome is completely off the skin.

   B. Using a Watson or Humby knife
   - The sharp edge of the knife is held to the skin with the knife at 45 degrees.
   - Small oscillating movements are made to advance the knife forward.

3. The graft is prepared by trimming it to size or by meshing (a process of placing slits in the graft to allow it to expand to cover larger areas (e.g. burn wounds). This can be performed manually or through a meshing machine).

4. The recipient site is prepared by rasping it with a scalpel or curette until it bleeds.

5. After bleeding is controlled, the skin graft is placed onto the wound bed with the dermal (shiny) side abutting the wound bed and secured with absorbable sutures.

6. The recipient site is closed, and sponge is secured with staples above the new graft to prevent graft shear.

7. The donor site is closed, and an alginate dressing (Kaltostat) is applied directly to the wound and bandaged in place. It is often soaked in local anaesthetic to reduce postoperative pain, but adhesive retention tape (e.g. Mefix) may also be used.

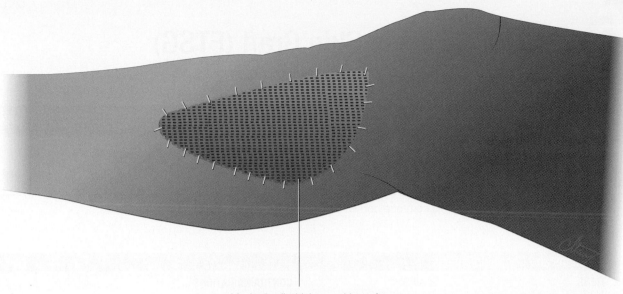

Meshed split-thickness skin graft
covering wound

Meshed split-thickness graft secured with staples.

Complications

EARLY

- Bruising, bleeding, and/or formation of ecchymosis.

INTERMEDIATE AND LATE

- Skin graft failure.
- Infection at either the donor or the recipient site.
- Altered sensation at the recipient site.
- Aberrant scarring at both donor and recipient sites.
- Poor cosmetic outcome due to pigment/texture mismatch and wound contraction (greater than with full-thickness graft)
- Delayed donor site healing.

Postoperative Care

RECIPIENT SITE

- Apply wet dressings twice daily until the graft has taken (approximately 2 weeks).
- The success of graft healing and complications can be assessed in the wound dressing clinic after 7 days.
- A well-healing graft assumes the colour of the surrounding skin and is well adherent to the wound bed.

DONOR SITE

- Remove dressing after 2 weeks to allow undisturbed reepithelialisation.

Surgeon's Favourite Question

Define and describe the process of 'graft take'.

Graft take is the process by which the graft adheres to the recipient site. Following transplantation, a fibrin network 'glues' the graft to the wound bed. The graft is initially nourished via imbibition, the process by which severed vessels within the graft dilate and draw nutrient-rich serous fluid into the graft. Inosculation (anastomosis of graft and wound bed vessels of similar diameter) occurs after 24–72 hours, providing a more secure nutrient source.

96 | Full-Thickness Skin Graft (FTSG)

Georgios Pafitanis

Definition

The harvesting of epidermis and dermis from one body area and transplantation onto another body part.

Indications and Contraindications

INDICATIONS
- Small defects in cosmetically and functionally sensitive areas such as the face and hands.
- Where local flaps or primary closure are not feasible or contraindicated.

CONTRAINDICATIONS
- Infected wound beds.
- Systemic disease resulting in unreliable vascularisation of the recipient bed.
- Bones and tendons stripped of periosteum and paratenon, respectively, should be avoided, as they have poor blood supply that will lead to failure of the graft to take.

Anatomy

- The skin is formed of two layers:
  1. Epidermis—superficial and avascular.
  2. Dermis.
- The epidermis:
  - Composed of stratified squamous epithelium and provides a physical barrier to the external environment.
  - Keratinocytes are the predominant epidermal cell type.
  - Since the epidermis is devoid of blood vessels, nutrients reach this layer via diffusion from the underlying dermis.

- The dermis:
  - The dermis is a complex layer containing structural components such as collagen, blood vessels, hair follicles, sweat glands, and cells, including fibroblasts and other immune cells.
  - The dermis is responsible for nourishing the epidermis, as harbouring epithelial cells are able to replenish the epidermis should the need arise (e.g. in the lining of hair follicles).
- Larger blood vessels and nerves, fat, and connective tissue compose the subcutaneous tissue layer.

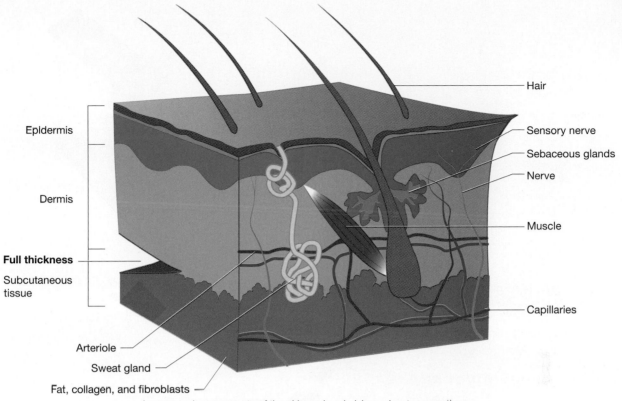

Layers and components of the skin and underlying subcutaneous tissue.

¹₂₃ STEP-BY-STEP OPERATION

Anaesthesia: general, regional, or local, dependant on whether skin grafting is being performed as a sole procedure or as part of a more complex operation (regional or general).

Position: dependant on the harvest and recipient site.

Considerations: Common areas for FTSG harvest include pre- and postauricular skin, supraclavicular skin, groin skin, or the inner arm or forearm.

Steps:

1. The graft is harvested by scoring the outline of an ellipse of appropriately sized skin with a scalpel.
2. The skin is then lifted from the corner with forceps and is separated under tension from the underlying subcutaneous fat using a scalpel.
3. The graft is prepared under tension by wrapping it around the surgeon's finger. Fat is then carefully removed using scissors.
4. Fenestrations are made to reduce the accumulation of exudates between the graft and the wound bed (FTSGs should not be finely meshed like split-thickness grafts).
5. The recipient site is prepared by rasping it with a scalpel or curette until it bleeds (making graft take and survival more likely).
6. After bleeding is controlled, the skin graft is placed onto the wound bed with the dermal (shiny) side abutting the wound bed.
7. The graft is then secured with absorbable sutures.
8. The recipient site is closed with sponge dressings being sutured above the new graft (these act as a 'bolster dressing' to prevent graft shear).
9. The donor site is closed with absorbable subcuticular sutures.

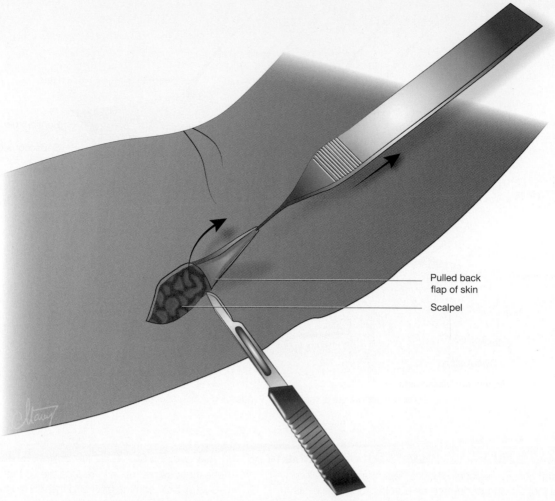

Pulled back
flap of skin

Scalpel

Lift and excision of a full-thickness skin graft under tension.

💬 Complications

EARLY
- Bleeding and/or haematoma formation.

INTERMEDIATE AND LATE
- Skin graft failure (greater risk than STSGs), since nutrients have a longer distance to diffuse.
- Infection at either the donor or the recipient site.
- Altered sensation at the recipient site.
- Aberrant scarring at both donor and recipient sites.
- Poor cosmetic outcome due to colour pigment/texture mismatch and wound contraction.

Postoperative Care

INPATIENT
- Recipient site:
  - Care should be taken to ensure no pressure of shearing forces is applied to the recipient site.
  - The recipient site should remain elevated and immobilised.
  - The initial dressing should not be removed for the first 3–7 days unless signs of complications, including pain, odour, or discharge occur.

OUTPATIENT
- Recipient site:
  - Graft take and complications can be assessed in the wound-dressing clinic within 7 days.
- Donor site:
  - Remove dressing (if applied) in the same dressing clinic.

❓ Surgeon's Favourite Question

What is the reconstructive ladder?

This describes wound management in increasing complexity.
1. 'Secondary intention': leaving the wound to heal from the bottom up.
2. 'Primary intention': approximating the wound edges.
3. Skin grafts.
4. Local tissue transfer such as local flaps, covering defects anatomically close to their origin.
5. Free flaps—flaps reattached from their original blood supply to vessels at the defect site.

Deep Inferior Epigastric Perforator (DIEP) Free-Flap for Breast Reconstruction

Georgios Pafitanis

Definition

An elective procedure to rebuild the breast mound following mastectomy, either as immediate or delayed reconstruction. Tissue that includes fat and skin with a vascular pedicle (a 'free-flap') is taken from the lower abdomen and transferred to the breast.

Indications and Contraindications

INDICATIONS

- Breast cancer reconstruction following mastectomy or wide local excision.
- Congenital syndromes of the breast (e.g. breast agenesis or Poland syndrome).

CONTRAINDICATIONS
Relative

- Previous abdominal liposuction.
- Active heavy smokers or those on nicotine replacement therapy (nicotine-induced vasoconstriction will compromise flap survival).
- Abdominal scars near the abdominal donor site.
- Radiotherapy to chest within previous 6 months.
- Thrombophilic conditions.
- Very obese patients.

Absolute

- Inadequate abdominal donor site (e.g. previous abdominal surgery with scar through the lower abdomen).
- Thin patients with insufficient skin and fat.

Anatomy

- The deep inferior epigastric artery (DIEA) and vein (DIEV) are branches of the external iliac vessels and run from lateral to medial, deep to or within the rectus abdominis muscle. The DIEA supplies the lower abdominal muscles, fat, and skin.
- The deep inferior epigastric (DIE) vessels branch either before entering the muscle or within it and then perforate through the muscle into the subcutaneous fat. These perforating vessels, 'perforators' of the DIE, range from 0.3 to 1.0 mm and form the vascular pedicle of the free-flap.

- The superficial inferior epigastric artery (SIEA) and vein (SIEV) originate from the external iliac vessels and contribute to the superficial vascular supply of the lower abdominal muscles, fat, and skin.
- Due to the bilateral vascular supply, two DIEP free-flaps can be raised from each side of the lower abdomen (this is done for bilateral breast reconstruction).
- The intercostal nerves T11 and T12 provide sensory innervation to the skin of the lower abdomen.

Local Flap Reconstruction of Soft Tissue Defects

Georgios Pafitanis

Definition

A local flap (an area of tissue with its own blood supply) that is moved to treat adjacent soft tissue defects.

 Indications and Contraindications

INDICATIONS
- Provide robust coverage in areas of tissue loss that cannot be closed directly.
- Provide an alternative to skin grafts in:
  1. Areas of exposed bone, tendon, or cartilage.
  2. Areas where grafts may fail due to shear forces.
  3. Areas where grafts may become traumatised/ulcerated.
  4. Areas where contraction must be avoided (e.g. over a joint and the hand dorsum).

CONTRAINDICATIONS
Relative
- Smoking.
- Peripheral arterial disease.

Absolute
- Active infection (delay coverage until this is resolved).
- Injured, poor-quality tissue around the defect and/or donor site.
- When raising a flap could compromise function (e.g. in the hand).

Anatomy

CORE CHARACTERISTICS OF A FLAP
1. Tissue composition:
   a. Cutaneous—skin only.
   b. Fasciocutaneous—fascia and skin.
   c. Musculocutaneous—muscle and skin.
   d. Muscle—muscle only.
   e. Osteocutaneous—bone, soft tissue, and skin.
2. Vascularity:
   - Random flaps—these are not based on a specific vessel. Their blood supply has a random pattern, derived from the subdermal plexus.
   - Axial flaps—these receive their blood supply from a specific known vessel (pedicle). This enables a larger area to be detached. These flaps tend to exhibit better survival, as they are more optimally perfused than random flaps.

3. Geometrical design/movement:
   - Advancement flap—the flap is advanced directly forward with no rotation or lateral movement (e.g. simple, bipedicled, or V-Y advancement flaps).
   - Rotational flap—these flaps are rounded in shape and are rotated about a pivot point. Their circumference should be five to eight times the width of the defect. The secondary defect can then be closed directly.
   - Transpositional flap—these flaps tend to be quadrilateral and are moved laterally about a pivot point. The flap becomes shorter as it is rotated. The resultant defect often needs wound coverage with a graft or a secondary local flap (e.g. rhomboid flap). Transpositional flaps are the most frequently utilised flap.
   - Interpolation flap—this flap is lifted off the donor site to cover a defect that is close but not adjacent, while maintaining its vascular pedicle. The flap often must be moved under or over an intervening soft tissue bridge.

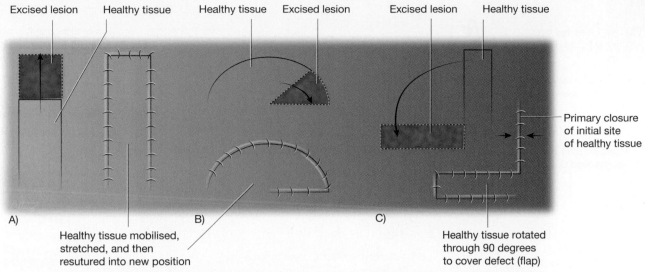

Geometric designs of a flap. (A) Advancement flap. (B) Rotational flap. (C) Transpositional flap.

¹²₃ STEP-BY-STEP OPERATION

Anaesthesia: general or regional.

Position: dependant on the harvest and recipient sites.

Considerations: In a V-Y advancement flap (as described in the following), the initial V-shaped incision is eventually converted into a Y-shaped scar (described here in relation to fingertip loss/coverage).

Steps:

1. A triangular Incision (the height of the triangle tends to be 1.5–2 times the base) is made from the edges of the wound (including skin and subcutaneous tissue). This becomes the 'flap' that will be moved to cover the defect. The triangle may need to have a curvilinear rather than a straight shape so that the incisions follow the natural skin creases ('Horn Flap').

2. The tissues surrounding the flap and laterally are undermined.

3. The apex and base of the flap are slightly undermined to further increase mobility and prevent tethering (care is taken to preserve a small amount of subcutaneous tissue and to not overly undermine the underlying subdermal plexus).

4. Any excess recipient subcutaneous tissue is removed to ensure that the original defect is the same thickness as the flap.

5. A skin hook is used to advance the flap base into position and to check there is no excessive tension.

6. The first securing suture is placed in the middle of the triangle base (or 'leading edge').

7. The remainder of the flap is then sutured into position.

8. The linear defect extending from the apex is then sutured directly.

9. The wound is dressed, ensuring there is adequate compression to prevent haematoma formation, but not so much as to compromise blood supply.

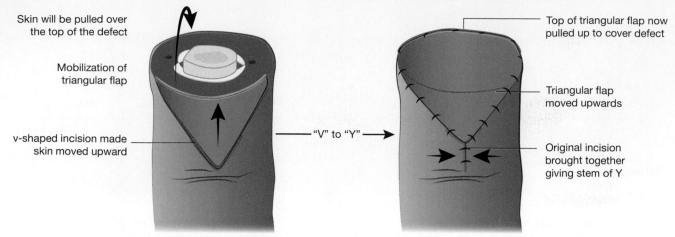

Skin will be pulled over the top of the defect

Mobilization of triangular flap

v-shaped incision made skin moved upward

"V" to "Y" →

Top of triangular flap now pulled up to cover defect

Triangular flap moved upwards

Original incision brought together giving stem of Y

V-Y advancement flap to cover fingertip loss.

 ## Complications

EARLY
- Haematoma and/or seroma formation.
- 'Dog-ears'—small triangular soft tissue bulges at the edge of a scar, which can be unsightly.

INTERMEDIATE AND LATE
- Compromised flap perfusion or flap necrosis due to:
  1. Tense closure.
  2. Insufficient length-to-width ratio.
  3. Flap raised outside of its pedicle's vascular territory.
  4. Excessive external pressure from dressings or a developing haematoma.
- Wound breakdown.
- Infection.

Postoperative Care

INPATIENT
- Large local flaps may require formal monitoring postoperatively for signs of vascular compromise and/or haematoma formation.

OUTPATIENT
- Wound check at 7–10 days in clinic to assess healing and to rule out infection.

? Surgeon's Favourite Question

Explain the difference between local, regional, and distant flaps.

Local: flap is adjacent to the defect. Regional: flap is composed of tissue from the same body region as the defect. Distant: the flap originates in a different area than the defect and can be pedicled or free.

Digital Tendon Repair

99

Georgios Pafitanis

Definition

Surgical repair of the digital flexor or extensor tendon(s) to restore function following tendon trauma.

Indications and Contraindications

INDICATIONS

Complete and partial tendon injuries (>30%), including:
- Laceration—traumatic or iatrogenic.
- Avulsion—usually a closed injury.
- Rupture secondary to:
  1. Trauma—unrepaired partial laceration.
  2. Failed repair.
  3. Inflammatory disease (e.g. rheumatoid arthritis).

CONTRAINDICATIONS

- Repair should be delayed until wound and soft tissues are optimised in:
  - Gross wound contamination or active infection.
  - Human-bite injuries.
  - Lack of soft tissue coverage.

Anatomy

- Tendons attach muscle to bone.
- Tendons are composed of dense, uniform connective tissue composed mainly of Type I collagen, elastin, and mucopolysaccharides.
- Flexor tendons:
  - Originate from:
    - Flexor digitorum profundus (FDP) and flexor digitorum superficialis (FDS) muscles, which flex the fingers.
    - Flexor pollicis longus (FPL) muscle, which flexes the thumb.
  - Tendons are enclosed within a protective flexor sheath that offers nourishment and enables smooth gliding.
  - Each FDS tendon starts superficial to the FDP, then divides on either side of it (over the proximal interphalangeal joint). These two slips then rejoin proximally, deep to the FDP.
  - FDS tendons insert into the middle phalanx and cause flexion across the proximal interphalangeal joints (PIPJs).
  - FDP tendons insert into the distal phalanx and cause flexion across the distal interphalangeal joints (DIPJs).

- Eight thickened areas known as pulleys (five annular and three cruciform) overlie the tendons and provide stability, preventing bow-stringing and increasing functional efficiency.
- Extensor tendons:
  - Extrinsic extension of the digits originates in the forearm and is influenced by the extensor digitorum communis (EDC), extensor indicis (EI), extensor digiti minimi (EDM), extensor pollicis longus (EPL), and extensor pollicis brevis (EPB).
  - Intrinsic extension of the digits originates in the hand via the seven interossei and four lumbrical muscles.
  - The extensor tendon divides into three, forming one central slip and two lateral bands.
  - The central slip inserts at the base of the middle phalanx and causes extension across the PIPJ.
  - The lateral slips combine with the lateral bands of the intrinsics, reuniting distally. Together they form the terminal extensor, which inserts into the distal phalangeal base and causes extension across the DIPJ.

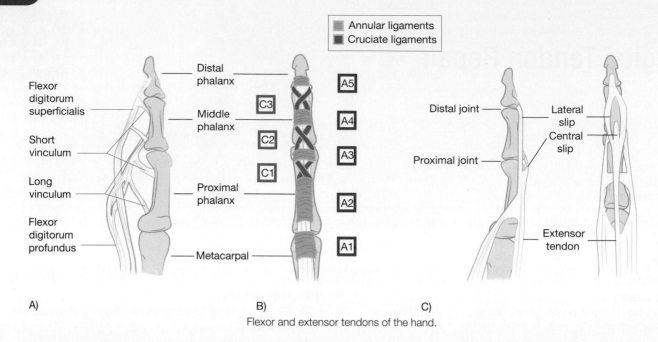

Annular ligaments
Cruciate ligaments

Flexor digitorum superficialis

Short vinculum

Long vinculum

Flexor digitorum profundus

Distal phalanx

Middle phalanx

Proximal phalanx

Metacarpal

C3

C2

C1

A5

A4

A3

A2

A1

A)

B)

Distal joint

Proximal joint

Lateral slip

Central slip

Extensor tendon

C)

Flexor and extensor tendons of the hand.

STEP-BY-STEP OPERATION

Anaesthesia: general, regional, or local (distal extensor injuries only).

Position: arm outstretched on an arm board.

Steps:

1. Extend the wound to allow both divided ends to be visualised and accessed (avoid longitudinal incisions across finger creases, as this may cause scar contractures and affect mobility).
2. The wound is irrigated and debrided.
3. The neurovascular bundle is located to assess for associated injury.
4. Both ends of the tendon are identified, assessed, and retrieved.
5. For the core repair, the 'Modified Kessler' with a two- or four-strand repair is employed using a 3/0 or 4/0 nonabsorbable monofilament suture. During the repair, the tendon ends are temporarily secured by pinning them in place with a hypodermic needle (in the Modified Kessler technique, the strength of the repair is proportional to the number of strands).
6. The epitendinous repair is then performed by placing a continuous running suture to the outer circumference of the tendon using a 5/0 or 6/0 suture (overly tight suturing can compromise the tendon's blood supply).
7. The wound is closed to ensure coverage of the repair.
8. The hand is placed in a splint.

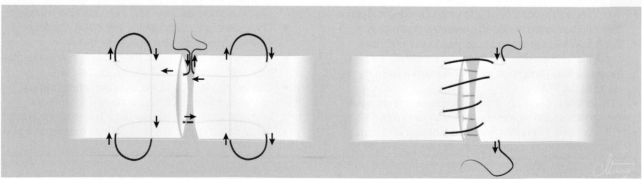

A) 2-strand modified Kessler repair

B) Epitendinous repair

Core and epitendinous stages of tendon repair.

Complications

EARLY
- Iatrogenic damage to the neurovascular bundle.
- Rupture of tendon repair.

INTERMEDIATE AND LATE
- Postoperative infection and/or wound breakdown.
- Poor mobility due to scarring, contractures, adhesions, poor repair, prolonged immobilisation, and noncompliance with therapy.
- Joint deformities—e.g. swan-neck, boutonniere (in extensor complications).
- Complex regional pain syndrome (CRPS)—a rare condition that can occur even after minor hand injuries.

Postoperative Care

INPATIENT
- Commonly performed as a day-case procedure.

OUTPATIENT
- Wound check at 7–10 days to assess for healing and infection.
- Hand therapy and rehabilitation by specialist hand physiotherapists—a vital component of successful tendon repair.
- Generally, early active mobilisation is advocated, although a short period of immobilisation may initially be required—duration of splinting is variable depending on type of injury.

? Surgeon's Favourite Question

When is a tendon repair at its weakest?

At around 10–12 days postoperatively, with most ruptures occurring at day 10.

100

Nail Bed Injury Repair

Georgios Pafitanis

Definition

Repair of a traumatic laceration involving the nail bed with the aim of ensuring continued nail growth and prevention of nail deformity.

Indications and Contraindications

INDICATIONS
- Repair of a nail bed laceration is done to ensure the best cosmetic outcome with regards to future nail growth in the following situations:
  - Crush injuries to nail bed.
  - Simple nail bed laceration.
  - Stellate lacerations of nail bed.
  - Avulsion of nail plate from nail fold.
  - Subungual haematoma >50% of visible nail.

CONTRAINDICATIONS
- Grossly contaminated or devitalised wound with complex underlying phalangeal fracture. These injuries may be more suitable for digital terminalisation and/or nail avulsion matrixectomy (removal of nail and germinal matrix to prevent nail regrowth).

Anatomy

- The nail plate is composed of hard, keratinised squamous cells attached to the nail bed inferiorly.
- The nail fold is where the nail plate proximally attaches to the underlying tissues and consists of the dorsal roof superiorly and the ventral floor inferiorly. The ventral floor is the site of the germinal matrix. The germinal matrix is responsible for the majority of nail production.
- The sterile matrix is the distal portion of the nail bed and is tightly adherent to both the overlying nail plate and the underlying periosteum. Along with the dorsal roof, it is a secondary site of nail production.
- The nail plate is loosely attached to the germinal matrix but is densely attached to the sterile matrix.
- The eponychium (cuticle) is the distal portion of the nail fold.
- The paronychium is the soft tissue along the lateral borders of the nail plate.
- Nails grow at roughly 3–4 mm per month (0.1 mm/day).

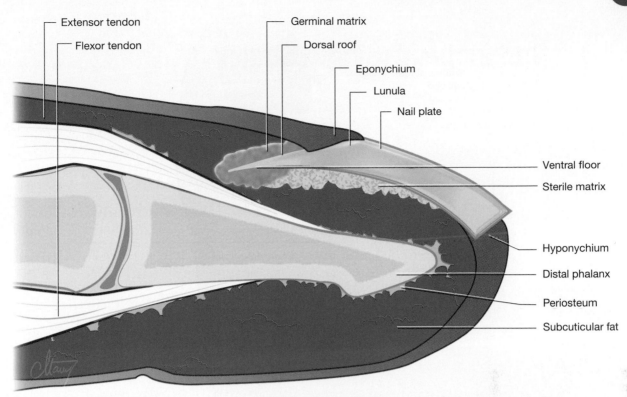

Anatomy of the nail bed.

Labels (clockwise): Extensor tendon, Flexor tendon, Germinal matrix, Dorsal roof, Eponychium, Lunula, Nail plate, Ventral floor, Sterile matrix, Hyponychium, Distal phalanx, Periosteum, Subcuticular fat

¹²₃ STEP-BY-STEP OPERATION

Anaesthesia: general with digital ring block (paediatrics), digital ring block only (adults). NB: local anaesthetic should not contain adrenaline due to the risk of avascular necrosis.

Position: arm and hand outstretched on an arm board.

Considerations: Apply a tourniquet to the digit to ensure a bloodless field for optimal visualisation of structures. Following hand trauma, these injuries may require additional surgical management, such as K-wire fixation.

Steps:

1. The nail plate is removed with a Kutz or Freer elevator and fine tenotomy scissors.
2. The nail bed is irrigated with saline.
3. Any grossly contaminated and nonviable tissue is excised.
4. Any associated finger pad laceration and/or distal phalanx injury is first repaired to minimise flailing of the distal segment.
5. Using fine absorbable sutures, the nail margin is then repaired to ensure anatomical alignment.
6. The nail bed is then sutured from the distal segment to proximal tissue.
7. The tourniquet is released and, using bipolar diathermy, haemostasis is achieved.
8. The removed nail plate acts as a dressing (often glued down over the nail bed repair). If the nail plate has been lost, Xeroform gauze or a silastic plate can be used.
9. A nonadherent dressing such as Mepitel, then gauze, tape, and a protective digital splint, is applied. Children require extensive bandaging of the hand ('boxing glove bandaging') to prevent picking or further injury.

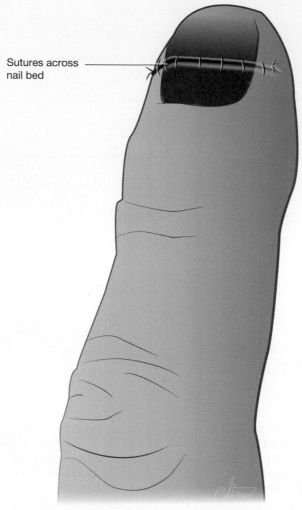

Sutures across nail bed

Suturing of a nail bed laceration.

 Complications

EARLY
- Bleeding.
- Pain and discomfort.

INTERMEDIATE AND LATE
- Infection.
- Absence of nail growth secondary to damage to the germinal matrix.
- Abnormal nail growth secondary to damage to the sterile matrix—ridged nail, hook nail, and nail spikes.
- Hypersensitivity—this can be transient or persistent.
- Complex regional pain syndrome—a rare condition that can occur even after minor hand injuries.

Postoperative Care

INPATIENT
- Commonly performed as a day-case procedure.
- Antibiotics in the case of contaminated wounds.

OUTPATIENT
- Dressing clinic in 7 days for removal of dressings and wound assessment.
- Protective splinting for 2 weeks.
- Outpatient follow-up in 6 weeks.
- Note: It takes approximately 100 days to grow a complete nail and see the final result of the nail bed repair.

? Surgeon's Favourite Question

What are the causes of a hook nail?

These are often caused by trauma to the nail bed—for example, in distal phalangeal bone loss resulting in poor support of the sterile matrix, causing a curved growth of the nail.

Ramstedt Pyloromyotomy

101

Mary Patrice Eastwood

Definition

A procedure to relieve outlet obstruction of the stomach caused by hypertrophy of the circular muscle of the pylorus.

Indications and Contraindications

INDICATIONS
- Hypertrophic pyloric stenosis.

CONTRAINDICATIONS
- Uncorrected metabolic abnormalities.

Anatomy

GROSS ANATOMY
- The stomach comprises of five parts:
  1. Cardia.
  2. Fundus.
  3. Body.
  4. Antrum.
  5. Pylorus.
- The stomach has two sphincters:
  1. Inferior oesophageal—this is a physiological sphincter created by the acute angle between the cardia and the oesophagus (the angle of His).
  2. Pyloric—an anatomical sphincter between the stomach and the duodenum made of a thick layer of circular smooth muscle. It is located at the level of the transpyloric plane (L1), 1 cm to the right of the midline.

NEUROVASCULATURE
- The parasympathetic nerve supply to the stomach arises from the vagus nerve.
- The sympathetic innervation of the stomach is derived from the coeliac, superior mesenteric, and inferior mesenteric ganglia.

- The blood supply to the stomach is from the coeliac trunk, which branches from the abdominal aorta at the level of T12.
- The left gastric artery (LGA), a direct branch of the coeliac trunk, supplies the superior lesser curvature of the stomach, whereas the right gastric artery (RGA), a branch of the common hepatic artery, supplies the inferior portion.
- The right gastro-epiploic (RGE) artery arises from the gastroduodenal artery and runs along the greater curvature from the distal aspect of the stomach.
- At the hilum of the spleen, the splenic artery divides into the short gastric arteries, which supply the fundus, and the left gastro-epiploic artery, which supplies the proximal greater curvature.
- The venous drainage of the stomach follows the arterial supply. An important vein to note in Ramstedt's pyloromyotomy is the pre-pyloric vein of Mayo, which runs anteriorly over the pylorus and drains into the right gastric vein.

102

Oesophageal Atresia/Tracheoesophageal Fistula Ligation With Repair

Mary Patrice Eastwood

Definition

A surgical procedure to correct and restore continuity of the oesophagus.

Indications and Contraindications

INDICATIONS

- Presence of oesophageal atresia (OA) with or without tracheoesophageal fistula (TOF).

CONTRAINDICATIONS

- Abdominal X-ray showing no air below the diaphragm signifies the absence of a distal TOF. In these cases, a gastrostomy is formed for feeding, and the primary repair is delayed.

Anatomy

EMBRYOLOGY

- Between the third and fourth gestational weeks, the foregut gives rise to a ventral diverticulum which becomes the respiratory primordium.
- The trachea is derived from the laryngotracheal diverticulum.
- Separation of the developing trachea and oesophagus (foregut) is tightly regulated within the developing embryo.
- OA occurs due to a failure in normal foregut development resulting in a failure of continuity of the oesophagus.

GROSS ANATOMY

- The trachea connects the pharynx and larynx to the lungs.
- The trachea comprises C-shaped cartilage with a posterior wall of muscle.
- The upper third of the oesophagus is composed of striated muscle that transitions to smooth muscle in the lower two-thirds.

NEUROVASCULATURE

- The trachea derives parasympathetic innervation from branches of the vagus nerve and the recurrent laryngeal nerve, and sympathetic innervation from the sympathetic trunk via the posterior and anterior pulmonary plexus.

- The oesophagus is parasympathetically innervated by the vagus nerve and sympathetically innervated by the thoracic spinal nerves.
- The trachea is perfused by branches of the subclavian, internal mammary, and brachiocephalic arteries.
- The upper third of the oesophagus is supplied by the inferior thyroid arteries.
- The middle third of the oesophagus is supplied by the oesophageal branches of the thoracic aorta.
- The lower third of the oesophagus is supplied by the left gastric artery and left inferior phrenic artery.

PATHOLOGY

- Gross classification is used to describe OA:
  - Type A—OA with no TOF (8%).
  - Type B—OA with TOF between the trachea and the upper portion of the oesophagus (1%).
  - Type C—OA with TOF between the trachea and the lower portion of the oesophagus (86%).
  - Type D—OA with TOF between the trachea and both the upper and lower portions of the oesophagus (1%).
  - Type E—TOF with no atresia of the oesophagus ('H-type') (4%).

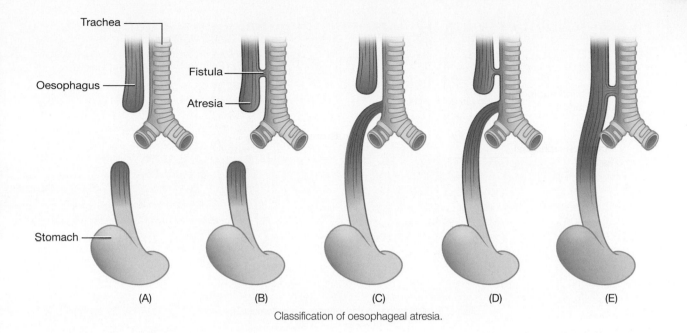

Classification of oesophageal atresia.

¹²₃ STEP-BY-STEP OPERATION

Anaesthesia: general.

Position: The patient is positioned on the left side with the right arm extended over the head.

Steps:

1. A thoracotomy incision (transverse) is made 1 cm below the right scapula extending across the midaxillary line. The muscle layers are split, and entry is made into the pleural cavity at the fourth to fifth intercostal space.
2. The right lung is gently retracted to visualise the oesophagus and trachea.
3. An extrapleural approach is attempted with posterior dissection of the pleural from the chest wall. The azygos vein is encountered running across the trachea and ligated.
4. The TOF is carefully dissected to avoid damage to the vagus nerve.

5. A loop is placed around the fistula and the lungs insufflated before separation to ensure the loop is not around the right main bronchus.
6. Sutures are placed across the oesophageal fistula close to the trachea, and the fistula is then divided distal to these sutures.
7. The distal end of the fistula is checked for patency and occasionally divided again a few centimetres distal from the first dissection to create a wider end for anastomosis.
8. The distal oesophagus (previously the fistula) is mobilised superiorly to meet the proximal oesophagus.
9. An end-to-end anastomosis is performed with care taken to include both mucosal and muscle layers.
10. A small nasogastric (NG) tube, also known as a trans-anastomotic tube (TAT), is placed to enable early NG feeding postoperatively. A chest drain is only necessary in cases of a difficult dissection. The chest wall is closed in layers.

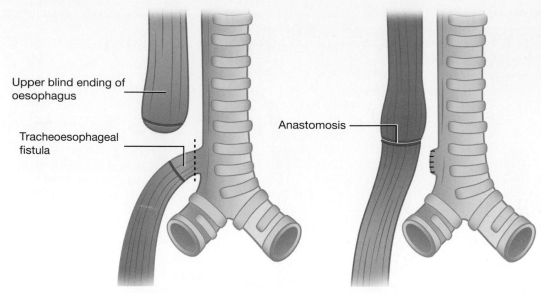

Upper blind ending of oesophagus

Tracheoesophageal fistula

Anastomosis

Sites of fistula ligation and oesophageal anastomosis.

 Complications

EARLY
- Anastomotic leak.

INTERMEDIATE AND LATE
- Anastomotic stricture.
- Recurrent TOF.

Postoperative Care

INPATIENT
- The patient is transferred to neonatal intensive care postoperatively.
- TAT feeds may commence on the second or third postoperative day, and oral feeding may be introduced gradually.
- Occasionally, an oesophageal contrast study may be performed to ensure no leak at the anastomotic site.

OUTPATIENT
- Omeprazole is prescribed for 1 year to minimise oesophageal reflux.

 Surgeon's Favourite Questions

What other abnormalities should be ruled out preoperatively in neonates with OA?

OA is associated with VACTERL syndrome (20%), encompassing vertebral, anal atresia, cardiovascular, tracheoesophageal, renal, and limb defects. It is particularly important to rule out a cardiac defect (20–50%), the most common being ventricular septal defect, as these are associated with a higher mortality rate.

Laparotomy for Necrotising Enterocolitis (NEC)

103

Mary Patrice Eastwood

Definition

Closure of isolated intestinal perforations and the resection of necrotic bowel and/or formation of a stoma.

Indications and Contraindications

INDICATIONS
- Intestinal perforation.
- Failure of NEC to respond to medical management.
- Abdominal mass with signs of intestinal obstruction or sepsis.

CONTRAINDICATIONS
- Total intestinal gangrene—treatment withdrawal should be considered.

Anatomy

EMBRYOLOGY
- The embryological development of the gut is derived from a primitive endodermal tube that is divided into three parts:
  1. Foregut—oesophagus to upper duodenum (d2) (supplied by the coeliac axis).
  2. Midgut—lower duodenum (d3) to proximal two-thirds of the transverse colon (supplied by the superior mesenteric artery).
  3. Hindgut—distal one-third of transverse colon to ectodermal part of the anal canal (supplied by the inferior mesenteric artery.

GROSS ANATOMY
- The small bowel starts at the duodenal jejunal (DJ) flexure (ligament of Treitz acts as the anatomical landmark) and travels obliquely and downwards towards the right sacro-iliac joint within the free edge of a mesentery attached to the posterior abdominal wall.
- The first two-fifths of the small intestine is termed the jejunum and the remainder the ileum; the distinction between the two is histological (Peyer's patches increased numbers in ileum).
- The colon comprises the caecum, ascending colon, transverse colon, descending colon, and sigmoid colon.
- The ascending colon extends upwards from the caecum to the under surface of the liver and at the hepatic flexure turns left to become the transverse colon.
- The transverse colon is covered completely by peritoneum (intraperitoneal) and runs from the hepatic flexure to the splenic flexure to become the descending colon.
- The descending colon passes from the splenic flexure to the sigmoid colon.
- The mesenteries of the ascending and descending colon blend with the posterior abdominal wall (retroperitoneal), except for the sigmoid colon (intraperitoneal).
- The pelvic brim marks the beginning of the sigmoid colon, which extends to the recto-sigmoid junction.
- Any part of the bowel may be affected by NEC, but the most frequent sites (respectively) are the terminal ileum, right hemi-colon, left hemi-colon, and sigmoid colon.

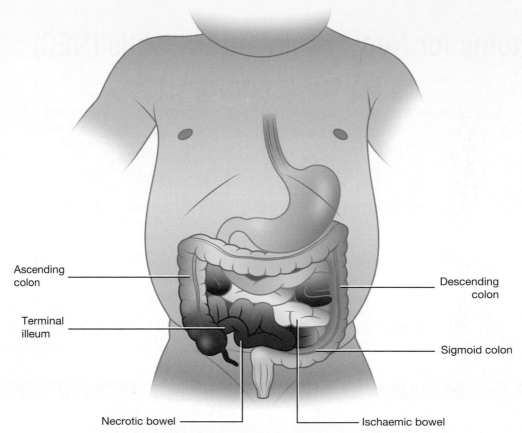

Necrotising enterocolitis in the gastrointestinal tract of a neonate.

Labels on image:
- Ascending colon
- Terminal illeum
- Descending colon
- Sigmoid colon
- Necrotic bowel
- Ischaemic bowel

1 2 3 STEP-BY-STEP OPERATION

Anaesthesia: general.

Position: supine.

Considerations: An exploratory laparotomy is conducted with the aim of controlling sepsis and removing areas of frankly necrotic bowel whilst preserving bowel length.

Steps:

1. A transverse supraumbilical incision is made (in preterm neonates, extra care should be taken not to damage the liver, which is extremely fragile; in these patients, a left-sided incision should be considered to avoid the liver).

2. Intraoperative options depend upon the amount of disease found:

   a. Isolated simple perforations—'focal NEC' (frequently occur in the terminal ileum) are closed with sutures placed transversely to prevent narrowing of the bowel lumen.

   b. Isolated necrotic or perforated segments (2 to 3 cm) with no involvement of the remaining bowel—are treated with resection and primary anastomosis. The intestine is cut at an angle of 30 to 45 degrees to increase the anastomotic circumference. Nonviable bowel is discarded, with healthy bowel ends anastomosed (anastomotic ends should bleed briskly when cut, indicating bowel viability).

   c. Multiple perforations and necrotic segments—can be treated with a combination of oversewing, resection with primary anastomosis, or 'clip and drop' in the case of an unstable neonate. 'Clip and drop' involves resecting and removing segments of necrotic bowel and closing the end independently using a LIGACLIP (metal clip) rather than performing a primary anastomosis. The most proximal piece of bowel can be formed into an enterostomy.

   d. Pan-intestinal NEC—usually results in the formation of a proximal jejunotomy. 'Clip and drop' is an option.

3. A defunctioning loop ileostomy or terminal stoma with distal mucosal fistula is formed.

4. Closure:

   a. Abdominal wound closure is performed in two fascial layers using a running absorbable suture.

   b. If the fascia is friable or difficult to identify, single-layer closure including both fascial layers and the rectus muscle is performed.

   c. In case of massive inflammation or difficulties in closing the abdominal cavity, a temporary patch should be considered to avoid the risk of compartment syndrome (raised intraabdominal pressure). A second-look operation may then be performed at 24 hours to check viability.

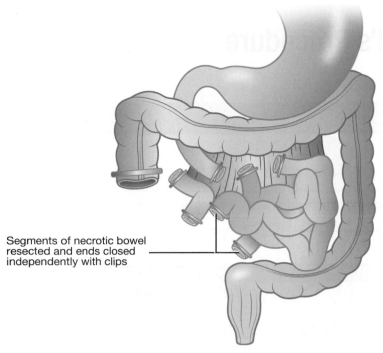

Segments of necrotic bowel resected and ends closed independently with clips

Sites of clip and drop in necrotising enterocolitis.

 Complications

EARLY

- Mortality is dependent on disease severity and gestational age at birth.

INTERMEDIATE AND LATE

- Neurodevelopmental delay.
- Stricture formation.
- Short gut syndrome.
- Vitamin B_{12} deficiency if ileal resection is required.

Postoperative Care

INPATIENT

- Postoperatively the patient is managed in the neonatal intensive care unit (NICU).
- Parental nutrition is commenced for feeding with complete bowel rest and intravenous antibiotics for at least 1 week.
- Future management depends on the surgical technique performed. Bowel continuity will need to be restored in the case of a 'clip and drop' when the neonate is stable and no longer septic.
- Total parenteral nutrition is established in cases where there may be a delay in enteral feeding (>5 days). When bowel continuity is restored, a trophic feed can be started and gradually built up as tolerated.
- Reanastomosis of a stoma is around the 8th to 12th postoperative week. A contrast enema is performed before reanastomosis to detect intestinal strictures that usually occur within the large bowel.

OUTPATIENT

- Children are followed up in the outpatient clinic and subsequently on a yearly basis to monitor for growth and late complications.
- In case of terminal ileum resection, long-term follow-up is needed to rule out possible vitamin B_{12} deficiency.

? Surgeon's Favourite Question

What are the radiographic findings in NEC?

Pneumatosis intestinalis is the pathognomonic radiographic finding. This signifies the presence of gas-producing organisms in the bowel wall. Other signs include a dilated bowel loop or a fixed loop 'signet sign', portal venous gas, and, importantly, pneumoperitoneum.

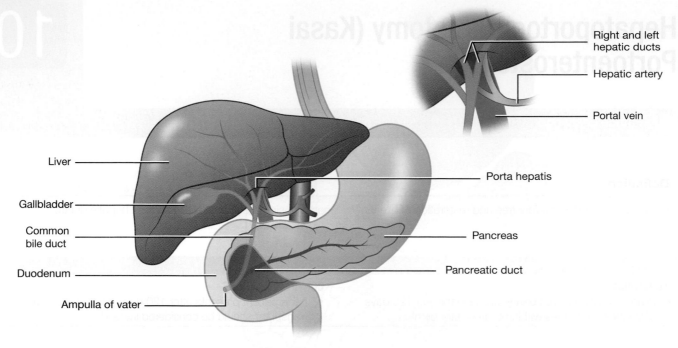

Right and left hepatic ducts

Hepatic artery

Portal vein

Liver

Porta hepatis

Gallbladder

Common bile duct

Pancreas

Duodenum

Pancreatic duct

Ampulla of vater

The biliary tree.

1 2 3 STEP-BY-STEP OPERATION

Anaesthesia: general.

Position: supine.

Considerations: A urinary catheter and a nasogastric (NG) tube are inserted. Prophylactic antibiotics are administered at induction. A portable image intensifier (II) is used to perform an on the table cholangiogram.

Steps:

1. A short subcostal incision is made in the hepatic area to facilitate an operative cholangiogram. A small catheter is secured in the gallbladder and contrast instilled to delineate the biliary tree (biliary atresia is confirmed when the on the table cholangiogram shows no passage of radiographic contrast media into the liver).

2. After confirming biliary atresia, the initial incision is extended to a full subcostal incision.

3. The falciform and coronary ligaments of the liver are divided to allow the liver to be brought out of the body and rotated so regions of fibrotic biliary tree can be dissected under direct vision whilst avoiding the vascular structures.

4. The fibrous bile duct is dissected, starting at the junction of the cystic duct.

5. The gallbladder is mobilised and removed.

6. Dissection then proceeds upwards until the porta hepatis is reached with the excision of any biliary remnants (care should be taken to ligate the small communicating branches of the portal vein if necessary).

7. Next, the jejunal Roux-en-Y loop is constructed. The jejunum is divided, and the distal end is brought up behind the transverse colon and anastomosed directly to the region of the porta hepatis, encompassing the bile ducts. The vascular structures at the porta hepatis must not be incorporated within this anastomosis.

8. The proximal end of the divided jejunum is anastomosed (end on side) to the Roux-en-Y loop of the jejunum.

9. The liver is replaced into the abdominal cavity; a drain may be placed.

10. The subcostal incision is closed in layers with absorbable sutures.

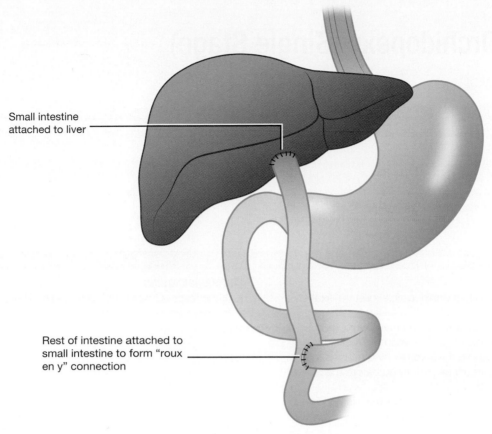

Small intestine attached to liver

Rest of intestine attached to small intestine to form "roux en y" connection

Anastomosis between the porta hepatis and the jejunum.

Complications

EARLY
- Failure to resolve/restore biliary drainage.

INTERMEDIATE AND LATE
- Cholangitis.
- Portal hypertension and oesophageal varices.

Postoperative Care

INPATIENT
- Monitoring of liver function.
- IV antibiotics are given to reduce the early risk of postoperative cholangitis. Oral antibiotic prophylaxis continues for 3 to 6 months.

OUTPATIENT
- Long-term oral ursodeoxycholic acid is given for its choleretic effect and to relieve symptoms of cholestasis, such as pruritus.
- Fat-soluble vitamin (A, D, E, and K) supplements should be continued until normal bilirubin has been achieved.
- Many patients will ultimately progress to at some point require a liver transplant.

Surgeon's Favourite Question

What is the most important initial investigation in a baby with prolonged jaundiced?

Split bilirubin, looking at the conjugated fraction of bilirubin.

106

Orchidopexy (Single Stage)

Mary Patrice Eastwood

Definition

Repositioning of the testis into the scrotum.

 Indications and Contraindications

INDICATIONS

- Testicular torsion with a viable testicle (bilateral fixation is required).
- To reduce the risk of infertility and malignancy in:
  - Congenital cryptorchidism—when the testicle has not descended into the scrotum by 6 months of age. Orchidopexy should be performed before the patient turns 1 year old.
  - Acquired cryptorchidism—orchidopexy is performed within 6 months of testicular ascent.

CONTRAINDICATIONS

- If the testis is impalpable, a two-staged procedure may be required.

Anatomy

EMBRYOLOGY

- The gonadal structures form in the urogenital ridge on the posterior abdominal wall at around 7 weeks in utero.
- The gonads descend from the abdominal cavity through the inguinal canal into the scrotum, guided by a fibrous structure called the gubernaculum.

GROSS ANATOMY

- The muscle and fascial layers of the anterior abdominal wall give rise to the layers of the spermatic cord.
- The spermatic cord contains the vas deferens, testicular and deferential arteries, a venous network (pampiniform plexus), testicular nerves, lymphatic vessels, and the tunica vaginalis.
- The layers of the scrotum, from skin to testes, are the skin, dartos fascia and muscle, external spermatic fascia (external oblique muscle), cremasteric muscle and fascia (internal oblique muscle), internal spermatic fascia (transversalis fascia), and parietal layer of the tunica vaginalis.

NEUROVASCULATURE

- The testis and the spermatic cord are innervated by sympathetic fibres from the thoracic spinal cord segments T1–12.
- The scrotum is mainly innervated by the posterior scrotal nerves (branches of the perineal nerve, arising from the pudendal nerve).
- The spermatic cord and testis derive their blood supply mainly from the testicular artery, which arises from the abdominal aorta. There is also collateral blood supply from the deferential artery and the cremasteric artery (internal and external iliac artery).
- The scrotum gets its blood supply from the anterior and posterior scrotal arteries.
- Venous drainage of the testis and spermatic cord is via the pampiniform plexus into the testicular vein. The left testicular vein drains into the left renal vein and the right testicular vein into the inferior vena cava.
- Blood is drained from the scrotum into the pudendal veins.
- The lymphatic vessels of the testis and spermatic cord drain into the para-aortic lymph nodes, while that of the scrotum drains into the superficial inguinal lymph nodes.

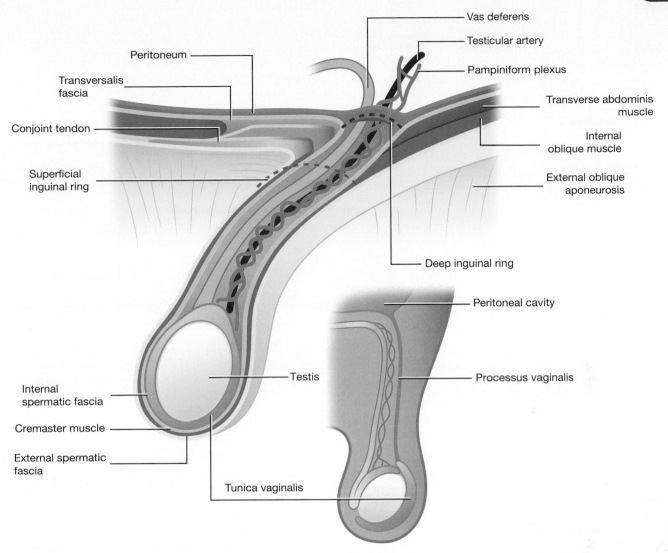

Layers of the spermatic cord.

1·2·3 STEP-BY-STEP OPERATION

Anaesthesia: general with a caudal block.
Position: supine.
Steps:

1. A transverse skin incision is made along the Langer's lines over the midinguinal point. The layers are separated to define Scarpa's fascia.

2. The external oblique aponeurosis is cleared, the reflection of the inguinal ligament and the external inguinal ring is identified, and an incision is made in the external oblique muscle and extended towards the external inguinal ring. The ilioinguinal nerve is identified and protected.

3. The spermatic cord superior to the testis is mobilised and delivered out of the incision.

4. The gubernaculum is detached and the spermatic cord is stripped of remaining cremasteric fibres.

5. To gain maximal length, the patent processus vaginalis or hernial sac is separated from the cord structures; care is taken to avoid injury to the vas deferens and vessels.

6. The hernial sac is divided and dissected from the cord structures to the level of the internal ring. It is twisted at the point of the internal ring, then transfixed and ligated.

7. A finger is passed from the incision into the scrotum, and a second horizontal incision is made over the fingertip in the ipsilateral scrotal skin. A sub-dartos pouch is developed just under the scrotal skin.

8. A pair of fine artery forceps is passed through the scrotal incision and guided into the inguinal incision as the fingertip is retracted.

9. The testis is brought through the opening of the fascia, ensuring the spermatic cord does not twist in the process. The testis is placed in the pouch and is fixed to the scrotum.

10. The scrotal skin is closed with absorbable sutures. The incisions, namely, the external oblique aponeurosis to the external ring, Scarpa's fascia, and the skin incision, are closed in layers.

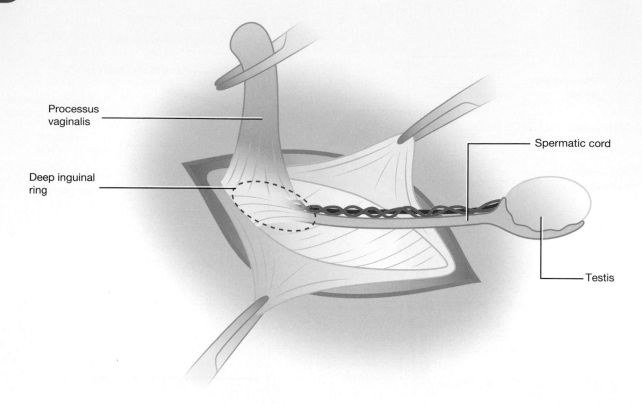

Separation of the processus vaginalis from the spermatic cord.

Complications

EARLY
- Scrotal haematoma.
- Injury to vas deferens (1–2%).

INTERMEDIATE AND LATE
- Wound infection.
- Testicular atrophy (<5%).
- Retraction of testis is dependent on testicular position—i.e. external ring, inguinal canal, or intra-abdominal (8–16%).

Postoperative Care

INPATIENT
- Commonly performed as a day-case procedure.

OUTPATIENT
- Vigorous or strenuous activities and straddle-type toys (e.g. bicycle) should be avoided for 2 weeks postoperatively.
- Clinic follow-up at 6 months to check for testicular atrophy or retraction.

Surgeon's Favourite Question

If the testis cannot reach the scrotum, what other techniques can be employed to gain extra length?

The retroperitoneal plane above the internal ring can be developed by pulling the peritoneal membrane anteriorly using a retractor. If the vas deferens is a limiting factor, the testis can be rerouted medially by dividing the inferior epigastric vessels to gain up to 1 cm in length.

Hysterectomy

107

Imogen Thomson, d'Arcy Ferris Baxter

Definition

Removal of the uterus either laparoscopically or via a laparotomy, or transvaginally. A hysterectomy can be:
- Total—removal of the uterus and the cervix.
- Subtotal—removal of the uterus but the cervix is preserved.
- Radical—removal of the cervix, upper third of the vagina, and the parametrium, including lymph nodes.

A hysterectomy does not imply removal of the fallopian tubes (salpingectomy) and ovaries (oophorectomy). These terms refer to separate procedural elements, although are frequently performed together.

Indications and Contraindications

INDICATIONS
General
- Malignancy (typically endometrial, cervical or ovarian).
- Dysfunctional uterine bleeding, such as due to adenomyosis.
- Severe endometriosis.
- Fibroids causing menorrhagia or pressure symptoms.
- Pelvic organ prolapse.
- Final life-saving option in massive postpartum haemorrhage.

CONTRAINDICATIONS
Relative
- Large or bulky uterus may make a laparoscopic approach more complex, and an open abdominal approach may be preferred.

Absolute
- Advanced uterine/cervical/ovarian malignancy where surgery is unlikely to improve symptoms or prognosis.

Anatomy

GROSS ANATOMY
- The uterus lies within the pelvis and is divided into the:
  - Fundus.
  - Cornua.
  - Corpus (body).
  - Cervix.
- The uterus is held within the broad ligament, which is continuous between the sides of the pelvis and comprises two leaves (anterior and posterior).
- The fallopian tubes arise from the cornua of the uterus, with the fimbrial ends opening to the peritoneal cavity adjacent (but not attached) to the ovaries.
- The ovaries are located on the posterior surface of the broad ligament. They are attached to the cornua of the uterus by the ovarian ligaments and to the pelvic side walls by the infundibulo-pelvic ligament (IP)/suspensory ligament. The suspensory ligament contains the ovarian blood vessels and nerves.
- The round ligaments travel anteriorly from the cornua to the inguinal canals.
- The uterosacral ligaments travel from the cervix to the second part of the sacrum.
- The cardinal ligaments travel from the cervix and upper vagina to the root of the internal iliac vessels and contain the nerves, arteries, and veins that travel from the pelvic sidewall to the genital tract.
- The uterus is connected through the cervix to the vagina, which lies immediately posterior to the urethra and bladder and anterior to the anal canal and rectum.

NEUROVASCULATURE
- Parasympathetic fibres of the uterus are derived from the pelvic splanchnic nerves (S2, S3, S4). Sympathetic fibres arise from the uterovaginal plexus, a division of the inferior hypogastric plexus. Afferent sensory fibres ascend through the inferior hypogastric plexus and enter the spinal cord at T10, T11, T12, and L1. Epidural analgesia therefore provides sensory block to these fibres.
- The main blood supply to the uterus is via the uterine arteries, which travel medially in the base of the broad ligament before ascending along the lateral aspect of the uterus and anastomosing with the ovarian arteries.

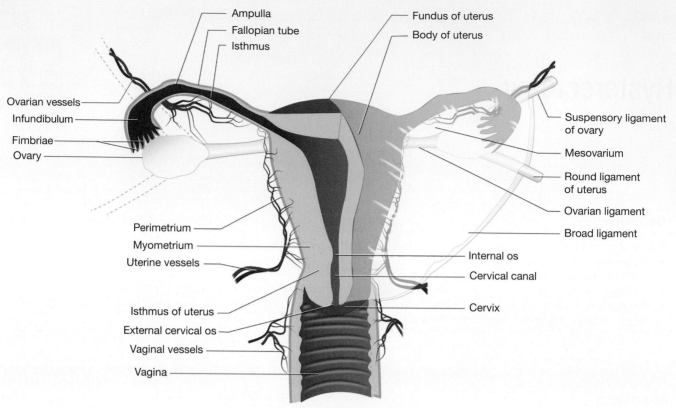

Gross anatomy and vasculature of the uterus, ovaries, and vagina.

1 2 3 STEP-BY-STEP OPERATION

Anaesthesia: general or regional (epidural or spinal).
Position: Trendelenburg for open and laparoscopic (described here) or lithotomy for transvaginal.
Considerations: An indwelling urinary catheter is inserted prior to laparoscopic entry.
Steps:
1. The cervix is dilated, and a uterine manipulator is inserted into the uterus.
2. Three to four laparoscopic trocars are positioned, and pneumoperitoneum is achieved via the Hasson technique:
   a. Umbilical ×1.
   b. Supra-pubic (optional) ×1.
   c. Medial to the anterior superior iliac spines ×2.
3. The uterus is mobilised to expose the round ligaments, which are then cut using bipolar diathermy.
4. Scissors are used to dissect the broad ligament's anterior leaf from the posterior leaf.
5. In ovarian conservation, the fallopian tube and utero-ovarian ligament are cut. However, in cases of salpingo-oophorectomy (removal of the fallopian tubes and ovaries), the infundibulopelvic ligament is cut.

6. The ureters are displaced laterally and posteriorly (where they are less susceptible to iatrogenic injury). The vesico-peritoneum is cut and elevated from the anterior uterine segment, and then the posterior leaf of the broad ligament is opened up to the uterosacral ligaments.
7. The vaginal mucosa is then cut near to the cervix and through the anterior section. Dissection is made caudally until the peritoneal cavity can be entered through the previous opening made in the vesico-peritoneum. The posterior vaginal mucosa is then incised just above the uterosacral ligaments to free the vagina.
8. The uterine arteries are clamped and ligated, and the uterus (±ovaries and fallopian tubes) is removed through the vagina.
9. The edges of the vaginal cuff are sutured and the vagina is returned to the pelvis. The uterosacral ligaments are plicated to ensure suspension of the vaginal cuff and to prevent prolapse. Drains may be inserted into the pelvis and exiting through the abdomen.
10. The abdomen is deflated, and port sites are closed with sutures.

Total hysterectomy

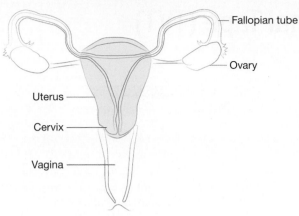

- Fallopian tube
- Ovary
- Uterus
- Cervix
- Vagina

Radical hysterectomy

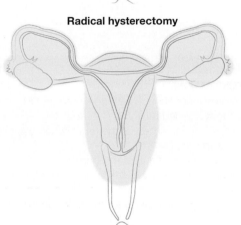

Total hysterectomy with unilateral salpingo-oopheractomy

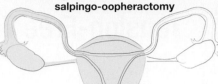

Total hysterectomy with bilateral salpingo-oopheractomy

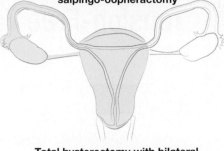

Subtotal hysterectomy

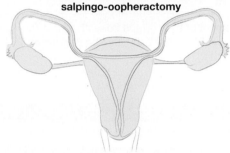

Subtypes of hysterectomy.

Complications

EARLY
- Bleeding.
- Injury—ureter, bladder, and bowel.
- Ileus.
- Urinary retention.

INTERMEDIATE AND LATE
- Infection—wound, vagina, urinary tract, intraabdominal.
- Vaginal cuff dehiscence.
- Abdominal adhesions—may cause bowel obstruction.
- Vaginal prolapse.

Postoperative Care

INPATIENT
- Patients can be discharged once mobile, passing urine after catheter removal, and any drains have been removed.
- Most patients are discharged home within 48 hours following surgery as long as no complications occur.

OUTPATIENT
- Consultant outpatient appointment 2 weeks postoperatively.
- Patients are advised to avoid heavy lifting.
- Vaginal intercourse is discouraged for 6 weeks postsurgery to facilitate healing and prevent infection.

Surgeon's Favourite Question

When would you choose open versus laparoscopic versus transvaginal hysterectomy?

Open hysterectomy:
- Multiple previous abdominal operations.
- Large uterus.
- Extensive disease.

Laparoscopic hysterectomy:
- Uterus equal in size to or smaller than that at 12 weeks' gestation.
- Anatomical barriers to transvaginal—narrow subpubic arch or a long and narrow vagina.

Transvaginal hysterectomy:
- Obesity—enhanced recovery compared to abdominal wound.
- General anaesthesia contraindicated, as can be performed under regional (spinal) anaesthesia.
- Vaginal prolapse.

108

Tension-Free Vaginal Tape (TVT)

Imogen Thomson, d'Arcy Ferris Baxter

Definition

The placement of a sling/tape beneath the urethra to provide support to the neck of the urethra in order to treat stress urinary incontinence (SUI). This can either be performed via the retropubic approach or the transobturator approach.

Indications and Contraindications

INDICATIONS

- SUI, the involuntary leakage of urine when pressure is applied to the bladder (e.g. on sneezing or coughing, or exertion) that affects quality of life and is unresponsive to conservative measures.

CONTRAINDICATIONS

- Pure urge incontinence with no element of SUI present (can be worsened by TVT).
- Previous hernia surgery in the groin (when using the retro-pubic approach).
- Vulval, vaginal, or cervical malignancy.
- Previous radiotherapy to the vulval, vaginal, or cervical tissue.
- Current pregnancy (plans for future pregnancy is a relative contraindication).

Anatomy

- The urethra and bladder lie posterior to the pubic symphysis and the space of Retzius (extraperitoneal space between the pubic symphysis and bladder) and anterior to the vagina.
- The female urethra is approximately 4 cm long and is embedded in the anterior vaginal wall immediately poste-rior to the pubic rami.
- The internal urethral sphincter (IUS) lies at the inferior end of the bladder and the proximal end of the urethra. It contains smooth muscle fibres in a horseshoe arrange-ment and is continuous with the detrusor muscle of the bladder. The IUS is controlled involuntarily though the autonomic nervous system.
- The external urethral sphincter (EUS) surrounds the urethra, is made up of striated muscle, and is under voluntary control. It includes three parts: the annular sphincter around the urethra (urethral sphincter), a part encircling both the vagina and the urethra (urethrovagi-nal sphincter), and a muscle attaching to the ischial rami and passing anterior to the urethra (compressor urethral muscle). It is innervated by the pudendal nerve (S2, S3, S4).
- At the bladder neck, the urethra is surrounded by multiple elastic fibres that also help to maintain urethral closure.
- The urethra passes through the levator ani muscles, which insert into the perineal body.
- The action of this group of muscles is to elevate the urethrovesical junction and to create an angle between the fixed lower portion and the flexible upper portion of the urethra. This also helps to maintain urinary continence.

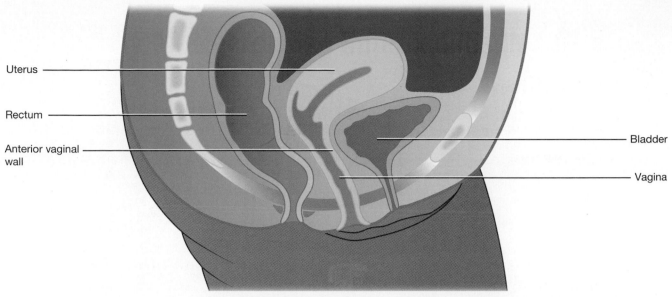

Cross-sectional anatomy of the female pelvis.

Uterus

Rectum

Anterior vaginal wall

Bladder

Vagina

STEP-BY-STEP OPERATION

Anaesthesia: general, regional (epidural or spinal), or local.
Position: lithotomy.
Steps:

1. The bladder is examined cystoscopically to ensure that there is no pathology within the bladder or within its walls, and a Foley catheter is then inserted into the bladder via the urethra.
2. Two exit sites are marked 2 cm immediately above and lateral to the pubic symphysis and at the level of the urethra. Local anaesthetic is injected submucosally.
3. At the two implant exit sites, a local anaesthetic solution mixed with adrenaline or plain saline is used to hydrodissect the bladder walls and the urethra off the surrounding tissue and organs. It is applied:
   a. Just above the pubic tubercle on both sides of the midline.
   b. To the anterior vaginal wall.
4. A sagittal incision is made at the urethral meatus, and dissection is performed paraurethrally towards the endopelvic fascia to dissect the urethra free of the anterior vaginal wall.
5. The bladder is drained, and a rigid catheter guide is inserted into the Foley catheter. The handle is pivoted to the left of the surgeon to expose the left endopelvic fascia.

6. The trochar is padded through the right paraurethral dissection. The right endopelvic fascia is punctured, and the trochar is then advanced through the space of Retzius and the anterior abdominal wall towards the right exit site. At the surface, the skin is incised to allow the needle to emerge.
7. The Foley catheter is removed, and a cystoscopy is performed to ensure bladder integrity. The Foley catheter is reinserted, along with the rigid catheter guide.
8. The procedure is repeated on the contralateral side, ensuring the sling/tape does not twist during insertion. The tape now forms a 'U' shape around the urethra. A further check via cystoscopy is performed.
9. The tape should be tension free. This is tested by filling the bladder with 250 mL of saline and applying pressure to the anterior abdominal wall. The sling/tape is pulled upwards gently on both sides until only a few drops leak out when pressure is applied.
10. The abdominal ends of the tape are cut, and the wounds are sutured. The vaginal wall is inspected, and the vaginal incision is sutured. If there has been significant bleeding, a vaginal gauze pack may be left in situ for 24 hours. A Foley catheter is placed.

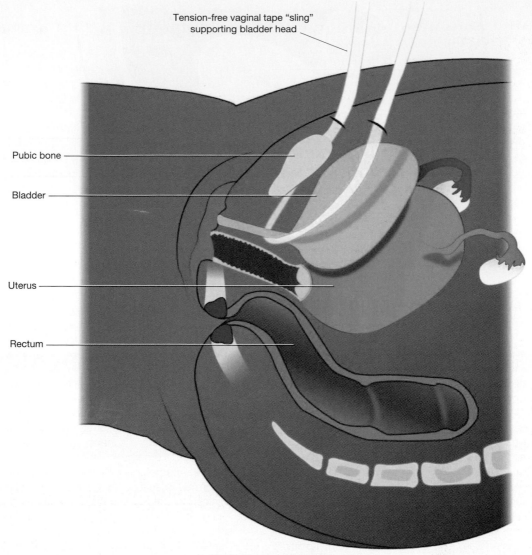

Tension-free vaginal tape "sling" supporting bladder head

Pubic bone

Bladder

Uterus

Rectum

Vaginal tension-free tape.

Complications

EARLY
- Bleeding.
- Urinary retention.
- Bladder perforation.

INTERMEDIATE AND LATE
- Infection.
- De novo or worsening urge incontinence.
- Voiding dysfunction.

Postoperative Care

INPATIENT
- Trial without catheterisation (TWOC) and, if passing urine, can be discharged home.

OUTPATIENT
- Outpatient appointment in 3 months to evaluate success of operation and check for wound healing and complications.

Surgeon's Favourite Question

What causes stress urinary incontinence?

SUI results from weakening of the pelvic floor muscles or displacement of the bladder neck. This can be caused by pregnancy (even if birth is by caesarean section and is due to the weight of the gravid uterus), vaginal delivery (operative and spontaneous), and menopause (lack of oestrogen atrophies the pelvic floor muscles). Additional risk factors include chronic cough, obesity, and constipation/straining. In all cases, there is damage to the pelvic floor and ligament support of the bladder neck and urethra, thus resulting in leakage when pressure is applied.

Imogen Thomson, d'Arcy Ferris Baxter

Definition

The diagnostic insertion of a camera (hysteroscope) through the cervix into the uterus. Can be combined with several therapeutic procedures.

Indications and Contraindications

INDICATIONS

- Diagnosis and management of abnormal uterine bleeding (AUB):
  - Endometrial biopsy for diagnosis of malignancy.
  - Polypectomy for uterine polyps.
  - Myomectomy for uterine fibroids.
  - Endometrial ablation therapy.
- To rule out, diagnose, and treat causes of subfertility:
  - Division of intrauterine adhesions (Asherman's syndrome).
  - Division of uterine septum.
  - Polypectomy.
- Removal of intrauterine devices (IUDs) if conservative attempts (e.g. ultrasound-guided removal) have failed.
- Removal of retained products of conception.

CONTRAINDICATIONS

Relative
- Active cervical or uterine infection.
- Known cervical or uterine cancer.

Absolute
- Viable intrauterine pregnancy.

Anatomy

GROSS ANATOMY
- The uterus lies within the pelvis and is divided into the:
  - Fundus.
  - Cornua.
  - Corpus (body).
  - Cervix.
- The uterus is held within the broad ligament, which is continuous between the sides of the pelvis and comprises two leaves (anterior and posterior).
- The fallopian tubes arise from the cornua of the uterus, with the fimbrial ends opening to the peritoneal cavity adjacent (but not attached) to the ovaries.
- The ovaries are located on the posterior surface of the broad ligament. They are attached to the cornua of the uterus by the ovarian ligaments and to the pelvic side walls by the infundibulo-pelvic ligament (IP)/suspensory ligament. The suspensory ligament contains the ovarian blood vessels and nerves.
- The round ligaments travel anteriorly from the cornua to the inguinal canals.
- The uterosacral ligaments travel from the cervix to the second part of the sacrum.
- The cardinal ligaments travel from the cervix and upper vagina to the root of the internal iliac vessels and contain the nerves, arteries, and veins that travel from the pelvic sidewall to the genital tract.
- The uterus is connected through the cervix to the vagina, which lies immediately posterior to the urethra and bladder and anterior to the anal canal and rectum.

NEUROVASCULATURE
- Parasympathetic fibres of the uterus are derived from the pelvic splanchnic nerves (S2, S3, S4). Sympathetic fibres arise from the uterovaginal plexus, a division of the inferior hypogastric plexus. Afferent sensory fibres ascend through the inferior hypogastric plexus and enter the spinal cord at T10, T11, T12, and L1. Epidural analgesia therefore provides sensory block to these fibres.
- The main blood supply to the uterus is via the uterine arteries, which travel medially in the base of the broad ligament before ascending along the lateral aspect of the uterus and anastomosing with the ovarian arteries.

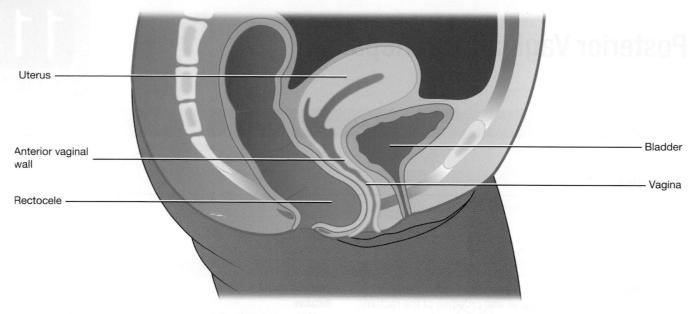

Uterus

Anterior vaginal
wall

Rectocele

Bladder

Vagina

Cross-sectional anatomy of the female pelvis with a rectocele.

1 2 3 STEP-BY-STEP OPERATION

Anaesthesia: general or regional (spinal or epidural).
Position: lithotomy.
Considerations: Under anaesthesia, a bimanual examination and examination of the perineal body are performed. A Foley catheter is inserted into the bladder.
Steps:
1. The posterior vaginal wall defect is exposed using vaginal wall retractors.
2. The posterior vaginal wall is then infiltrated with a mixture of local anaesthetic solution with adrenaline or simply with normal saline in order to hydrodissect the rectum off the vaginal wall.
3. The posterior vaginal mucosa is clamped at the mucocutaneous junction of the vaginal opening and at the maximum apex point of the rectocele (this may reach up to the vaginal vault).
4. A longitudinal incision is made on the posterior vaginal wall between the two clamps, and the posterior vaginal mucosa is then dissected away from the rectovaginal fascia (the dissection should continue to a point slightly above the defect and transversely as far as the sidewalls).
5. If perineorrhaphy (repair of the perineum) is to be incorporated, a triangular section of skin overlying the perineal body is removed to expose the aponeurosis of the superficial transverse muscle of the perineum and the bulbocavernosus muscle.

6. The exposure of the rectovaginal fascia and perineal body allows for visualisation of any defects. The edges are grasped and brought into position in the midline. Absorbable sutures are used to bring the left and right sides of the fascial defects together.
7. Depending on the location of the defect, the rectovaginal fascia may be attached to the remaining portion of the uterosacral ligaments at the top of the vagina or to the superficial transverse perinei muscle at the base.
8. Following repair of the rectovaginal fascia, the vaginal mucosa is closed over, and the perineal body should be reconstructed using two to three long-acting absorbable sutures (the sutures should be placed into the separated ends of the perineal muscle group on the left and the right and brought together in the midline).
9. The vaginal mucosa should be carefully aligned and be trimmed with caution. A suture at the top of the vaginal wall can be tied to that at the level of the hymen to pull the vagina posteriorly and into a more anatomical position. The remainder of the vagina is then sutured.
10. A vaginal exam should be performed to exclude narrowing of the orifice, and a rectal exam to ensure no sutures are palpable in the rectum. A vaginal pack is inserted at the end of the operation.

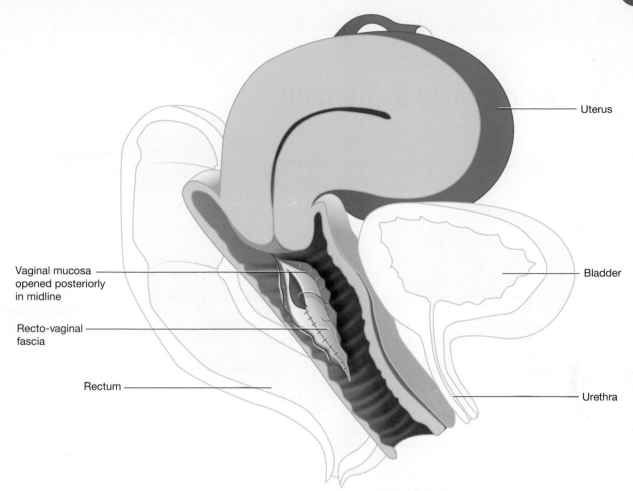

- Uterus
- Bladder
- Urethra
- Vaginal mucosa opened posteriorly in midline
- Recto-vaginal fascia
- Rectum

Suturing of the recto-vaginal fascia in a posterior vaginal wall repair.

Complications

EARLY
- Bleeding.
- Damage to local structures—rectum and small bowel.
- Urinary retention.

INTERMEDIATE AND LATE
- Infection—bladder, vagina, or pelvis.
- Dyspareunia (painful sexual intercourse).
- Bowel and defecatory dysfunction (e.g. faecal impaction or faecal incontinence).
- Rectovaginal or rectoperineal fistula.

Postoperative Care

INPATIENT
- The vaginal pack and urinary catheter are usually removed the day after surgery.

OUTPATIENT
- Follow-up at 6 weeks to 3 months after the operation; women are advised to prevent putting undue stress on the pelvic floor.

Surgeon's Favourite Question

What alternative surgical procedures are available for posterior vaginal wall prolapse?

In those in whom the vaginal vault is also affected, a vaginal procedure to hitch the posterior vaginal wall onto the sacro-spinous ligament (known as sacro-spinous fixation) may be used to improve the support of the entire wall. In those in whom a prior vaginal procedure has failed, a laparoscopic/open sacro-colpopexy may be used to support the posterior vaginal wall and the vaginal vault by utilising native tissue reconstruction or applying a nonabsorbable mesh and securing it onto the sacral promontory. If offering nonabsorbable mesh, consent must include risks/benefits, including the permanence of the mesh, the alternatives, and mesh complications which may not be resolved if the mesh is removed.

114

Angioplasty ± Stenting

Laura Cormack

Definition

The introduction of a balloon, ± a stent, into a blood vessel to widen or open a pathological narrowing.

Indications and Contraindications

INDICATIONS

- Atherosclerosis of the coronary arteries.
- Carotid artery disease (causing significant stenosis or neurological sequelae).
- Peripheral arterial disease (refractory to medical treatment, causing life-limiting claudication, rest pain, or ischaemic ulceration).
- Renovascular hypertension secondary to atherosclerosis of the renal artery or fibromuscular dysplasia (in selected cases).

CONTRAINDICATIONS
Relative

- Chronic kidney disease or acute kidney injury—care must be taken in patients with poor renal function if iodinated contrast is being used (it is used in most cases).
- Allergy to iodinated contrast media (depending on severity of prior reaction).
- Inability of the patient to lie flat and still.
- Uncorrected bleeding disorder or anticoagulation/antiplatelet therapy.
- Long segment of multifocal stenoses.
- Eccentric, calcified stenosis.
- Stents may not be used in patients where dual antiplatelet therapy is contraindicated.

Anatomy

- In the vascular tree, there are:
  - Arteries.
  - Arterioles.
  - Capillaries.
  - Venules.
  - Veins.
- Arteries and veins have three layers:
  - Tunica intima—one layer thick and is made up of squamous epithelium and internal elastic lamina forming connective tissue.

- Tunica media—thicker in arteries than in veins and contains smooth muscle that can contract to change the diameter of the vessel. It also contains the external elastic lamina.
- Tunica adventitia—thicker in veins and consists purely of connective tissue. In larger vessels, this layer contains the vasa vasorum (the vessels supplying the vessel wall).
- Capillaries are one cell layer of endothelium thick.

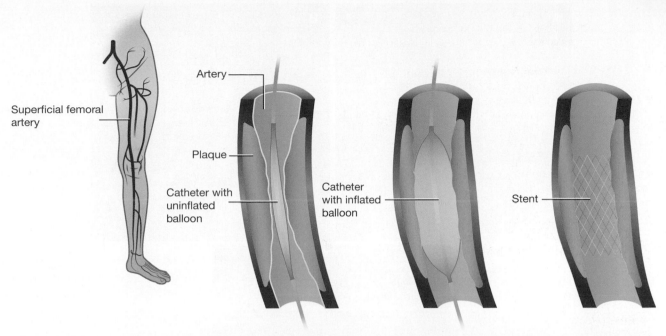

Superficial femoral artery

Artery

Plaque

Catheter with uninflated balloon

Catheter with inflated balloon

Stent

Balloon angioplasty and stenting of an atherosclerotic narrowing of the superficial femoral artery.

1 2 3 STEP-BY-STEP OPERATION

Anaesthesia: general or local with IV sedation.
Position: supine.
Steps:

1. Using ultrasound guidance, the desired vessel is cannulated (commonly the right common femoral artery).
2. Via a short introducer sheath (usually 4, 5, or 6 French), using a catheter for support, a guide wire is inserted and, under fluoroscopic guidance, is passed along the vessel beyond the stenosis.
3. The catheter is then threaded over the guide wire and through the stenosis (the Seldinger technique).
4. The catheter can be used to measure the pre- and poststenotic pressure and calculate the pressure gradient.
5. Using angiography or preprocedure imaging, the diameter of the normal vessel is measured, and an appropriately sized balloon is selected.

6. After removing the catheter, the angioplasty balloon is passed through the sheath over the wire so that it bridges the stenosis.
7. The angioplasty balloon is inflated with a mixture of contrast and saline (inflation time varies from a few seconds to a few minutes).
8. The angioplasty balloon is deflated, and the poststenosis pressure gradient can be measured (in the arterial system a gradient of less than 20 mm Hg is acceptable).
9. Depending on the pressure gradient and/or angiographic appearance, a stent may be deployed to achieve vessel patency.
10. Angiography is then used to confirm the success of the procedure. The guide wire and introducer sheath are removed and haemostasis at the sheath insertion site achieved with either compression or an arterial closure device.

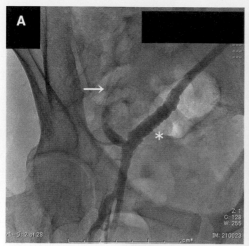
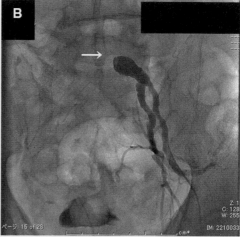
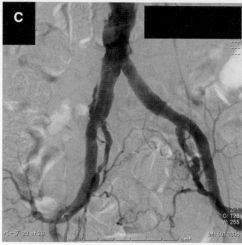

Digital subtraction angiography of A: the right femoral artery. The asterisk indicates a Dacron graft; the arrow indicates occlusion of native external iliac artery. B: The left femoral artery. The arrow indicates total occlusion of native common iliac artery. C: Post-stenting digital subtraction angiography demonstrating recanalization of the common and external iliac arteries.

(Source: *Suematsu, Y., Morizumi, S., Okamura, K. and Kawata, M., 2015. A rare case of axillobifemoral bypass graft infection caused by Helicobacter cinaedi. Journal of Vascular Surgery, 61(1), pp. 231-233.*)

 Complications

EARLY
- Allergic reaction to iodine-based contrast.
- Bleeding/haematoma at the vascular sheath insertion site.
- Dissection/rupture of the target vessel.
- Embolisation of atheroma or thrombus into distal vessels.

INTERMEDIATE AND LATE
- Recurrence of the stenosis.
- Pseudoaneurysm.
- Stent thrombosis.
- In-stent stenosis.
- Stent fracture.

Postoperative Care

INPATIENT
- Usually a day-case procedure, with patients discharged home on the same day provided there are no complications. Mobilisation is encouraged.

OUTPATIENT
- Patients are usually given a long-term single antiplatelet agent such as aspirin (75 to 100 mg/day) or clopidogrel (75 mg/day).
- Follow-up, if required, is either via the interventional radiologist or the vascular surgeon 4–6 weeks postprocedure.
- Patients are advised to seek urgent medical attention if ischaemic symptoms reoccur (pain, pallor).

? Surgeon's Favourite Question

How do you differentiate veins from arteries on ultrasound?

1. By anatomical knowledge (e.g. nerve-artery-vein in the femoral sheath).
2. Pulse: arteries are pulsatile, veins are not.
3. Compressibility: veins are more readily compressible compared to arteries (the most important feature).
4. Colour mode Doppler: while flow towards the transducer is red and away is blue by convention, this distinction is relative to the position of the probe. The flow waveform can also help distinguish arteries from veins.

Transjugular Intrahepatic Portosystemic Shunt (TIPSS)

115

Laura Cormack

Definition

Creation of a tract between the portal vein and the hepatic vein to shunt blood away from the portal venous system, reducing portal venous pressure.

Indications and Contraindications

INDICATIONS
- Indications are the sequelae of decompensated liver disease:
  - Uncontrolled variceal haemorrhage (usually secondary to oesophageal varices).
  - Refractory ascites.
  - Hepatic pleural effusion (hydrothorax).
- TIPSS may also be beneficial in Budd-Chiari syndrome and hepatorenal syndrome.

CONTRAINDICATIONS
Relative Contraindications
- Uncorrected bleeding disorder or anticoagulation/anti-platelet therapy.
- Obstructing neoplasm.

Absolute Contraindications
- Severe liver failure (those with a model for end-stage liver disease (MELD) score >40 and have a 71% 3-month mortality after TIPSS).
- Severe encephalopathy.
- Polycystic liver disease.
- Severe right-sided heart failure.

Anatomy

- The internal jugular vein (IJV):
  - The IJV forms at the jugular foramen and drains the inferior petrosal sinus, the sigmoid sinus, and the veins of the face.
  - The IJV lies superficially in the neck and descends within the carotid sheath. Within the sheath, it sits lateral to the carotid artery; the vagus nerve sits posteriorly between the two vessels.
  - This superficial position makes the IJV amenable to cannulation. However, its close proximity to the vagus nerve and carotid artery means that these structures are at risk of iatrogenic damage during TIPSS.
- Vasculature of the liver:
  - The liver has a dual vascular supply: the hepatic artery (25%) and the portal vein (75%). Together, these vessels supply the liver with approximately 1.5 L of blood per minute.

- The common hepatic artery is a branch of the coeliac trunk. It gives off the gastroduodenal and right gastric branches and then becomes the hepatic artery proper. At the hilum of the liver, the cystic artery branches from the hepatic artery proper, which then further divides into the right and left hepatic arteries.
- The portal vein is formed by the convergence of the superior mesenteric and splenic veins posterior to the neck of the pancreas. The portal vein is responsible for carrying the nutrients absorbed from the intestines for 'first-pass' metabolism. At the hilum of the liver, the portal vein divides into right and left branches.
- Blood drains from the liver via the right, left, and inter-mediate (middle) hepatic veins directly into the IVC.
- The portal triad consists of the hepatic portal vein, the hepatic artery proper, and the common bile duct. The portal triad enters the liver at the porta hepatis and is bounded by a fibrous capsule (Glisson's capsule).

Stent

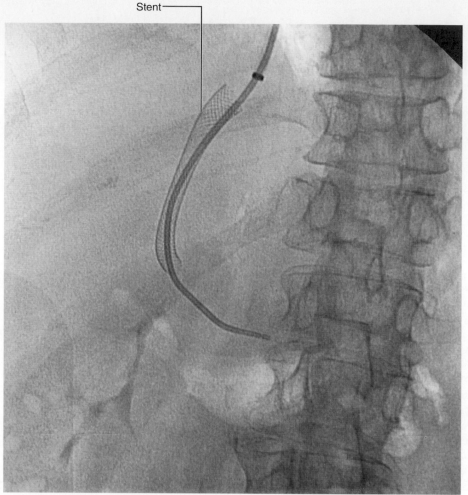

Position of a trans-jugular intrahepatic portosystemic shunt stent radiograph.
(Source: Veeramani, R., 2023. Gray's Anatomy for Students, 3rd South Asia Edition-Two-Volume Set. Elsevier.)

123 STEP-BY-STEP OPERATION

Anaesthesia: general.
Position: supine.
Steps:

1. Ultrasound guidance is used to cannulate the right IJV.
2. A long sheath is inserted into the right atrium, and the right atrial pressure is measured.
3. Under fluoroscopic guidance, a guide wire is advanced into the inferior vena cava and then into the right hepatic vein. A stiff catheter is then inserted over the guide wire into the right hepatic vein.
4. A needle is advanced through the stiff sheath and is passed from the right hepatic vein towards the right portal vein (ultrasound is used for guidance).
5. Once the right portal vein has been punctured, access is secured by advancing a wire over which the sheath can then be advanced into the right portal vein. The pressure is then measured using a catheter.
6. In cases of variceal bleeding, the varices can be embolised with coils through a catheter.
7. The tract from the right hepatic vein to the right portal vein is dilated with a balloon, and a covered stent (TIPSS stent) is inserted through the tract.
8. A portogram is performed to confirm the TIPSS is working. The pressure in the main portal vein and right atrium are remeasured. The portosystemic gradient is calculated and compared with the pre-TIPSS value.
9. The sheath is removed, and haemostasis at the neck is achieved with manual compression.

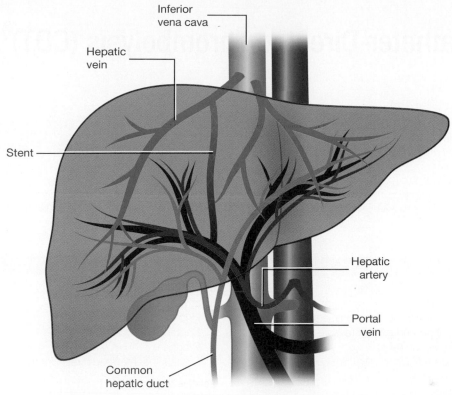

Intrahepatic shunting between the hepatic vein and portal vein.

Complications

EARLY
- Bleeding.
- Bile leak causing chemical peritonitis.

INTERMEDIATE AND LATE
- Infection.
- Encephalopathy—due to the reduction in first pass metabolism
- In-stent stenosis, thrombosis, or occlusion.
- Hepatic ischaemia.
- Mortality.

Postoperative Care

INPATIENT
- In the case of variceal bleeding, the central venous pressure should be kept as low as possible (right atrial pressure is transmitted into the varices through the TIPSS).

OUTPATIENT
- Ultrasound follow-up can be used to ensure the TIPSS remains patent.

Surgeon's Favourite Question

What are the signs of decompensated liver failure?

Ascites, encephalopathy, and variceal bleeding.

Definition

Catheter-directed thrombolysis (CDT) is a technique whereby tissue plasminogen activator (tPA) is injected through a catheter directly into a thrombus.

Indications and Contraindications

INDICATIONS

- Acute critical limb ischaemia where symptoms have been present for <14 days and the predicted time to reestablish anterograde flow is short enough to preserve limb viability.
- Acute myocardial infarction (AMI).
- Deep vein thrombosis (DVT).
- Pulmonary embolism (PE).
- Acute ischaemic stroke (AIS).
- CDT versus systemic thrombolysis may be considered in patients at high risk of bleeding and with persistent hemodynamic instability despite systemic thrombolysis. Those at risk of death before systemic thrombolysis can manifest effectiveness.

CONTRAINDICATIONS
Relative Minor

- Hepatic failure.
- Bacterial endocarditis.
- Pregnancy.
- Diabetic haemorrhagic retinopathy.

Relative Major

- Cardiopulmonary resuscitation within the last 10 days.
- Major nonvascular surgery or trauma within the last 10 days.
- Severe uncontrolled hypertension: >200 mm Hg systolic or >110 mm Hg diastolic.
- Intracranial tumour.
- Recent eye surgery.

Absolute

- Established cerebrovascular event (including transient ischaemic attacks within the last 2 months).
- Active bleeding diathesis.
- Recent gastrointestinal bleeding (<10 days).
- Neurosurgery (intracranial and spinal) within the last 3 months.
- Intracranial trauma within the last 3 months.

Anatomy

- The femoral triangle (Scarpa's triangle) is an anatomical space of the upper thigh. It is of particular importance, as vascular access is often obtained through the femoral artery or vein (both of which are located within the triangle).
- The borders of the femoral triangle are:
  - Superiorly—the inguinal ligament running from the pubic tubercle to the anterior superior iliac spine (ASIS).
  - Medially—adductor longus originating at the pubic body inserting into the linea aspera of the femur.
  - Laterally—sartorius running from the ASIS to form part of the pes anserinus, which inserts into the anteromedial tibia.
  - The floor—pectineus (a quadrangular muscle running from the pectineal line of the pubic tubercle to the pectineal line of the femur) and adductor longus.

- The roof—fascia lata (a thick fascia that envelops the fascial compartments of the leg; laterally, it thickens to form the iliotibial tract).
- Contents of the femoral triangle (from lateral to medial, nerve, artery, vein; 'NAV-Y-fronts'):
  - The femoral nerve originates from L2, L3, and L4 and passes into the femoral triangle deep to the inguinal ligament. It descends the thigh in the femoral canal, innervating the anterior compartment of the thigh.
  - The external iliac artery becomes the common femoral artery at the inguinal ligament.
  - The common femoral vein drains the popliteal vein and becomes the external iliac vein at the inguinal ligament.
  - Deep inguinal lymph nodes and associated lymphatic vessels.

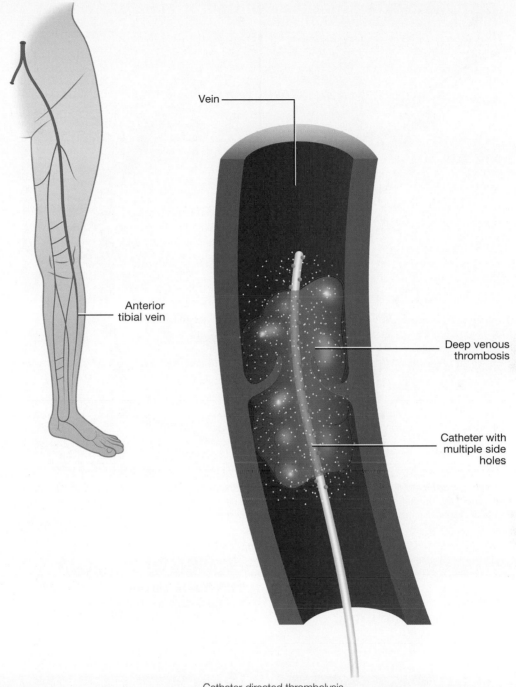

Catheter-directed thrombolysis.

Labels:
Vein
Anterior tibial vein
Deep venous thrombosis
Catheter with multiple side holes

1 2 3 STEP-BY-STEP OPERATION

Anaesthesia: IV sedation.

Position: supine.

Considerations: While this section will focus on CDT for acute lower limb ischaemia, the technique is similar for thrombolysis elsewhere in the arterial and venous system.

Steps:

1. Using ultrasound guidance, the common femoral artery is cannulated.
2. A diagnostic angiogram is performed by injecting contrast through the catheter.
3. Fluoroscopic imaging is used to ascertain the location of the occlusion (it will appear as a filling defect in the vessel).
4. Under fluoroscopic guidance, the occlusion is probed with a soft guide wire. Caution must be used, especially with autologous vessel grafts, as there is a risk of damage to the vessel wall.
5. The occlusion is traversed, and a catheter is pushed beyond the most distal aspect of the occlusion. If this is not possible, thrombolysis can be initiated from the proximal end of the occlusion. The thrombolysis catheter has side holes to allow for the tPA to be dispersed throughout the thrombus.
6. The thrombolytic agent is infused continuously (for a period of time that varies with severity, time of symptom onset, and patient weight). Alternatively, a series of boluses can be used.
7. Postprocedure imaging is used to determine the success of the procedure.

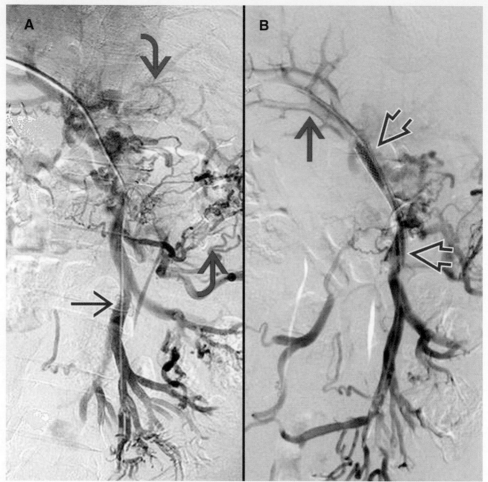

Step-by-Step: Portal Thrombolysis (Post-TIPS Creation and Thrombolysis). A: Sheath placed through the occlusion (blue arrow) and pharmacomechanical thrombolysis performed. B: After successful thrombolysis. TIPS was created with a stent extending from the initially placed SMV stent. *(Source: Wible, B.C., 2023. Diagnostic Imaging: Interventional Radiology. Elsevier.)*

 ## Complications

EARLY
- Intracranial haemorrhage.
- Major bleeding requiring transfusion or surgery.
- Distal embolisation.

INTERMEDIATE AND LATE
- Compartment syndrome.

Postoperative Care

INPATIENT
- Patients remain as an inpatient under the appropriate team until the cause and complications of their acute critical limb ischaemia, AMI, DVT, PE, or AIS have been managed.
- On discharge, the patient should be advised to monitor for the return of ischaemic symptoms and for bleeding complications.

OUTPATIENT
- The patent should be followed up by the appropriate team according to their presenting thrombotic pathology.

? Surgeon's Favourite Question

What are the six P's of acute ischaemia?

Pain, paralysis, paraesthesia, pulselessness, pallor, and perishingly cold.

Embolisation

Laura Cormack

Definition

Embolisation is an intravascular technique used to occlude blood vessels with the deposition of embolic materials.

Indications and Contraindications

INDICATIONS

- Haemorrhage—gastrointestinal (GI), epistaxis, trauma, postpartum, aneurysms, and pseudoaneurysms.
- Vascular anomalies—arteriovenous malformations (AVMs).
- Others—tumours, uterine fibroids, varicoceles, and prostatic arteries (for benign prostatic hyperplasia).

CONTRAINDICATIONS

Absolute

- In the context of uterine artery embolisation, concurrent pregnancy is an absolute contraindication unless there is a life-threatening bleed.

Relative

- Coagulopathy should be corrected prior to embolisation (depending on clinical urgency).
- Pregnancy.
- Wanting future pregnancies (for uterine artery embolisation).
- Contrast agent allergy.

Anatomy

- For the purposes of this chapter, the procedure will focus on embolisation therapy for uterine fibroids.
- The uterus is supplied by branches of the paired ovarian arteries and the uterine arteries.
- Within the broad ligament of the uterus is an extensive anastomosis between the two arterial supplies.
- The ovarian arteries:
  - The ovarian arteries are the main blood supply to the ovaries.
  - The ovarian arteries arise from the abdominal aorta distal to the origin of the renal arteries; they then descend into the pelvis in the uterine suspensory ligament to enter the mesovarium.
- The uterine arteries:
  - The uterine arteries are the major blood supply to the uterus.
  - The paired uterine arteries originate from the internal iliac arteries and travel to the uterus in the cardinal ligament, where they then enter the inferior broad ligament of the uterus.
  - An important anatomical relation to note is that the uterine arteries cross anterior to the ureters (water passes under the bridge).
  - Blood volume through the uterine arteries increase significantly during pregnancy.

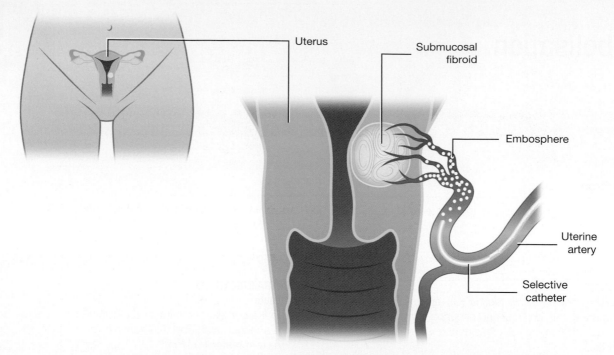

Delivery of proembolic material via the uterine artery into the blood supply of a submucosal fibroid.

1 2 3 STEP-BY-STEP OPERATION

Anaesthesia: local anaesthetic ± IV sedation (sometimes combined with epidural anaesthesia for postoperative pain relief).

Position: supine.

Considerations: While this section will focus on embolisation for uterine fibroids, the technique is similar for elsewhere in the body.

Steps:

1. Using ultrasound guidance, the right common femoral artery is punctured and using the Seldinger technique, an introducer sheath is inserted.
2. The guide wire is manoeuvred into the left uterine artery and is followed by the catheter.
3. Uterine supply is confirmed by fluoroscopy and contrast injection, and assessment is made for other vessels that should be excluded from embolisation.
4. Once the catheter has been correctly and safely positioned in the left uterine artery (proximal to the uterus), the selected embolisation material is deployed (usually plastic beads or gelatine sponge particles). Other embolic materials that can be used in procedures elsewhere in the body include platinum coils, glue, Onyx, lipiodol, and vascular plug devices.
5. This embolisation procedure is then repeated for the right uterine artery.
6. If there is significant fibroid supply from an ovarian artery, embolisation may be considered, depending on the patient's desire to minimise the risk of reduced fertility.
7. The catheter and introducer are then removed and common femoral artery haemostasis is achieved with either manual compression or a vascular closure device.
8. A dressing is applied.

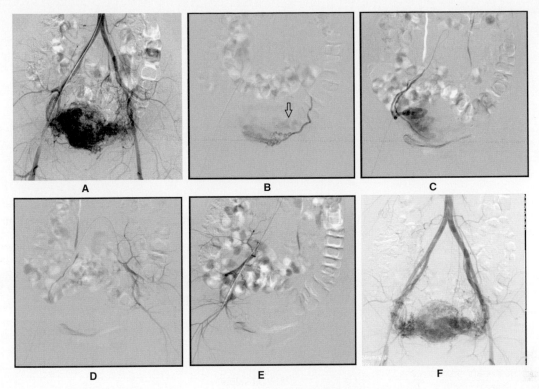

GTN in a 24-year-old woman. She was admitted to the emergency department as a result of massive uterine bleeding. A: Non-selective pelvic arteriogram outlined the main blood supply to the GTN from the uterine arteries. Selective left (b) and right (c) uterine angiography confirmed the bilaterally hypertrophied uterine arteries and early opacification of the pelvic vein due to fistula. After embolisation, there is no opacification of the hypervascular tangle after selective injection of the left (d) or right (e) internal iliac artery. This patient required repeat embolisation for recurrence of massive bleeding 30 months after the first embolisation procedure. F: Angiography showed uterine AVM.
(Source: Wang, Z., Li, X., Pan, J., Chen, J., Shi, H., Zhang, X., Liu, W., Yang, N., Jin, Z. and Xiang, Y., 2017. Bleeding from gestational trophoblastic neoplasia: embolotherapy efficacy and tumour response to chemotherapy. Clinical Radiology, 72(11), pp. 992-e7.)

Complications

EARLY
- Allergic reaction to iodine-based contrast.
- Bleeding/haematoma at the arterial sheath insertion site.
- Pseudoaneurysm.
- Dissection/rupture of the target vessel.
- Nontarget embolisation (embolic material going where not intended).
- Postembolisation syndrome: a combination of fever, nausea and vomiting, and pain.

INTERMEDIATE AND LATE
- Premature menopause.
- Vaginal discharge—usually self-limiting, but if purulent with fever needs assessment ± antibiotics.
- Amenorrhea.
- Ovarian failure.
- Failure to improve symptoms.

Postoperative Care

INPATIENT
- Patients are usually admitted overnight following fibroid embolisation.
- The arterial puncture site and vital signs are monitored.
- There can be significant postprocedural pain, which is often managed with a PCA pump or epidural (if still in place).
- Once the patient's pain is controlled by simple oral analgesia, they can be discharged.

OUTPATIENT
- Shrinkage of fibroids usually continues for 3–6 months, and therefore, clinical consultation and repeat imaging can be undertaken after 3–6 months to assess response to therapy.

Surgeon's Favourite Question

What is postembolisation syndrome?

A syndrome that comprises fever, nausea/vomiting, and other flu-like symptoms. It usually occurs within the first 72 hours, is usually self-limiting, and does not predict infection.

Laura Cormack

Definition

An inferior vena cava (IVC) filter is placed in a patient with lower limb deep vein thrombosis (DVT) to prevent mobilisation of clots causing pulmonary embolism (PE) or stroke if patent foramen ovale (PFO) is present.

Indications and Contraindications

INDICATIONS

- Where systemic anticoagulation is contraindicated or has failed.
- Massive PE with residual DVT at risk for further PE.
- Free-floating ilio-femoral or IVC thrombus.
- Severe cardiopulmonary disease with DVT.
- Prophylactic indications include severe trauma (i.e. closed head injury, spinal cord injury, and/or multiple long bone or pelvic fractures).

CONTRAINDICATIONS

Relative

- The presence of an IVC thrombus that carries a risk of iatrogenic PE.
- Sepsis or bacteraemia.

Absolute

- Inaccessible IVC (for example, compression by tumour).
- IVC too small or too large to accommodate a filter.

Anatomy

GROSS ANATOMY

- The deep veins of the leg begin in the calf and unite as the popliteal vein. The popliteal vein becomes the superficial femoral vein and then the common femoral vein within the thigh.
- The common femoral vein passes under the inguinal ligament, medial to the common femoral artery, and enters the abdomen as the external iliac vein.
- The external iliac vein travels superiorly, receiving the internal iliac vein (which drains the pelvis) to then form the common iliac vein.
- The IVC is formed by the confluence of the left and right common iliac veins at L4/5 and acts as the major source of venous drainage from the abdomen and lower limbs.

- The renal veins drain into the IVC at approximately L2. During the deployment of an IVC filter, it is preferable that it be placed below the renal veins.
- The IVC enters the thorax through the caval opening of the diaphragm at T8 and continues to travel superiorly to the right of the midline and empty into the inferior aspect of the right atrium.

PATHOLOGY

- A lower limb DVT is an intraluminal clot formed in the deep veins of the leg.
- A DVT has the potential to travel through the venous system to enter the right atrium and then continue through to the right ventricle to embolise in a pulmonary artery, resulting in PE. In the presence of a PFO, a PE can cross the heart and travel directly to the brain, causing stroke.

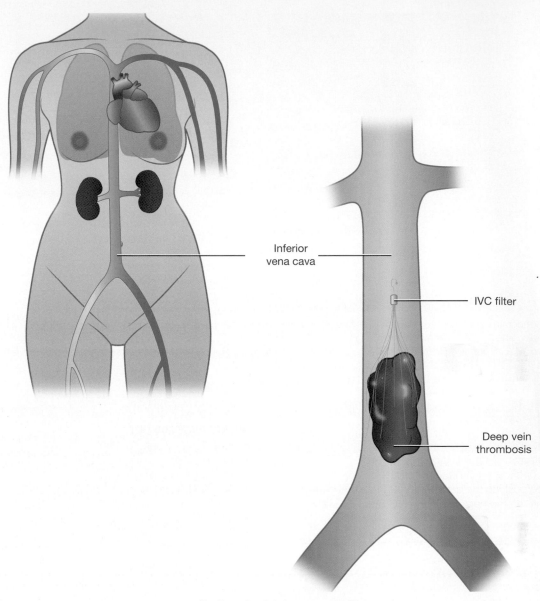

Inferior
vena cava

IVC filter

Deep vein
thrombosis

Position of an inferior vena cava filter.

¹²₃ STEP-BY-STEP OPERATION

Anaesthesia: local anaesthetic with IV sedation.
Position: supine.
Considerations: This procedure can be performed using either the jugular or femoral approach. Two general types of filter are available: permanent and retrievable.

Steps:

1. Ultrasound is used to locate the vein; local anaesthetic is infiltrated.
2. The skin and soft tissue overlying the target vessel are incised.
3. Using ultrasound guidance, the vein is punctured, and an introducer sheath is inserted into the vein using the Seldinger technique.
4. A guidewire and catheter are advanced into the IVC.
5. A cavogram is performed by injecting contrast through the catheter, and the patency and size of the IVC are evaluated.
6. The position of the renal veins is identified.
7. The IVC filter is then inserted through a sheath and deployed in the desired position (commonly in the infrarenal IVC).
8. A final venogram is performed to check the position of the filter.
9. The insertion sheath is removed.
10. Haemostasis is achieved with manual compression.

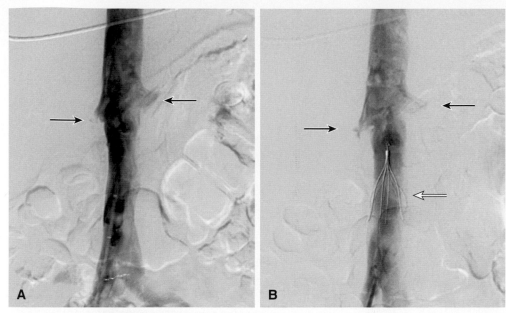

Conventional venograms of inferior vena cava (IVC) before (A) and after (B) IVC filter insertion. Note location of renal veins (black arrows), important landmarks for placement of IVC filter (white arrow) in (B).
(Source: Mauro, M.A., Murphy, K.P., Thomson, K.R., Venbrux, A.C. and Morgan, R.A., 2020. Image-guided interventions. Elsevier.)

Complications

EARLY
- Allergy to contrast material.
- Pneumothorax (if jugular approach is used).
- Bruising or bleeding at puncture site.
- PE due to pushing the catheter through an embolus.
- Guide wire entrapment within the IVC filter.

INTERMEDIATE AND LATE
- Infection of wound or filter.
- Failed procedure (i.e. passage of clots through the filter to the lungs, resulting in a PE).
- IVC obstruction because the filter becomes clogged with clots—commonly results in lower limb oedema.
- Filter migration, erosion, or fracture.
- Chronic thrombosis/recurrent thromboembolism.
- Retrievable filters may scar and become stuck, meaning they become permanent.

Postoperative Care

INPATIENT
- For well patients, ensuring there are no complications, this is commonly a day-case procedure.

OUTPATIENT
- Patients who have undergone the femoral approach should avoid heavy lifting and straining activities for 48 hours.
- Retrievable IVC filters should be removed when no longer indicated.

❓ Surgeon's Favourite Question

Explain the mechanism of action of common anticoagulants.

- Warfarin—inhibits vitamin K-dependant clotting factors (II, VII, IX, X).
- Heparin—potentiates the action of antithrombin III.
- Abciximab, clopidogrel, aspirin—antiplatelet agents.
- Rivaroxaban—direct factor Xa inhibitor.
- Dabigatran—direct thrombin inhibitor.
- Alteplase—tissue plasminogen activator.

119

Percutaneous Biliary Drainage

Laura Cormack

Definition

Access to and drainage of the biliary system using the Seldinger technique with ultrasound and fluoroscopic guidance.

 Indications and Contraindications

INDICATIONS
- To relieve biliary obstruction secondary to:
  - Gallstones.
  - Head of pancreas tumour.
  - Biliary strictures due to surgery or primary sclerosing cholangitis.
  - Cholangiocarcinoma.

CONTRAINDICATIONS
Relative
- Contrast allergy—depends on severity.
- Uncorrected bleeding disorder or anticoagulation/antiplatelet therapy.
- Multifocal obstruction—multiple points of obstruction may limit the success of the procedure.
- Ascites—paracentesis could be considered.

Absolute
- No safe access to bile ducts—e.g. overlying bowel.

Anatomy

- Biliary drainage of the liver:
  - Bile is produced in the liver's bile canaliculi, which come together to form intrahepatic bile ducts (within the portal triad).
  - The portal triad consists of a branch of the hepatic artery, a branch of the portal vein, and an intrahepatic bile duct.
  - The intrahepatic ducts converge to form interlobular ducts. These form the right and left hepatic ducts, which then merge to form the common hepatic duct.
- The gallbladder:
  - Bile is stored and concentrated in the gallbladder.
  - The gallbladder consists of a rounded distal portion called the fundus, the body, and the neck, which empties into the cystic duct. The cystic duct merges with the common hepatic duct to form the common bile duct (CBD).
  - The gallbladder is supplied by the cystic artery (commonly a branch of the right hepatic artery).
- The biliary tree:
  - The CBD merges with the pancreatic duct to form the ampulla of Vater, which at the major duodenal papilla empties into the duodenum through the sphincter of Oddi.
  - The head of the pancreas and its uncinate process are in close proximity to the CBD; a malignant lesion here can cause obstruction of the CBD.

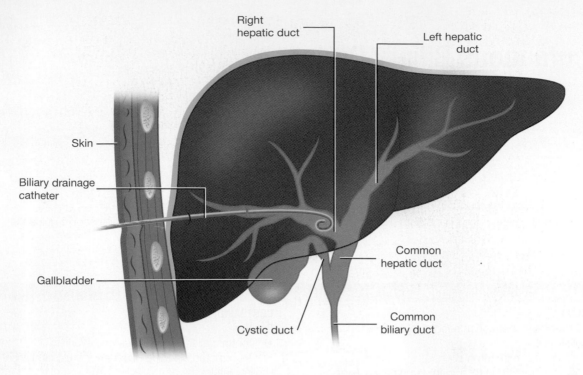

Right
hepatic duct

Left hepatic
duct

Skin

Biliary drainage
catheter

Gallbladder

Common
hepatic duct

Cystic duct

Common
biliary duct

Percutaneous insertion of a drain into the biliary tree.

⑫③ STEP-BY-STEP OPERATION

Anaesthesia: general or IV sedation with local anaesthetic infiltration.

Position: supine.

Considerations: Antibiotic prophylaxis is administered. Preoperative imaging is reviewed to decide the preferred drain insertion site.

Steps:

1. The procedural site is infiltrated with local anaesthetic.
2. Ultrasound guidance is used to guide the puncture needle into the biliary tree.
3. Contrast and fluoroscopy are used to confirm the needle position within the biliary tree.
4. A guide wire is inserted through the needle to secure access.
5. An introducer sheath is inserted over a wire into the bile duct.
6. A wire and catheter are advanced through the sheath more centrally towards the liver hilum and, if possible, into the duodenum.
7. A drainage catheter is then fed over the guide wire to allow drainage of bile.
8. The guide wire is then removed, and the drainage catheter is connected to a drainage bag.
9. The drain is secured with dressings and a suture.

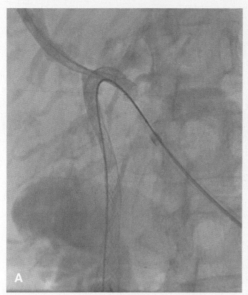
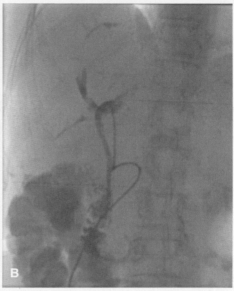

(A) Percutaneous transhepatic cholangiogram guided external biliary drainage with deployment of biliary stents. A catheter wire was initially traversed across the hilar occlusion into the duodenum. A second catheter wire was traversed from the left to the right hepatic duct. A 10 mm x 9 cm stent was deployed from the left duct across the ampulla and dilated. A cholangiogram demonstrated contrast flow through the stent. An internal external drain was left in situ through the left-sided hepatic duct stent and left on free drainage. (B) Three days following the primary procedure, the external drains were removed. A repeat cholangiogram demonstrates excellent patency of the biliary tree and contrast flowing freely into the duodenum.

(Source: Khurram, R., Khamar, R., Husain, A.A., Khawaja, Z. and Lunat, R., 2021. Multifocal pancreatobiliary malignancies: A diagnostic and therapeutic challenge. Radiology Case Reports, 16(2), pp. 289-294.)

Complications

EARLY
- Failure to access a bile duct.
- Bleeding.
- Intraperitoneal bile leak.
- Puncture of pleura causing a pneumothorax or pleural bile leak.

INTERMEDIATE AND LATE
- Sepsis (typically cholangitis) is a major complication.
- Failure to relieve blockage.
- Obstruction/displacement of drain.

Postoperative Care

INPATIENT
- Biliary output through the drain should be monitored to confirm relief of the obstruction.
- If the drain output is not adequate, a diagnostic cholangiogram can be performed to check drain position and patency.

OUTPATIENT
- The patient is educated on how to care for the catheter, including how to flush the drain with saline daily and how to set the catheter to drain externally should they develop a fever (in the case of long 'internal/external' biliary drains passing into the duodenum).
- The catheter should be replaced every few months (in cases of long-term drainage).

Surgeon's Favourite Question

What are the most common complications of gallstone disease?

In the gallbladder:
- Biliary colic
- Acute cholecystitis
- Mucocele
- Empyema
- Perforation of gallbladder
- Gallbladder carcinoma
- Pericholecystic abscess
- Mirizzi syndrome

In the CBD:
- Obstructive jaundice
- Pancreatitis
- Cholangitis

In the gut:
- Gallstone ileus

120

Percutaneous Nephrostomy

Laura Cormack

Definition

Insertion of a drain into the renal collecting system using the Seldinger technique with the aid of ultrasound and fluoroscopic guidance.

 Indications and Contraindications

INDICATIONS

- Complicated urinary tract obstruction (e.g. stone, tumour, trauma, retroperitoneal fibrosis where stenting is not possible).
- Urinary diversion—ureteric injury and urinary leak.
- Access for percutaneous procedures—stone treatment or ureteric stenting.
- Diagnostic testing—antegrade pyelography (rare).

CONTRAINDICATIONS
Relative

- Uncorrected bleeding disorder or anticoagulation/antiplatelet therapy.
- Ureteral stenting may be preferred in simple obstruction.

Anatomy

GROSS ANATOMY

- The kidneys lie on either side of the vertebral column in the retroperitoneum.
- The renal pelvis is formed from the convergence of the major calices of the kidney.
- The renal pelvis progressively narrows as it travels inferiorly and out of the hilum of the kidney.
- At the ureteropelvic junction (the narrowest point), the renal pelvis transitions to become the ureter, which descends into the pelvis to drain into the bladder.

NEUROVASCULATURE

- The right and left renal arteries arise as branches of the abdominal aorta just inferior to the origin of the superior mesenteric artery. The left renal artery commonly arises superior to the right renal artery. The right renal artery is longer and passes posterior to the inferior vena cava.

- As the renal artery courses towards the hilum of the kidneys, it gives off two branches: the ureteric branch of the renal artery and the inferior suprarenal artery. Within the hilum, these then divide into four branches: superior, anterior, posterior, and inferior segmental branches.
- The posterior portion of the kidney is the least vascular, the 'avascular plane of Brodel', and therefore is the safest point for access.
- Within the renal pelvis, interlobar/interlobular veins converge to form the renal vein, which runs anterior to the renal artery.
- The left renal vein crosses the midline anterior to the abdominal aorta. Both renal veins drain into the inferior vena cava.

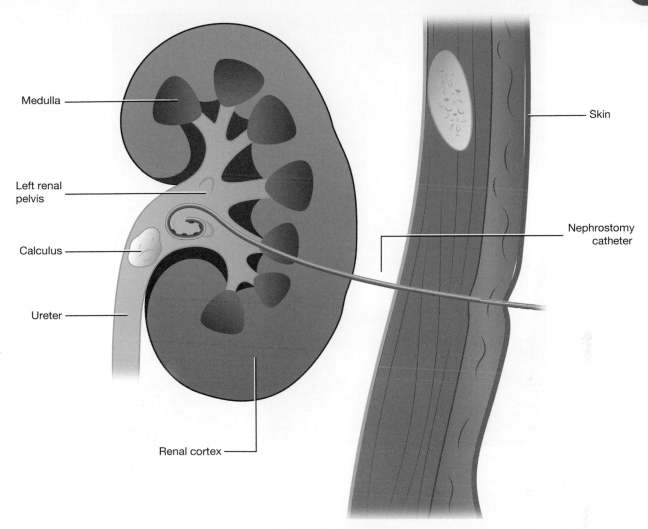

Medulla

Left renal pelvis

Calculus

Ureter

Renal cortex

Skin

Nephrostomy catheter

Percutaneous nephrostomy.

STEP-BY-STEP OPERATION

Anaesthesia: local with IV sedation.
Position: prone, lateral decubitus, or supine.
Steps:

1. Using ultrasound guidance, the plane of Brodel is located.
2. Using an 18-gauge needle, a posterior minor calix in the plane of Brodel is punctured and a small amount of urine aspirated (this may be sent for analysis). The process of puncturing the calix is easier when the renal collecting system is dilated.
3. To confirm the position of the needle, a small volume of contrast is injected into the collecting system, and fluoroscopy is performed.
4. A guidewire is then passed through the needle and into the renal collecting system to secure access.
5. A series of dilators of increasing diameter are then passed over the wire to progressively widen the tract into the collecting system.
6. Once a tract is wide enough, an 8.5F or 10F pigtail catheter (depending on operator preference) is passed over the wire.
7. The pigtail catheter is then locked into position.
8. The pigtail catheter is connected to the draining catheter bag.
9. The insertion site is dressed.

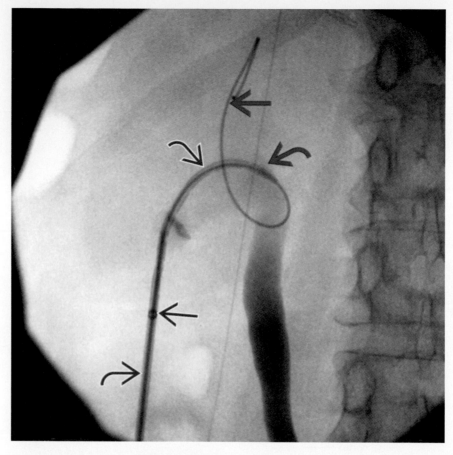

Percutaneous Nephrostomy: Catheter Placement. After the inner stiffener is unscrewed, it is held in a stationary position, and the catheter (curved black arrows) is advanced over the guidewire (blue arrows) further into the collecting system. A radiopaque marker (straight black arrow) demonstrates the last side-hole of the nephrostomy catheter, which should reside within the collecting system.
(Source: Foster, B.R. and Fananapazir, G., 2022. Diagnostic Imaging: Genitourinary. Elsevier.)

 Complications

EARLY
- Haemorrhage—severe cases may require renal artery embolisation.
- Bowel injury and peritonitis.
- Urine leak.

INTERMEDIATE AND LATE
- Infection—can progress to septic shock.
- Uncontrollable hypertension.
- Catheter displacement.

Postoperative Care

INPATIENT
- A day-case procedure if a well patient with no complications.

OUTPATIENT
- The nephrostomy tube should be changed every 3 months.
- Removal of the nephrostomy tube depends upon the indication and reversibility of obstruction.

Surgeon's Favourite Question

Explain the mechanism by which a parenchymal bleed can cause hypertension.

Bleeding into the renal parenchyma increases the intracapsular pressure. This can cause constriction of the renal vasculature, resulting in reduced perfusion of the renal parenchyma. Reduced perfusion activates the renin-angiotensin-aldosterone system, resulting in constriction of the renal artery and increasing blood pressure. Increased blood pressure then leads to further bleeding, beginning a vicious cycle intxo uncontrollable hypertension.

Radiologically Inserted Gastrostomy (RIG) or Gastrojejunostomy (RIGJ)

121

Laura Cormack

Definition

The insertion of an enteral feeding tube into the stomach percutaneously using ultrasound and fluoroscopic guidance.

Indications and Contraindications

INDICATIONS
- Enteral access is usually considered when it is anticipated that a patient will not be able to meet their nutritional needs by mouth for more than 7 days.

CONTRAINDICATIONS
- Uncorrected bleeding disorder or anticoagulation/anti-platelet therapy.
- Abdominal wall abnormalities (e.g. anterior abdominal varices).
- Organomegaly obstructing access to the stomach/jejunum.
- Large volume ascites.

Anatomy

GROSS ANATOMY
- The stomach has two curvatures (lesser and greater) and five parts (cardia, fundus, body, antrum, and pylorus).
- The acute angle between the cardia and the oesophagus is known as the cardiac notch or angle of His. It is formed by the fibres of the collar sling and the circular muscles surrounding the gastro-oesophageal junction. It forms a sphincter that prevents reflux.
- The stomach is attached to other structures by a series of ligaments:
  - Gastrocolic ligament—part of the greater omentum, connects the greater curvature of the stomach and the transverse colon.
  - Gastrosplenic ligament—connects the greater curva-ture of the stomach and the hilum of the spleen.
  - Gastrophrenic ligament—connects the fundus of the stomach to the diaphragm.
  - Hepatogastric ligament—connects the liver to the lesser curve of the stomach, forms part of the lesser omentum.

HISTOLOGY
- The gastric mucosa contains:
  - Numerous gastric glands.
  - A two- or three-layer muscularis mucosa (aids in emptying the glands).
  - An intervening lamina propria.
- The smooth muscle of the muscularis externa is arranged in three layers:
  - Outer longitudinal.
  - Middle circular.
  - Inner oblique.
- When the stomach is empty and contracted, the mucosa and underlying submucosa are thrown into irregular, temporary folds called rugae. These rugae flatten when the stomach is full.

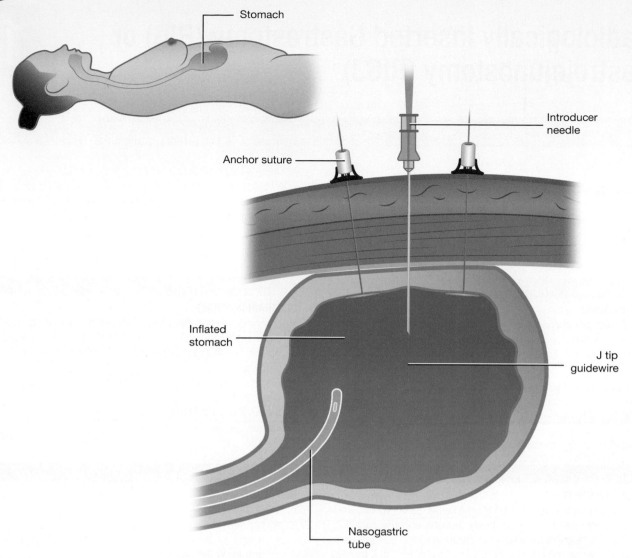

Radiologically inserted gastrostomy.

123 STEP-BY-STEP OPERATION

Anaesthesia: IV sedation. Buscopan or glucagon may also be given to promote gastric distension.

Position: supine.

Considerations: Oral barium may be administered the night before to visualise the colon. Here we describe the retrograde nonbarium approach to a gastrostomy tube insertion.

Steps:

1. Using a preinserted nasogastric tube, the stomach is inflated with air.
2. Lateral fluoroscopy can be used to identify a safe puncture site with no intervening transverse colon.
3. Using a needle through the anterior abdominal wall, the inflated stomach is punctured.
4. The position of the needle in the stomach is then confirmed by injecting contrast.
5. A gastropexy suture is inserted through the needle. This is repeated for a total of two to four sutures to ensure that the stomach is flush and fixed against the abdominal wall.
6. Another needle is inserted into the inflated stomach at the gastropexy site.
7. A gastrostomy tube is then inserted into the stomach and a balloon inflated to keep it in position.
8. In the case of gastrojejunostomy tube insertion, a wire is passed through the gastrostomy site and is advanced into the jejunum. A long gastrojejunostomy tube can then be inserted over the wire.
9. The site of insertion is then cleaned and dressed.

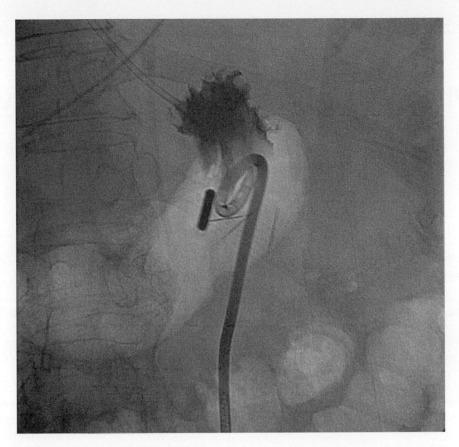

Image showing gastrostomy tube coiled in the gastric fundus. The nasogastric tube is still in position and contrast outlines the normal gastric folds (rugae). There is also a visible T-tack anchor; this is a metal bar within an introducer needle that is used to secure the stomach to the anterior abdominal wall during the procedure.
(Source: Valji, K., 2012. The Practice of Interventional Radiology, with Online Cases and Video. Elsevier.)

Complications

EARLY

- Gastric haemorrhage.
- Peritoneal leak around gastrostomy.
- Misplacement of tube outside stomach.
- Injury to liver, small or large intestine.

INTERMEDIATE AND LATE

- Tube extrusion or accidental removal.
- Aspiration pneumonia after feeding gastrostomy.
- Gastro-cutaneous fistula.

Postoperative Care

INPATIENT

- Patients must be monitored for signs of peritonitis (fever, severe abdominal pain, rigidity). This can occur if administered feeds or medications leak into the peritoneum.
- Feeding through the tube is normally initiated slowly, often beginning after 24 hours and increasing feeds by 50 mL hourly.
- Tube sites need to be checked daily for infection and patency.

OUTPATIENT

- Routine tube changes every 3–6 months.
- Patient/family education on tube inspection and monitoring.

? Surgeon's Favourite Question

What is the immediate management if a long-term gastrostomy falls out?

For long-term gastrostomies, there will be an established tract. If the tube falls out, insertion of a Foley catheter (without inflation of the balloon) will maintain the tract until a formal gastrostomy catheter can be reinserted.

122

Phacoemulsification (Cataract Surgery)

Farihah Tariq, Oliver Riley

Definition

Removal of an opacified crystalline lens by emulsification (using ultrasound to break up the lens into smaller pieces) and subsequent implantation of an artificial intraocular lens.

 Indications and Contraindications

INDICATIONS

No minimum level of vision is required to have a cataract operation. However, surgery is indicated when:

- Symptoms of cataracts such as reduced vision, glare, and monocular diplopia interfere with the patient's activities of daily living.
- Cataract hinders monitoring and treatment of a coexistent posterior segment pathology such as diabetic retinopathy.
- Lens-induced disease:
  - Large cataracts pushing forward the iris thereby causing secondary acute angle-closure glaucoma (phacomorphic glaucoma).
  - Leakage of lens material from a hypermature cataract which obstructs the trabecular meshwork causing secondary open angle glaucoma (phacolytic glaucoma).
  - An inflammatory response to the lens proteins causing phacoanaphylactic uveitis.
- Second eye surgery to balance the refractive power of both eyes (reduce anisometropia) and improve stereopsis.

CONTRAINDICATIONS

Relative

- Active inflammatory conditions.
- Infections (e.g. untreated blepharitis).
- Unstable diabetic retinopathy.
- Recent cataract surgery to the other eye; a delay by at least 1 month should occur before performing cataract on second eye to ensure healing and reduce risk of complications.

Absolute

- Nil.

Anatomy

GROSS ANATOMY

- The lens and cornea function to focus light onto the retina.
- The lens accounts for 30% of the eye's refractive power, 15 dioptres (a diotrope is the unit of measurement of optical power of a lens or curved mirror), whilst the cornea is responsible for the remainder, 43 dioptres.
- The lens is a transparent, ellipsoid biconvex-shaped structure that sits posterior to the iris and anterior to the vitreous body in a depression called the hyloid fossa.
- The lens is suspended via the zonular fibres, which connects to the ciliary body.
- Contraction of the ciliary muscles allows the lens to adapt its shape, enabling the eye to change focus from distance to near (accommodation).
- The lens consists of lens fibres that form the inner nucleus and outer cortex enveloped in an elastic capsule.

NEUROVASCULATURE

- The lens is an epithelial structure with no direct innervation by nerves or blood vessels. It obtains its nutrients from the aqueous humour by passive diffusion.

PATHOLOGY

- Several types of cataract exist, including age related, traumatic, and metabolic. Age related is the most prevalent, with its aetiology being not completely understood but is believed by be multifactorial. A traumatic cataract can occur following both blunt and penetrating eye injuries, electrocution, chemical burns, and exposure to radiation. Metabolic cataracts occur in in diabetes, Wilson's disease, and myotonic dystrophy.
- As age related is the most common type, it is divided into three subtypes using an anatomical classification within the lens:
  - Nuclear sclerotic.
  - Cortical.
  - Posterior subcapsular cataracts.

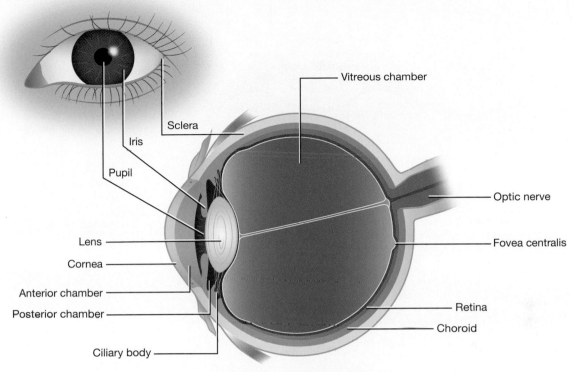

Gross anatomy of the eye.

STEP-BY-STEP OPERATION

Anaesthesia: general or local (topical or regional orbital block, e.g. sub-Tenon's, peribulbar or retrobulbar block)
Position: supine.
Considerations: The eye and surrounding structures are washed with 5% povidone-iodine, dried, and draped ensuring no lashes are in the surgical field. A speculum is inserted to keep the eye open.

Steps:

1. The primary phaco incision is made using a keratome at the corneal margin, placed either temporally (laterally) or superiorly, approximately 3 mm in width whilst stabilising the globe with a micro-grooved forceps.
2. A viscous gel is inserted into the anterior chamber (stabilising the anterior chamber during the next step, and protecting the corneal endothelium from intraoperative trauma).
3. A smaller secondary incision known as paracentesis is made to accommodate additional instruments.
4. Next, capsulorhexis is performed, where a circular opening in the anterior capsule is made using a cystotome or rehixis forceps.
5. A balanced salt solution is injected between the lens and capsule edge separating the nucleus from the cortex known (hydrodissection).
6. Using a phaco probe and chopper instrument, the cataract is broken into smaller pieces using ultrasound energy (phacoemulsification). These fragments and other remaining soft lens matter adherent to the capsule are aspirated and removed.
7. The viscous gel is inserted into the capsular bag to open up the bag, creating space for the artificial lens. The patient-specific lens is then inserted.
8. The viscoelastic gel is removed, and the anterior chamber is refilled with the balanced salt solution.
9. Antibiotics are given intracamerally (into the anterior chamber of the eye). Sutures are typically not required as the wounds are self-healing.
10. A clear shield is placed over the orbit to protect the eye.

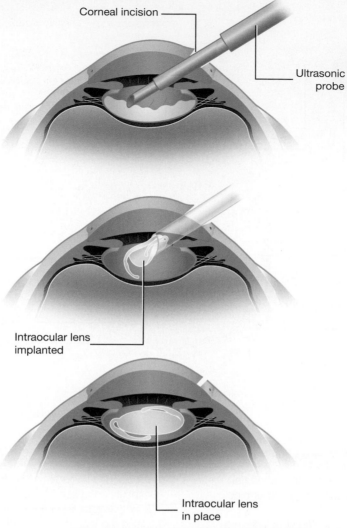

Corneal incision

Ultrasonic probe

Intraocular lens implanted

Intraocular lens in place

Phacoemulsification and artificial lens implantation.

Complications

EARLY

- Rupture of posterior lens capsule with or without vitreous loss.
- Damage to the anterior capsule.
- Zonular dehiscence causing the capsule to become unstable.
- Loss of nuclear (lens) fragments into the vitreous chamber.
- Suprachoroidal haemorrhage—accumulation of blood between the choroid and the sclera.
- Corneal oedema—swelling of cornea.
- Uveitis—inflammation of the uveal tract usually anterior.
- Increased intraocular pressure.
- Wound leak due to poorly constructed wounds.
- Iris prolapse.
- Endophthalmitis—inflammation of the intraocular cavity which may cause visual loss.

INTERMEDIATE AND LATE

- Cystoid macular oedema—fluid accumulation in the retina at the macula.
- Rhegmatogenous retinal detachment—break or tear in the retina causing fluid accumulation between the neurosensory retina and the underlying retinal pigment epithelium.
- Corneal decompensation.
- Endophthalmitis.
- Lens-related problems, e.g. decentred, subluxed, or unstable.
- Posterior capsular opacification, where there is thickening of the residual posterior lens capsule, which may occur months to years following surgery. This is easily treated with Nd:YAG laser posterior capsulotomy.
- Visual loss.

Postoperative Care

INPATIENT

- This procedure is typically performed as a day-case procedure.
- Eye shield on the postoperative eye should be worn at night for five nights to protect the eye from injury.

OUTPATIENT

- Immediate resumption of activities of daily living.
- Strenuous activity, e.g. sports, gardening, and heavy lifting, should be avoided for 2 weeks to decrease risk of complications associated with raised intraocular pressure.
- Patients should avoid swimming for 2 weeks to in order to reduce the risk of infection.
- Patients should avoid applying eye makeup during the immediate postoperative period.
- Day 1 postoperative reviews are only required if there are complications during surgery, or if there is concurrent pathology; otherwise, patients are reviewed in clinic at 4 weeks or seen by their local optometrist.
- A course of tapering steroids, e.g. dexamethasone 0.1% (one drop four times a day for 4 weeks).
- A course of topical antibiotic drops, e.g. chloramphenicol 0.5% (one drop four times daily for 2–4 weeks).
- Patients should visit the optometrist 6 to 8 weeks postoperatively for refraction (new prescription for spectacles).

 Surgeon's Favourite Question

What are the latest advances in cataract surgery?

Laser-assisted surgery, and intraoperative aberrometry (ORA), is a new emergency technique which takes an additional measurement of the eye during surgery that allows for more accurate measurement of the synthetic lens.

123 | Vitrectomy

Farihah Tariq, Oliver Riley

Definition

Removal of the vitreous gel from the posterior segment and replacement with sterile saline or a tamponade such as gas or silicone oil.

Indications and Contraindications

INDICATIONS

The extent of vitrectomy (pars plana vitrectomy) is determined by the indication of vitrectomy, retinal pathology, lens status, and goals of the surgery. It is performed when access to the posterior segment of the eye is necessary in the following circumstances:

- Retinal detachment.
- Proliferative diabetic retinopathy.
- Nonclearing vitreous haemorrhage.
- Peeling of macular internal limiting membrane or epiretinal membrane.
- Vitreomacular traction (when the vitreous within an aging eye fails to completely detach from the macula).
- Endophthalmitis (inflammation of the intraocular cavity usually secondary to infection).
- Removal of retained lens fragments or a displaced intraocular lens following cataract surgery.
- Intraocular foreign bodies secondary to trauma.
- Severe inflammatory changes within the vitreous.
- Tumour biopsy.

CONTRAINDICATIONS

- Established nonreversible severe visual impairment or blindness.
- Retinoblastoma or choroidal melanoma (to avoid seeding).

Anatomy

GROSS ANATOMY

- The vitreous is a transparent gel-like structure occupying two-thirds of the globe. Its role is to maintain both the spherical shape of the globe of the eye and to keep the retina correctly positioned (by maintaining a pressure).
- The outer zone is a denser collagenous layer and forms the anterior and posterior hyaloid face.
- The central zone constitutes the vitreous humour.
- The vitreous is strongly adherent to the retina at the margins of the vitreous base, the optic disc, the retinal vessels, and the posterior lens capsule.
- The pars plana is part of the ciliary body and is found posterior to where the iris and sclera meet. This is a relatively avascular structure, thus making it a good point of entry for instruments during vitrectomy surgery.

NEUROVASCULATURE

- The choroid is the vascular layer of the posterior segment and provides nutrients to the retina.

HISTOLOGY

- The retina is a complex 10-layered photosensory structure. The photoreceptors (rods and cones) convert light signal into electrical signal.
- Ganglion cells from the retina give rise to the optic nerve which deliver the signals ultimately to the occipital cortex.

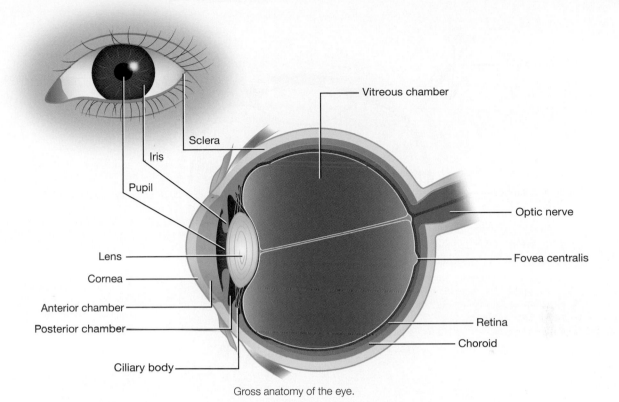

Gross anatomy of the eye.

123 STEP-BY-STEP OPERATION

Anaesthesia: local.

Position: supine.

Considerations: The eye and surrounding structures are washed with povidone-iodine 5%, dried, and draped to ensure that lashes do not obscure the surgical field.

Steps:

1. Access to the posterior segment is achieved using a trochar to pierce the sclera and choroid (sclerotomy). The sclerotomies are placed at three port sites via the pars plana (to minimise disruption to the eye):
   a. For the infusion cannula.
   b. For the light source.
   c. For the vitrectomy cutter (or vitrector)
2. An irrigating solution is infused into the eye to maintain both globe shape and intraocular pressure.
3. The vitrector and light source are then introduced. The infusion cannula maintains positive pressure of the globe by infusing fluid into the posterior chamber whilst the surgeon uses one hand to hold the light source and the other to hold the vitrector.
4. The vitrector is aimed towards the centre of the vitreous to achieve a core vitrectomy.
5. The vitrector is then placed lower into the posterior vitreous cavity to achieve a posterior vitrectomy. The light source is manoeuvred carefully with the other hand to ensure a good view at all times (infusion pressure must be monitored carefully, as vitrector use without adequate infusion will cause the eye to collapse).
6. Once the posterior vitreous is removed, the vitreous base is shaved (as its adherence to the retina prevents total removal)—this step is key in vitrectomy for a retinal detachment. Dye is utilised to help visualise any remaining vitreous.
7. Sterile saline (balanced salt solution—BSS), a tamponade (usually gas—octafluoropropane), or silicone oil is introduced.
8. The instruments are then removed.
9. Most 23-gauge and 25-gauge sclerotomies are self-sealing but require careful inspection. To prevent postoperative hypotony and reduce the risk of infection, it is important to ensure no fluid leaks.
10. Subconjunctival antibiotics are injected, and the eye is shielded.

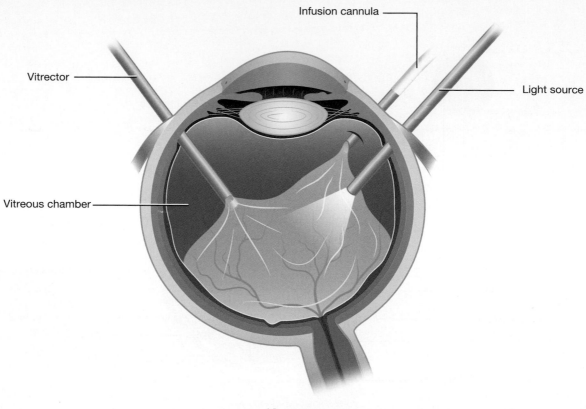

Infusion cannula

Vitrector

Light source

Vitreous chamber

Vitrectomy.

Complications

EARLY
- Iatrogenic retinal breaks or detachment.
- Choroidal haemorrhage.
- Endophthalmitis.

INTERMEDIATE AND LATE
- Cataract.
- Glaucoma.
- Tamponade-associated problems—increased intraocular pressure and central retinal artery occlusion.
- Sympathetic ophthalmia—a bilateral, granulomatous uveitis that occurs after trauma to the eye.

Postoperative Care

INPATIENT
- This procedure is typically performed as a day-case procedure.

OUTPATIENT
- Patients who have had air or gas inserted will need to maintain a head-down posture for as long as possible over the following 7 days.
- Patients are reviewed in clinic on day 1 postoperatively and as needed thereafter.
- Antibiotic and mydriatic eye drops for 7 days with a tapering course of steroids eye drops for 3–4 weeks.
- Patients with air or gas bubbles in vitreous cavity should be warned against air travel for the following 7 days.

Surgeon's Favourite Question

Why does the patient need to maintain a head-down posture postoperatively when a gas or air bubble is introduced?

Holding a head-down position will allow the air or gas bubble to rise and settle adjacent to the retina. This will help to hold the retina flat (drain/prevent the reaccumulation of subretinal fluid before the retinopexy seals the break) and promote optimal healing.

Trabeculectomy

Farihah Tariq, Oliver Riley

Definition

Creation of a fistula between the anterior chamber and the subconjunctival space to facilitate aqueous outflow from the eye to lower intraocular pressure.

Indications and Contraindications

INDICATIONS

Trabeculectomy, also known as filtration surgery, is performed for chronic glaucoma in the following circumstances:

- If intraocular pressure is not controlled with maximal medical therapy.
- If intraocular pressure is not controlled following previous laser therapy (in clinical trials, trabeculectomy has proven consistently more successful at lowering intraocular pressure than either medication or laser).
- In patients where laser therapy is contraindicated, such as severe glaucoma, rapid progression, or previous unsuccessful laser treatment.
- Patients who are noncompliant with medical therapy.
- Patients with progressive glaucomatous optic nerve damage and/or loss of visual field.
- Ocular surface disease, e.g. side effect of eye drops.

CONTRAINDICATIONS

- Severe scarring on conjunctiva.
- Active neovascular glaucoma.
- Uveitic glaucoma.
- Active intraocular inflammation.
- Severe visual impairment.

Anatomy

GROSS ANATOMY

- The conjunctiva, a thin transparent mucous membrane, lines the sclera (bulbar conjunctiva) and the inside of the eyelid (palpebral conjunctiva). The junction between the bulbar and palpebral conjunctiva forms a fold known as the conjunctival fornix.
- The sclera is the white outer fibrous coat of the globe. As it continues anteriorly, it becomes transparent (the cornea). The junction between the cornea and sclera is the limbus.
- The iridocorneal angle lies between the iris and the cornea. This drainage angle is where aqueous humour flows from the eye and into the trabecular meshwork.
- The trabecular meshwork is an array of collagenous tunnels overlying Schlemm's canal and involved in the drainage of the aqueous humour.
- Schlemm's canal is collecting ducts which channel the aqueous humour from the anterior chamber into the venous system via the episcleral vessels.
- The ciliary body is composed of the ciliary muscles and epithelium. This is the site of aqueous humour production. Contraction of the ciliary muscle facilitates outflow via the trabecular meshwork.

NEUROVASCULATURE

- The short ciliary nerve, a branch of the ciliary ganglion, contains parasympathetic fibres that innervate the sphincter pupillae and ciliary muscle and sympathetic fibres that innervate the dilator pupillae muscle.
- The long ciliary nerve, a branch of the nasociliary nerve (a branch of the ophthalmic division of the trigeminal nerve), provides sensory innervation to the eyeball and cornea. It accompanies the short ciliary nerve from the ciliary ganglion.
- The eye is supplied by the central retinal artery, the anterior ciliary arteries, and the short and long posterior ciliary arteries. All are branches of the ophthalmic artery, a branch of the internal carotid artery.
- The cornea has no blood vessels and receives nutrients from passive diffusion from tear fluid and the aqueous humor.
- The venous drainage is primarily via the vortex and central retinal veins, which merge with the inferior and superior ophthalmic veins that drain posteriorly into the cavernous sinus.

HISTOLOGY

The cornea is a specialised mucous membrane that covers the anterior part of the eye and is composed of five histologically distinct layers, from superficial to deep:

- The epithelium is a thin layer of nonkeratinised stratified squamous epithelium of approximately five cells thick. It is highly innervated by pain fibres.
- Bowman's membrane is a thick acellular layer and is composed of type I collagen fibres.
- The stroma is the largest layer, making approximately 90% of the cornea. It is composed of bundles of type I collagen fibres interspersed with fibroblasts and elastic fibres.

- Descemet's membrane is the basement membrane of the corneal endothelium.
- Endothelium lines the posterior surface of the cornea and is a single layer of simple squamous to simple cuboidal cells. The cells have sodium pumps within their membranes that allow sodium ions into the anterior chamber, followed passively by negatively charged chloride ions and water molecules. This allows the stroma to remain relatively dehydrated and maintain its transparency.

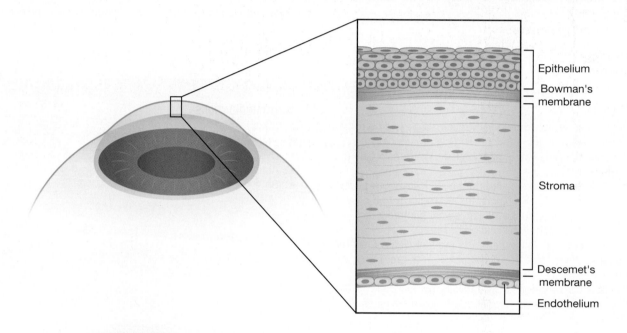

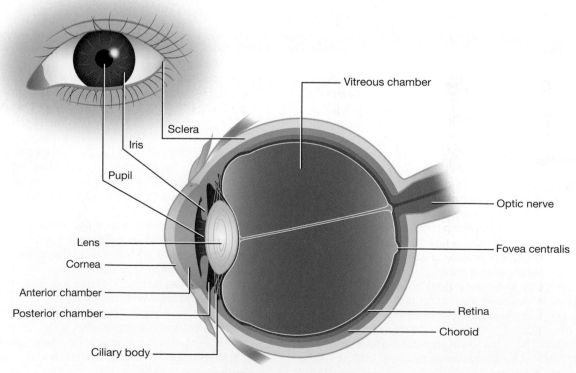

Layers of the sclera and cornea and gross anatomy of the eye.